肩胛骨障碍及其在肩损伤中的作用：临床评估和康复指南

[美] W. 本·基布勒（W. Ben Kibler）
[美] 亚伦·D. 西亚西亚（Aaron D. Sciascia） 主编
王芗斌 何红晨 主译

电子工业出版社
Publishing House of Electronics Industry
北京·BEIJING

First published in English under the title
Disorders of the Scapula and Their Role in Shoulder Injury: A Clinical Guide to Evaluation and Management
edited by W. Ben Kibler and Aaron D. Sciascia
Copyright © Springer International Publishing AG, 2017
This edition has been translated and published under licence from Springer Nature Switzerland AG.

本书中文简体字版授予电子工业出版社独家出版发行。未经书面许可，不得以任何方式抄袭、复制或节录本书中的任何内容。

版权贸易合同登记号　图字：01-2020-2896

图书在版编目（CIP）数据

肩胛骨障碍及其在肩损伤中的作用：临床评估和康复指南／（美）W. 本·基布勒（W. Ben Kibler），（美）亚伦·D. 西亚西亚（Aaron D. Sciascia）主编；王芗斌，何红晨主译．—北京：电子工业出版社，2022.1
书名原文：Disorders of the Scapula and Their Role in Shoulder Injury: A Clinical Guide to Evaluation and Management
ISBN 978-7-121-42355-0

Ⅰ. ①肩⋯　Ⅱ. ①W⋯　②亚⋯　③王⋯　④何⋯　Ⅲ. ①肩胛骨－骨疾病－诊疗　②肩胛骨－骨疾病－康复　Ⅳ. ① R681.7

中国版本图书馆 CIP 数据核字（2021）第 231406 号

责任编辑：郝喜娟
印　　刷：中国电影出版社印刷厂
装　　订：中国电影出版社印刷厂
出版发行：电子工业出版社
　　　　　北京市海淀区万寿路 173 信箱　邮编：100036
开　　本：787×1092　1/16　印张：14.25　字数：296 千字
版　　次：2022 年 1 月第 1 版
印　　次：2022 年 1 月第 1 次印刷
定　　价：158.00 元

凡所购买电子工业出版社图书有缺损问题，请向购买书店调换。若书店售缺，请与本社发行部联系，联系及邮购电话：(010) 88254888，88258888。
质量投诉请发邮件至 zlts@phei.com.cn，盗版侵权举报请发邮件至 dbqq@phei.com.cn。
本书咨询联系方式：haoxijuan@phei.com.cn

译者名单

主译：
　　王艻斌　福建中医药大学
　　何红晨　四川大学华西医院

副主译：
　　马　钊　北京医院
　　孙　扬　上海体育学院
　　刘燕平　福建中医药大学附属康复医院
　　连晓文　福建中医药大学附属康复医院
　　张　鑫　同济大学
　　苟艳芸　福建中医药大学
　　陈倩倩　福建中医药大学
　　陈　翰　陆军军医大学第一附属医院

前言 1

为什么写这本书

随着肩部病理解剖学的明晰，肩胛骨在这种复杂关系中的动态角色也更加明显。但是，一直到最近，肩胛骨仍然未被考虑完全[1]。很明显，必须充分了解肩胛骨，才能有效优化各种肩损伤的治疗。作为一名执业外科医生，能意识到这点，对于在门诊检查患者、计划肩损伤手术，以及帮助患者康复都是非常重要的。的确，资深人士认为矫正肩胛骨位置和运动轨迹是保证所有肩部手术长期成功的一个关键。有肩部疾病的患者都存在一定形式的肩胛骨功能异常，如果没有被识别并适当治疗，会影响检查、影像、手术和保守治疗的准确性。因此，准确识别、诊断、治疗肩胛骨障碍，对于任何希望成功治疗肩损伤的外科医生来说，都是势在必行的。

识别

肩胛骨运动障碍可以在临床查体中确定，因此需要临床人员有能力识别异常，懂得适当治疗[2]。本书的写作目的正在于此。肩胛骨运动障碍可能是内部因素（固有肌力量弱或神经血管损伤）造成的，也可能是外部因素（肩锁关节、盂肱关节损伤或软组织损伤）造成的。外科医生必须能够识别肩胛骨障碍的原因，以成功治疗肩损伤[2]。不仅肩损伤可导致肩胛骨功能障碍，固有的肩胛骨病理也可导致更严重的肩部疾病[1]。肩胛骨和肩部疾病之间存在复杂的平衡关系，彻底了解肩胛骨障碍，可使医生对肩损伤的理解更加全面，并指导合理治疗，包括手术和保守治疗。本书的后续章节收集了相关信息，以备执业外科医生使用。

与肩胛骨障碍有关的肩部病变主要有几类，后续章节会深入讨论。对这些特定损伤的简要概述，显示出了解肩胛骨–肩关系对成功治疗肩损伤的重要性。

肩袖问题

肩袖撕裂患者的解剖学研究显示肩胛骨上旋增加。目前还不明确这种肩胛骨位置是肩袖撕裂的原因还是结果，但它确实影响了患者的肩功能[1]。肩胛骨前伸会降低肩袖的最大力量输出，虽然实际力量正常，但显示出的肌力是下降的[1,2]。因此，肩胛骨运动障碍的康复应当是患者首次完整治疗的一部分。对于有肩袖病变和肩胛骨运动障碍的患者来说，治疗肩部应先注重纠正肩胛骨运动异常，再集中康复肩袖[1]。肩胛骨功能正常，才能准确评估肩袖肌力和肩袖完整性。不对肩胛骨障碍进行适当的康复和治疗，将难以明确肩袖损伤的性质，可能导致不当治疗。

肩锁关节和锁骨问题

识别出肩锁关节分离患者有严重的肩胛骨运动障碍，常提示保守治疗会成功。是否能纠正下斜、肩胛骨功能失调从而减少脱位肩锁关节的畸形，是决定患者是否需要手术治疗肩锁关节分离的重要因素[1,2]。锁骨将肩胛骨连接到中轴骨上，从而为肩胛骨移动和旋转提供了锚点。与锁骨分离会导致肩胛骨出现明显的功能损害，包括肩袖力量缺失和肩关节撞击综合征[1,2]。肩锁关节分离导致肩胛骨运动障碍，若早期治疗方案失败，可能需要手术固定肩锁关节，改善肩胛骨运动障碍。若患者肩锁关节分离后无肩胛骨运动障碍，通常保守治疗结局良好[1]。因此，肩锁关节分离造成的肩胛骨疾病可决定手术治疗与非手术治疗，这要求外科医生能识别和理解肩胛骨损伤和肩损伤之间的关系。

如同肩锁关节分离所见的，因锁骨骨折而失去锁骨的支撑功能也可改变中轴骨和肩胛骨的关系。这同样会导致肩胛骨不适当地前伸，继而改变盂肱关节的生物力学，潜在导致肩袖变弱、活动缺失和撞击[2]。这些改变明显影响患者的主观功能评分。缩短 1.5 cm 的骨折就可以导致明显的肩胛骨功能失调，因此，肩胛骨功能失调是肩损伤的结果，但它会传导损伤，改变肩关节的运动学。锁骨骨折伴肩胛骨运动障碍患者应考虑手术固定，实现对锁骨长度、对位及旋转的修复[1]。若能在肩胛骨骨折时识别出肩胛骨运动障碍，会使外科医生考虑手术固定的潜在需要，而不是保守治疗。

不稳定问题

上盂唇前后部损伤（SLAP损伤）：在诊断上盂唇撕裂时，识别肩胛骨运动障碍也是重要的。早期内旋和前倾的肩胛骨运动障碍使应力落在肩前部韧带[1,2]。这种病理性应力造成盂唇撞击，导致上盂唇撕裂[1]。因此，当肩胛骨障碍影响肩部疾病发展时，在治疗中矫正运动障碍是至关重要的。另外，若早期识别并矫正肩胛骨运动障碍，可阻止后续上盂唇撕裂的发展。因此，外科医生若能在没有肩部病变时准确识别肩胛骨运动障碍，便可以对患者进行合理治疗，预防这些损伤发生[1]。

投掷类项目运动员：与SLAP损伤相关的整体肩胛骨功能失调问题在过头投掷类项目运动员群体中最常见。大部分有SLAP损伤的投掷类项目运动员不需要手术，只要通过简单的肩胛骨复位即可矫正他们的不平衡，继而返回比赛。过头投掷类项目运动员的肩胛骨位置不良，导致内部撞击加重、盂肱关节内旋不足增加、胸小肌挛缩、肩峰下撞击症状和肩袖肌腱炎，加大了治疗难度。

多向不稳定（MDI）：伴随多向不稳定的有症状患者常有严重的肩胛骨运动障碍，这限制了肩袖把肱骨头维持在盂窝中的能力，增加了半脱位、撞击和肌腱炎发生的可能性。严重的运动异常导致关节盂生物力学对位不良，关节盂位置改变使肱骨头更容易脱位[1, 2]。识别MDI中的肩胛骨运动障碍可使治疗适当瞄准正确肌群。通过合适的肌力训练和稳定训练，可使关节盂对位回归正常，减少脱位复发的风险。通过识别MDI中存在的多种因素，包括肩胛骨病理，外科医生可以出具适当的、有效的治疗处方。的确，若患者的肩胛骨不能早期复位，治疗不仅无效，而且非常痛苦。

前后向不稳定：肩胛骨在单向盂肱关节不稳定中也扮演着重要角色。肩胛骨骨运动障碍会造成潜在的异常肩部生物力学，会在盂肱关节不稳定中表现出来[3]。肩关节不稳定中的肩胛骨运动障碍源自多种可见的不稳定因素，包括肌肉协调性下降、由于骨骼肌肉损伤引起的关节疼痛导致运动学改变、肌肉力量变弱或疲劳[3]。因创伤继发不稳定的患者通常有结构性损伤，在解剖病理未矫正前运动障碍无法纠正。因微创伤和慢性关节盂损伤继发不稳定的患者，其肩胛骨运动障碍多在肌肉力量变弱后出现，对运动障碍的康复常常也是对不稳定的治疗[1]。特别是在后向不稳定中，翼状肩胛会导致肱骨头脱位[4]。自发性后向脱位患者须重现这种因运动障碍才出现的脱位。因此，在单向不稳定中，了解病因很重要，以便对同时出现的运动障碍进行适当治疗。

如在与肩胛骨病变相关的肩损伤例子中所示，识别肩胛骨运动障碍的重要性显而易见。然而，外科医生不仅需要精通肩胛骨的病理诊断，还要理解肩损伤和肩胛骨运动障碍之间的关系。在某些情况下，肩胛骨异常可能是肩损伤的原因，反过来的情况也有，或者在其他情况下这种因果关系可能不成立。若肩损伤引起了肩胛骨运动障碍，在检查中又发现运动障碍需要治疗，那么外科医生理解这些关系对他们出具治疗肩损伤的整体方案是很重要的。只治疗肩损伤忽视肩胛骨运动障碍，或者反过来，都会导致结局不良，无论手术做得好不好、治疗方案是否得当。这两种损伤必须一起考虑，它们之间的因果关系很重要。这本书对强调这些关系有重要作用，同时帮助读者理解针对这些损伤的适当的治疗方案，是非常有价值的资源。我们强烈推荐这本书给所有需要处理肩功能失调的医务人员。

作为外科医生，我们可以诚实地说，Kibler博士的理论使我们对患者的治疗取得了更好的效果。

Felix H. Savoie 3rd

Emily Wild

参考文献

1. Kibler WB, Ludewig PM, McClure PW, et al. Clinical implications of scapular dyskinesis in shoulder injury: the 2013 consensus statement from the "scapular summit". Br J Sports Med, 2013, 47(14): 877–885.
2. Kibler WB, Sciascia AD. Current concepts: scapular dyskinesis. Br J Sports Med, 2009, 44(5): 300–305.
3. Kibler WB, Sciascia AD. The role of the scapula in preventing and treating shoulder instability. Knee Surg Sports Traumatol Arthrosc, 2015, 24(2): 390–397.
4. Pande P, Hawkins R, Peat M. Electromyography in voluntary posterior instability of the shoulder. Am J Sports Med, 1989, 17(5): 644–648.

前言 2

治疗骨骼肌肉和运动损伤需要了解脊柱各节段是如何共同工作来实现特定生物力学过程的。投掷棒球需要将足部的地面反作用力通过脊柱向上传递,使球从以精准方式握持的手中抛出。各关节所有肌肉的激活和时序对优化功能至关重要。了解脊柱各节段的复杂工作是理解身体正常生理和生物力学及运动损伤病理生理学的基础。肩胛骨是个绝佳的例子,它的位置极具"战略性",影响了即便不是大部分,也是很多的上肢体育运动。终于有本书来探讨肩胛骨的方方面面,以及它对运动康复的诸多启示。

对于面对大量脊柱、肩、上肢损伤的康复科医生和非手术治疗运动损伤的医生来说,了解肩胛骨的功能、动作和它与其他骨骼肌肉系统之间的相互作用是很关键的。30多年前,我对肩部所有的关注几乎都集中在盂肱关节、肩袖对维持旋转瞬时中心的影响[1-3]。我记得 Kibler 在 1998 年的一篇文章里描述了肩胛骨位置的重要性,关节盂为旋转的肱骨提供了稳定的窝,并且是肩旋转的瞬时中心。突然间,除了单纯的肩袖,肩部活动有了新内容。后来有文章描述了肩胛骨运动障碍,这是肩胛骨处在非优化的功能异常时的显著临床表现,对肩袖有重要影响[5]。对我而言,肩胛骨的概念更清晰了,它构成了3处骨连接(锁骨、肱骨和胸椎),是18条肌肉的起点和止点附着,并对很多运动专项动作显示出巨大影响,如投掷动作和网球发球。显著的力量产生、转移和衰减都是通过肩胛骨及其周围组织良好的协调动作而获得的。肩胛骨在身体上的位置与很多我们治疗的主要肩部病变(如肩袖疾病、盂唇撕裂等)有一定距离,因此容易忽视它其实是上肢损伤因果关系中的一个重要部分。之后,人们又进一步发现肩胛骨与颈椎、胸椎相互作用的重要性,它参与了上肢和脊柱上段的相关损伤。

从实践角度讲,我对任何有上肢、脊柱上段问题的患者都会进行肩胛骨位置和运动评估。幸运的是,肩胛骨相对容易触诊、视诊和观察。只要看一下颈椎、胸椎和肩胛骨位置的相互关系，以及上臂和手在休息时的位置，就得到了很多信息，如哪些结构过度负荷或张力过大。

除了肩胛骨视诊，也可定量测量肩胛骨相对于脊柱的位置。Kibler在1998年的文章里描述了肩胛骨滑动的测量方法，它简便易行，能很好地评估肩胛骨的静态和动态位置[4]。在使用肩胛骨滑动测量方法作为临床工具多年后，我发现肩胛骨滑动在肩部病变患者中是非常普遍的，特别是肩袖撞击。进行适当的康复，待症状缓解后，肩胛骨滑动常常也有改善。

其他的肩胛骨临床测试也是我对上肢问题进行查体的常规部分。Kibler[4]设计了肩胛骨辅助试验来确定撞击是否是由于缺乏肩峰主动抬高造成的。一个明显的撞击征象是主动或被动抬高手臂至60°～130°的疼痛弧，提示肩峰下空间被挤压和激惹。肩袖在测试时可能表现为因疼痛而肌力减弱，伴随弹响、撞击症状。肩胛骨辅助试验使撞击症状正常化，提示肩胛骨功能失调与撞击综合征相关。测试包括患者在肩胛骨平面上抬手臂时，将肩胛骨内下缘向外、向上推，同时稳定肩胛骨内上缘，模拟上抬的前锯肌和下斜方肌力偶。若撞击与这些肌肉抑制有关，撞击症状会减少或消失。这项测试是非常重要的评估有撞击症状的患者的方法。

肩胛骨后缩/复位测试（SRT）也是评估肩袖撞击的一项重要、有用的测试。Kibler在2006年和Tate在2008年描述了肩胛骨后缩/复位测试。撞击测试阳性时，可再做一次，同时用SRT做肩胛骨手法复位。进行SRT时，抓住肩胛骨，手指在前方接触肩锁关节，手掌和大鱼际在后方接触肩胛冈，前臂斜向肩胛骨下角，给内侧缘额外支持。以这种方式，检查者的手和前臂施加中度力量使患者的肩胛骨后缩（后缩测试），或后倾和外旋，将肩胛骨靠近胸廓中部位置。肩胛骨复位测试具备可靠性，在进行测试时患者可以表现出更大的肩袖力量，并报告疼痛减轻[6,7]。

给颈、肩、手臂疼痛患者提供适当的康复方案时，医生对肩胛骨的了解尤为重要[8]。如果肩胛骨位置不当（如过度前伸），在前屈、外展时上抬手臂会更加困难。而且，由于肩胛骨过度前伸，胸肌和斜角肌会处于紧张、短缩的状态，中斜方肌和下斜方肌被拉长。这将导致头前伸，迫使上斜方肌过度工作来保证头不往前掉。这种肩胛骨在胸椎上的位置，以及头前伸的姿势，即使不是大多数，也是很多颈椎异常的核心原因。尽管有点怪，但在处理很多颈椎问题时，我们会先处理肩胛骨并使之复位。

我认为这是一本独一无二的书，它讨论了运动医学中一个关键的解剖结构，提供了肩胛骨知识的点点滴滴，能加强医生诊断和治疗上肢和脊柱的运动障碍及骨骼肌肉损伤的能力。本书布局合理，按照临床相关性和实用性进行排序。我日常都会使用本书介绍的概念为患者进行评估和治疗。它是运动医生的必备书，不管是外科医生还是其他医生。

Joel Press

参考文献

1. de Duca CJ, Forrest WJ. Force analysis of individual muscles acting simultaneously on the shoulder joint during isometric abduction. J Biomech, 1973, 6(4): 385–393.
2. Poppen NK, Walker PS. Normal and abnormal motion of the shoulder. J Bone Joint Surg Am, 1976, 58(2): 195–201.
3. Shoup TE. Optical measurement of the center of rotation for human joints. J Biomech, 1976, 9(4): 241–242.
4. Kibler WB. The role of the scapula in athletic shoulder function. Am J Sports Med, 1998, 26(2): 325–337.
5. Kibler WB, McMullen J. Scapular dyskinesis and its relation to shoulder pain. J Am Acad Orthop Surg, 2003, 11(2): 142–151.
6. Kibler WB, Sciascia AD, Dome D. Evaluation of apparent and absolute supraspinatus strength in patients with shoulder injury using the scapular retraction test. AM J Sports Med, 2006, 34: 1643–1647.
7. Tate A, McClure P, Kareha S, et al. Effect of the scapula reposition test on shoulder impingement symptoms and elevation strength in overhead athletes. J Ortho Sports Phys Ther, 2008, 38: 4–11.
8. Voight ML, Thomson BC. The role of the scapula in rehabilitation of shoulder injuries. J Athl Train, 2000, 35(3): 364–372.

序言

肩胛骨是一块神奇的骨头，它的作用广泛，能促进、优化几乎所有人类活动中的肩臂功能。它位于肩后部，被皮下组织和肌肉组织覆盖。它的活动度很大，一直以来，在考虑肩功能和损伤的过程中都未被充分重视和评估。但是，现代学术研究显示肩胛骨在促进肩功能的过程中有多重关键作用，凸显了肩胛骨静态位置和动态运动改变在多种肩病理和损伤中的角色。

当肩胛骨功能正常时，它是增加肌肉力量的好伙伴，移动肩峰为活动的手臂腾出空间，是手臂运动的基石，可以优化力量和爆发力的产生机制。肩胛骨的作用通过整个手臂来显现。但当肩胛骨无法正常工作时，它就变成了难应付的对手，使肩的力量下降，造成或加剧关节不稳定，加剧活动时的疼痛。它的负面作用遍及肩和手臂。临床检查肩胛骨可能有困难，治疗方案可能很复杂。这需要精确、全面地评估影响肩功能的所有因素。总体来说，由于缺乏对肩胛骨的医学教育，医生在治疗此类患者时需要更多的努力。

我也不例外。经过医学院教育和住院医生培训后，我对肩胛骨的了解寥寥无几。我个人对肩胛骨的学习是从30年前开始的，当时我注意到一位肩撞击患者存在翼状肩胛，她对传统治疗的反应不好。在手法复位后，她的症状立刻好转了，这使我踏上了学习肩胛骨的道路。我在这条路上持续很久，走走停停，也遇见了很多"死胡同"。我尝试理解它的基本动作及二维和三维的功能，然后形成几类动作评估及描述，最后与临床紧密结合：这些活动在肩功能和损伤中的角色是什么样的？最好的治疗方案是什么？……并且，需要有相同想法、愿意分享、有研究能力和临床能力的人员联合起来，共同发展肩胛骨的基础知识和临床应用。

这些努力促成了一系列的"肩胛骨峰会"，我们将相关人员组织起来，整理知识，聚焦未来研究和应用方向，为感兴趣的人们创造更大的联系网络。这些会议和在会议中发表的共识声明，刺激产生了一个大的知识体，这些知识大部分都在本书中体现。Phil

McClure、Paula Ludewig、Ann M. Cools 和 Tim L. Uhl 从一开始就参与进来，打造了基础知识的核心。另外，Jed Kuhn、Robin、Cromwell、Dave Ebaugh、Lori Michener 和 Marty Kelley 为扩展基础知识做出了宝贵的贡献。我要特别感谢 Aaron D. Sciascia，他在建立肩胛骨数据库、拟定临床治疗及康复方案和确定本书结构时起到了关键作用。

这本书是经过长期发展与实践获得的成果，它占据了我职业生涯的一大部分。我要感谢肯塔基肩中心的 David Dome、Pete W. Hester、Trevor Wilkes 和 Brent Morris，他们承担了很多临床工作，使研究得以开展，他们也撰写了本书的部分章节。

投身于本书的努力也影响了我的个人生活。我最坚实的后盾和最佳顾问总是 Betty Kibler——和我结婚47年的妻子。她对我生活方方面面的帮助早已超越眼睛能看见或人们所知道的，我永远都会向她寻求帮助、指导和建议。

肩胛骨是人体这台精密"仪器"的一个不可思议的部分。它的构造非常精妙，它的各部分即使在解剖学上相互独立，但却如此完美地相互合作完成功能。我感谢上帝让我对这个奇迹般的作品有所洞察，也希望可以继续解开人体的谜团，帮助那些有肩损伤和功能失调的人们。

最后我想向评估和治疗过的所有肩胛骨患者表示感谢。由于医生对肩胛骨的知识相对缺乏，他们常得不到及时的治疗，导致产生挫败感和肩功能问题。他们坚持寻求治疗，志愿参加研究，帮助我们对肩胛骨运动障碍的了解更深入。这是激励我们更新知识、改进照护方法的一大因素。我可以真诚地说，他们是这本书的合伙人。

是时候撰写本书了。我们已经积累了足够的科学知识，包括肩胛骨功能和失能情况的理论基础、足够的临床经验、足够的康复知识，以及验证肩胛骨功能/失能与各种肩损伤相关性的足够的临床知识。各章节的作者对相关领域非常精通，多是该领域知识建立的先驱者。本书不是了解肩胛骨的终点，而是一个非常好的起点。

请畅阅。

W. Ben Kibler

译者序

本书承蒙美国物理治疗师 Dr. Wendy S. Burke 的引介，在与美国南加州大学合作的高级临床培训项目中，我们有幸得到她的悉心教导和手把手的临床带教。Wendy 对康复理论和方法的评判性思想帮助我们拓展、更新了肌骨康复的整体理论，她清晰的临床推理思路也让我们在临床思辨和技能方面得到很大的提升。Wendy 作为肩关节康复领域的专家，向我们推荐了本书。在受益于本书对临床康复的指导作用后，我们翻译此书的热情被激发了。

本书围绕肩胛骨运动障碍这个较新的概念，系统说明了相关的解剖学和生物力学理论基础、肩胛骨障碍在各种常见肩损伤中的作用，以及运动障碍的评估方法和康复治疗方案。另外，书中汇总了详尽的科研资料，体现了循证实践的特点，也启发了后续的临床和科研思路。

本书还提供了丰富、清晰的图片，方便读者理解相关的解剖知识、运动学特点、运动障碍表现及评估和训练的方法等，让本书具有更强的实用价值。相信读者能够借助此书，在治疗肩胛骨运动障碍时取得更好的疗效，为患者提供更大的帮助。

感谢本书全体译者，以专业、敬业、精业的态度完成了翻译工作，让我们得以将此书推广给更多从事肩关节康复的同业。本书在翻译过程中，还得到了肩关节外科同业关于手术术语的指导，在此一并感谢。另外，我们在尽量忠于原文的基础上，对书中的一些用词根据中文习惯做了少许的调整，可能在翻译过程中还存在一些用法的不同或偏差，也恳请读者在阅读时批评指正。正如本书主编 Dr. Kibler 在序言中提及的，我们同样相信本书不是了解肩胛骨的终点，而是一个非常好的起点。

欢迎共同交流探讨！

王芗斌
何红晨

贡献者名单

Ann M. Cools, PhD, PT Faculty of Medicine and Health Sciences, Department of Rehabilitation Sciences and Physiotherapy, Ghent University, Ghent, Belgium

Robin Cromwell, PT Shoulder Center of Kentucky, Lexington, KY, USA

David Dome, MD Department of Orthopedics, Lexington Clinic Orthopedics—Sports Medicine Center, The Shoulder Center of Kentucky, Lexington, KY, USA

David Ebaugh, PT, PhD Department of Health Sciences, Department of Physical Therapy and Rehabilitation Sciences, College of Nursing and Health Professions, Drexel University, Philadelphia, PA, USA

T. Bradley Edwards, MD Department of Shoulder Surgery, Texas Orthopedic Hospital, Houston, TX, USA

Todd S. Ellenbecker, PT Physiotherapy Associates Scottsdale Sports Clinic, Scottsdale, AZ, USA

Margaret Finley, PT, PhD Department of Physical Therapy and Rehabilitation Sciences, College of Nursing and Health Professions, Drexel University, Philadelphia, PA, USA

Peter W. Hester, MD Orthopedics-Sports Medicine, Lexington Clinic, Lexington, KY, USA

Zaamin B. Hussain, BA Steadman Philippon Research Institute, Vail, CO, USA

Martin J. Kelley, PT, DPT, OCS Department of Orthopaedic Surgery, Good Shepherd Penn Partners, University of Pennsylvania, Philadelphia, PA, USA

John D. Kelly 4th, MD Department of Ortho, University of Pennsylvania, Philadelphia, PA, USA

W. Ben Kibler, MD Department of Orthopedics, Lexington Clinic Orthopedics—Sports Medicine Center, The Shoulder Center of Kentucky, Lexington, KY, USA

John E. Kuhn, MD, MS Vanderbilt University Medical Center, Nashville, TN, USA

Rebekah L. Lawrence, DPT, PT, OCS Division of Rehabilitation Science, Department of Rehabilitation Medicine, Medical School, The University of Minnesota, Minneapolis, MN, USA

George F. Lebus, MD Steadman Philippon Research Institute, Vail, CO, USA The Steadman Clinic, Vail, CO, USA

Donald Lee, MD Department of Orthopaedic Surgery, Vanderbilt University Medical Center, Nashville, TN, USA

Paula M. Ludewig, PhD, PT, FAPTA Divisions of Physical Therapy and Rehabilitation Science, Department of Rehabilitation Medicine, Medical School, The University of Minnesota, Minneapolis, MN, USA

Phil McClure, PT, PhD, FAPTA Department of Physical Therapy, Arcadia University, Glenside, PA, USA

Lori A. Michener, PhD, PT, ATC Division of Biokinesiology and Physical Therapy, University of Southern California, Los Angeles, CA, USA

Peter J. Millett, MD, MSc Steadman Philippon Research Institute, Vail, CO, USA
The Steadman Clinic, Vail, CO, USA

Brent J. Morris, MD Department of Orthopedics, Lexington Clinic Orthopedics –Sports Medicine Center, The Shoulder Center of Kentucky, Lexington, KY, USA

Michael T. Piercey, PT, DPT, OCS, Cert. MDT, CMP, CSCS Good Shepherd Penn Partners, University of Pennsylvania, Philadelphia, PA, USA

Jonas Pogorzelski, MD, MHBA Steadman Philippon Research Institute, Vail, CO, USA

Katherine E. Reuther, PhD Department of Biomedical Engineering, Columbia University, New York, NY, USA

Aaron D. Sciascia, PhD, ATC, PES Assistant Professor, Athletic Training Education Program, Eastern Kentucky University, Richmond, KY, USA

Stephen J. Thomas, PhD, ATC Department of Kinesiology, Temple University, Philadelphia, PA, USA
Penn Throwing Clinic, Philadelphia, PA, USA

Tim L. Uhl, PhD, ATC, PT, FNATA Division of Athletic Training, Department of Rehabilitation Sciences, College of Health Sciences, University of Kentucky, Lexington, KY, USA

Trevor Wilkes, MD Department of Orthopedics, Lexington Clinic Orthopedics—Sports Medicine Center, The Shoulder Center of Kentucky, Lexington, KY, USA

Thomas W. Wright, MD Department of Orthopaedics and Rehabilitation, University of Florida, Gainesville, FL, USA

缩略语表

胸腹简明外伤量表　abbreviated injury scale，AIS
美国肩肘外科医生评分　American shoulder and elbow surgeons score，ASES
复合肌肉动作电位　compound muscle action potential，CMAP
计算机断层扫描　computed tomography，CT
上肢功能　disability of arm shoulder and hand，DASH
动态盂唇剪切　dynamic labral shear，DLS
盂肱关节内旋不足　glenohumeral internal rotation deficit，GIRD
创伤严重度评分　injury severity score，ISS
肩胛骨外侧悬吊系统　lateral scapular suspension system，LSSS
胸长神经麻痹　long thoracic nerve palsy，LTNP
磁共振成像　magnetic resonance imaging，MRI
自主运动单元电位　motor unit potentials，MUPs
神经肌肉电刺激疗法　neuromuscular electrical stimulation，NMES
切开复位内固定术　open reduction and internal fixation，ORIF
疼痛灾难化程度量表　pain catastrophizing scale，PCS
反向肩关节置换手术　reverse shoulder arthroplasty，RSA
副神经麻痹　spinal accessory nerve palsy，SANP
肩胛骨辅助试验　scapular assistance test，SAT
肩肱节律　scapulohumeral rhythm，SHR
肩胛骨错位、下内侧缘突出、喙突痛和肩胛骨运动障碍　scapula malposition/inferior medial border prominence/coracoid pain/scapular dyskinesis，SICK
上盂唇前后部　superior labral anterior to posterior，SLAP

肩胛骨后缩/复位测试　scapular retraction or reposition test，SRT

肩部症状调整手段　shoulder symptom modification procedure，SSMP

肩胛骨弹响综合征　snapping scapula syndrome，SSS

肩上方悬吊复合体　superior shoulder suspension complex，SSSC

简单肩关节测试　simple shoulder test，SST

尺侧副韧带　ulnar collateral ligament，UCL

目录

第一部分 基础

第 1 章 肩胛骨解剖   2
Trevor Wilkes, W. Ben Kibler, Aaron D. Sciascia

第 2 章 肩胛骨力学在肩功能和功能障碍中的作用   6
Paula M. Ludewig, Rebekah L. Lawrence

第 3 章 与肩胛骨功能和功能障碍相关的肌肉激活   24
David Ebaugh, Margaret Finley

第 4 章 肩胛骨检查   33
Phil McClure, Aaron D. Sciascia, Tim L. Uhl

第二部分 肩胛骨和肩部病变

第 5 章 撞击综合征和肩袖疾病   48
Katherine E. Reuther, Brent J. Morris, John E. Kuhn

第 6 章 投掷类、过头类项目运动员的肩胛骨   57
Stephen J. Thomas, John D. Kelly 4th

第 7 章 肩胛骨运动障碍和盂肱关节不稳定   79
W. Ben Kibler, Aaron D. Sciascia

| 第 8 章 | 锁骨骨折 | 90 |

Peter W. Hester, W. Ben Kibler

| 第 9 章 | 肩锁关节分离及关节炎 | 98 |

Brent J. Morris, David Dome, Aaron D. Sciascia, W. Ben Kibler

| 第 10 章 | 肩骨关节炎 | 107 |

Brent J. Morris, T. Bradley Edwards, Thomas W. Wright

| 第 11 章 | 肩胛骨肌肉撕脱 | 113 |

W. Ben Kibler, Aaron D. Sciascia

| 第 12 章 | 神经损伤和翼状肩胛 | 122 |

John E. Kuhn

| 第 13 章 | 神经问题的康复方案 | 131 |

Martin J. Kelley, Michael T. Piercey

| 第 14 章 | 肩胛骨弹响综合征 | 145 |

George F. Lebus, Zaamin B. Hussain, Jonas Pogorzelski, Peter J. Millett

| 第 15 章 | 肩胛骨骨折 | 158 |

Donald Lee, Schuyler Halverson

| 第 16 章 | 肩胛骨运动障碍的康复 | 177 |

Ann M. Cools, Todd S. Ellenbecker, Lori A. Michener

| 第 17 章 | 复杂型肩胛骨功能障碍的康复：考虑疼痛和运动模式改变 | 189 |

Aaron D. Sciascia, Robin Cromwell, Tim L. Uhl

第一部分

基础

第1章 肩胛骨解剖

Trevor Wilkes, W. Ben Kibler, Aaron D. Sciascia

引言

理想的肩胛骨功能反映了肩胛骨复杂的解剖结构,并且它是所有肩功能的基础。肩胛骨扮演着许多角色。在解剖学上,它是盂肱关节中的关节盂部分,也是肩锁关节中的肩峰部分。在生理上,它是肩肱节律肩的部分,肩胛骨和上肢协同运动,使上肢处于完成各种动作最理想的位置上。在生物力学方面,肩胛骨是肌肉激活的稳定基础,是维持球窝运动的移动平台,是躯干和上肢的有效连接——躯干产生力量,上肢传导并发出力量。上述一系列运动的关键就是正常的肩胛骨活动。

深入掌握肩胛骨解剖结构对于理解肩胛骨复杂的生物力学至关重要。

众所周知,各种肩部病理改变均会体现在肩运动的改变上。通常评估肩胛骨的肌肉附着点、神经支配、运动和位置可以为治疗和康复提供关键信息。肩胛骨的功能及临床意义均基于肩胛骨的解剖结构,本章将简要介绍肩胛骨的解剖学相关知识。

解剖

肩胛骨的解剖揭示了其运动发育的优势,如抓握和过头动作。这反映在原始人的肩胛骨随着时间推移发生的几个主要变化中。首先,肩峰变宽并侧向化,使三角肌发挥力学优势[1]。喙突增大,理论上有助于预防肩关节在外展90°时前脱位[2, 3]。最后,冈下肌和小圆肌的力矢量的扩大和改变,增加了外旋强度和肱骨头下压[4]。

肩胛骨是一个大的扁平骨,由一组间质细胞形成[5]。它在胚胎发育第5周时即显示出骨化迹象[5]。肩胛骨遵循既定程序从颈椎旁区域下降到胸廓。这个过程的失败会导致Sprengel畸形[6]。到第7周,肩胛骨已经下降到最终位置,这时很容易识别关节盂。

肩胛骨主要通过膜内成骨形成。肢体和脊柱在出生时骨化,随后遵循预期的模式成长。然而,有几个值得注意的、具有临床意义的例外。喙突由2个骨化中心形成,一般在15岁时融合。极少数情况下,在尖端的第3个骨化中心可以持续存在并与骨折混淆[7]。关节盂也由2个独立的骨化中心形成，一个位于喙突的底部，另一个在其下方呈马蹄形轮廓[7]，通常在15岁之前融合。最后，多达8%的人可能有肩峰小骨，这是有2或3个骨化中心的结果，这些骨化中心在青春期出现，并且未能在预期的22岁时融合[8]。各种融合失败会导致以下异常结构，从前到后依次为：前肩峰、中肩峰（最常见）、偏肩峰和基础肩峰。

总体来说，肩胛骨是一块薄薄的骨头，它是肌肉附着的关键部位。血液供应主要是通过骨膜的血管网络，血液自肌肉附着点进入骨。肩胛骨的骨质在肩胛骨外侧缘及上、下角增厚。肩胛骨腹侧凹面在肋骨上形成光滑的关节面。腹侧存在小的斜嵴，为肩胛下肌提供附着点[5]。与之类似，背侧存在小的纤维隔，用来附着和分隔冈下肌、小圆肌和大圆肌。肩胛冈在肩胛骨背侧表面横穿两个凹陷，形成冈上窝和冈下窝。这些凹窝内侧的2/3发出冈上肌和冈下肌。肩胛冈包含两个重要的切迹。喙突底部的肩胛上切迹包含肩胛上神经，此位置受压迫将影响冈上肌和冈下肌[3, 9]。冈盂切迹存在于肩胛冈的外侧边缘[3]。各种原因也可导致这里的肩胛上神经受压，产生单纯冈下肌萎缩。

通常人们对肩胛骨解剖结构中的喙突、肩峰或关节盂较有兴趣。喙突的英文"coracoid"源自希腊语"korakodes"，意思是"像乌鸦的喙"[3]。喙突弯曲的形状类似于手指指向关节盂。希腊词"akros"的意

思是点，而肩峰（英文"acromion"）就是肩部的顶点。肩峰的形态研究是最多的。大量的尸体研究都是针对Bigliani[1]提出的1至3型肩峰的相对多发情况和假定原因。然而，肩峰形状与撞击综合征或肩袖撕裂之间的关系在文献中并未得到证实。关节盂也已成为被深入研究的主题，研究者着重探索肩部不稳定的骨骼解剖原因[7, 10-13]。关节盂的平均尺寸为高35 mm、宽25 mm，但存在相当大的变异性；因此如果想精确定义骨质流失，需要与对侧进行比较。关节盂倾斜角也是不定的，后倾最常见，多达6°，在75%的人口中可见。但是也有前倾多达2°的报道[14-18]。

肩胛骨的功能取决于18块附着其上的肌肉的复杂募集模式[19]。这些肌肉通常可分为中轴肩胛骨肌群、肩胛肱骨肌群和上臂肌群（喙肱肌、肱二头肌和肱三头肌）[20, 21]。

中轴肩胛骨肌群用于固定肩胛骨，而肩胛骨是肩部的基石。此外，它们引导肩胛骨进行必要活动。这些肌肉包括前锯肌、肩胛提肌、胸小肌、菱形肌和斜方肌。斜方肌是最大和最浅表的中轴肩胛肌，起自枕骨、项韧带和$C_7 \sim T_{12}$棘突[20]。上斜方肌止于锁骨远端1/3和肩峰处。中斜方肌止于肩胛冈和冈底部下方。宽阔的肌肉可通过不同的激活模式使肩胛骨完成复杂的后缩、上抬和后倾功能。通常上斜方肌和下斜方肌是各自激活的。第11对脑神经，即副神经支配斜方肌[3]。菱形肌分为大菱形肌和小菱形肌。小菱形肌起于C_7和T_1的棘突，止于肩胛骨内侧缘[20]。大菱形

肌起于 $T_2 \sim T_5$ 棘突，止于肩胛骨内侧缘后方。这样的肌肉走行在肩胛骨后缩中起重要作用。肩胛背神经（C_5）提供神经支配。

前锯肌由3个分支组成，起自第1～9肋的前外侧。支配前锯肌的神经是胸长神经。前锯肌为使肩胛骨前伸和上旋及使上肢前屈和抬高的几乎所有位置提供重要的稳定功能，并能防止过多的肩胛骨内旋。

肩胛提肌与前锯肌密切相关，起到抬高和上旋肩胛骨的作用。肩胛提肌起自 $C_1 \sim C_3$ 横突，有时至 C_4，止于肩胛骨上角，神经支配来自 C_3 和 C_4 的深层分支。胸小肌对肩胛骨位置的作用经常被忽视，它起自第3～5肋，走向外上方止于肩胛骨喙突。该肌慢性紧张可导致肩胛骨处于前伸和前倾位[22-24]。

肩胛肱骨肌群由三角肌、冈上肌、冈下肌、肩胛下肌、小圆肌和大圆肌组成，产生盂肱关节运动。三角肌起于肩峰和肩胛冈，止于肱骨三角肌粗隆，这种结构允许它在多个平面提供有利的上抬动作。如前所述，冈上肌和冈下肌起自它们各自窝的内侧2/3，同时以较复杂的排列方式止于肱骨大结节。肩胛下肌起自肩胛骨前侧并附着在肱骨小结节上。小圆肌起于肩胛骨外侧的中间部分，受腋神经后支支配。大圆肌位于肩胛骨外侧的更下方，并且在二头肌沟的内侧与背阔肌形成共同肌腱，它们均由肩胛下神经支配，功能为使肱骨内旋、内收和伸展。

肩胛骨周围存在两个主要的滑囊，下锯滑囊位于前锯肌和胸壁之间，上锯滑囊位于肩胛下肌和前锯肌之间。此外，还有一些小的滑囊分布在肩胛骨内上缘。这些滑囊可能因过度使用和力学方面的细微异常而持续存在炎症。

（陈翰）

参考文献

1. Bigliani LU. The morphology of the acromion and its relationship to rotator cuff tears. Orthop Trans, 1986, 10: 228.

2. Lal H, Bansal P, Sabharwal VK, et al. Recurrent shoulder dislocations secondary to coracoid process fracture: a case report. J Orthop Surg, 2012, 20(1): 121–125.

3. Moore KL, Dalley AF. Clinically oriented anatomy. Baltimore: Lippincott Williams & Wilkins, 1999.

4. Baumgartner D, Tomas D, Gossweiler L, et al. Towards the development of a novel experimental shoulder simulator with rotating scapula and individually controlled muscle forces simulating the rotator cuff. Med Biol Eng Comput, 2014, 52: 293–299.

5. Huang R, Christ B, Patel K. Regulation of scapula development. Anat Embryol, 2006, 211(Suppl 1): 65–71.

6. Schrock RD. Congenital elevation of the scapula. J Bone Joint Surg, 1926, 8: 207–215.

7. O'Brien SJ, Arnoczky SP, Warren RF, et al. The shoulder. Philadelphia: W. B. Saunders Company, 1990.

8. Nicholson GP, Goodman DA, Flatow EL, et al. The acromion: morphologic condition and agerelated changes. A study of 420 scapulas. J Shoulder Elbow Surg, 1996, 5(1): 1–11.

9. Lorei MP, Hershman EB. Peripheral nerve injuries in athletes: Treatment and prevention. Sports Med, 1993, 16(2): 130–147.
10. Cain PR, Mutschler TA, Fu FH, et al. Anterior instability of the glenohumeral joint: a dynamic model. Am J Sports Med, 1987, 15(2): 144–148.
11. Howell SM, Galinat BJ. The glenoid-labral socket, a constrained articular surface. Clin Orthop Relat Res, 1989, 243: 122–125.
12. Prodromos CC, Perry JA, Schiller AL, et al. Histological studies of the glenoid labrum from fetal life to old age. J Bone Joint Surg (Am Vol), 1990, 72(9): 1344–1348.
13. Zarins B, Rowe CR. Current concepts in the diagnosis and treatment of shoulder instability in athletes. Med Sci Sports Exerc, 1984, 16(5): 444–448.
14. Kronberg M, Brostrom L, Soderlund V. Retroversion of the humeral head in the normal shoulder and its relationship to the normal range of motion. Clin Orthop Relat Res, 1990, 253: 113–117.
15. Osbahr DC, Cannon DL, Speer KP. Retroversion of the humerus in the throwing shoulder of college baseball pitchers. Am J Sports Med, 2002, 30: 347–353.
16. Reagan KM, Meister K, Horodyski M, et al. Humeral retroversion and its relationship to glenohumeral rotation in the shoulder of college baseball players. Am J Sports Med, 2002, 30(3): 354–360.
17. Robertson DD, Yuan J, Bigliani LU, et al. Three-dimensional analysis of the proximal part of the humerus: relevance to arthroplasty. J Bone Joint Surg Am, 2000, 82(11): 1594–1602.
18. Soderlund V, Kronberg M, Brostrom L. Radiologic assessment of humeral head retroversion. Acta Radiol, 1989, 30(5): 501–505.
19. Kibler WB, Sciascia AD. Current concepts: scapular dyskinesis. Br J Sports Med, 2010, 44(5): 300–305.
20. de Vita A, Kibler WB, Pouliart N, et al. Atlas of functional shoulder anatomy. Milan: Springer, 2008.
21. Pu Q, Huang R, Brand-Saberi B. Development of the shoulder girdle musculature. Dev Dyn, 2016, 245: 342–350.
22. Borstad JD. Measurement of pectoralis minor muscle length: validation and clinical application. J Orthop Sports Phys Ther, 2008, 38: 169–174.
23. Borstad JD, Ludewig PM. Comparison of three stretches for the pectoralis minor muscle. J Shoulder Elbow Surg, 2006, 15(3): 324–330.
24. Borstad JD, Ludewig PM. The effect of long versus short pectoralis minor resting length on scapular kinematics in healthy individuals. J Orthop Sports Phys Ther, 2005, 35(4): 227–238.

第 2 章　肩胛骨力学在肩功能和功能障碍中的作用

Paula M. Ludewig, Rebekah L. Lawrence

引言

肩的作用是使手可以跨越很大的空间范围或有功能性工作空间。因此，盂肱关节是人体活动范围最大的关节，用来满足肩部活动的需求。肩胛骨（关节盂）作为肩关节的近端部件，在使手能触及最大范围的同时，仍在保持盂肱关节的完整性方面起着至关重要的作用。本章回顾了在上肢运动期间肩胛骨的正常位置和运动的现有知识，并概述了肩胛骨运动异常将如何导致肩疼痛和功能障碍。我们认识到，随着研究推进，持续更新对肩功能和功能障碍的理解的重要性。

关节运动成分和肩胛骨功能概述

虽然肩胛胸壁在定义上不是真正的关节，但在临床和科学文献中经常用它来描述整个肩胛骨在胸部的位置和运动（即肩胛胸壁的位置和运动），而不描述为胸锁关节和肩锁关节的位置和运动。这在一定程度上是由于观察和测量肩胛胸壁的位置和运动更容易。本章将提供与肩胛胸壁有关的知识，以及目前已知的胸锁关节和肩锁关节的具体功能。作为连接的节段，如果胸锁关节和肩锁关节没有运动，肩胛骨就不可能在胸部产生运动。最常见的是，胸锁关节和肩锁关节都发生运动[1, 2]。胸廓表面为肩胛骨可能的位置和运动提供了额外的约束。胸廓、锁骨、肩胛骨及其相关关节通常被统称为肩胛带。因此，肩胛胸壁运动实际上是组合了肩胛带复合体的运动。

总的来说，肩胛骨在胸部移动和重新定位的能力对肩功能的多个方面都很重要。正如已经提到的，肩胛胸壁的复杂运动使手的活动范围最大化时，肱骨头仍保持在肩胛骨关节盂中至关重要[3]。图 2.1 直观地说明了没有肩胛骨运动时的大致功能活动空间，以及通过肩胛骨和肱骨组合运动可获得的额外活动范围。此外，盂肱关节拥有较大的活动度，使得三角肌在解剖学上的单关节肌群中具有独特性，即当肱骨相对于胸部抬高时可能会发生主动功能不足[4]。通过肩胛骨运动（特别是向上旋转），三角肌的近侧肩胛骨附着点移动维持

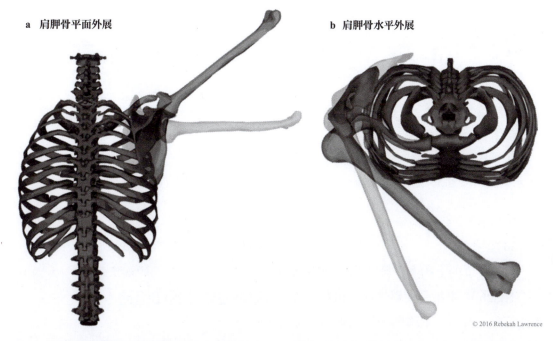

图 2.1　肩胛骨运动对整个肩运动的贡献。透明骨骼表示无肩胛胸壁贡献时预期的活动范围，不透明骨骼表示盂肱关节和肩胛胸壁一起贡献时的活动范围（经 Rebakah L. Lawrance 许可转载）

了更稳健的长度-张力关系。更好地维持长度-张力关系可以使三角肌产生更大的力量，使盂肱关节达到需要抬高的角度。肩胛骨的位置和运动被认为是既能保持盂肱关节的稳定性和功能性，又能使肌肉和关节结构（如肩袖、盂唇、肱二头肌长头、肩锁关节及盂肱关节的关节囊和韧带、喙肩韧带和肩峰下表面等）的额外应力最小化的关键。本章将总结并进一步讨论异常肩胛骨位置和运动或运动障碍对组织和关节应力的影响。

胸锁关节位置和运动

胸锁关节由锁骨的胸骨端和胸骨柄的锁骨切迹组成（图 2.2）。在国际上，有许多不同的动作命名存在，但我们将胸锁关节的三类旋转动作称为上抬和下降、前伸和后缩，以及绕长轴前旋和后旋。除了骨运动学的旋转运动，少量的平移可以在关节的三个平面发生。这些平移运动和相关的关节运动在其他文献中[5]有描述，并不是本章的重点。

胸锁关节的前伸和后缩接近于垂直轴（图 2.2a）。前伸使锁骨远端向前运动，而后缩使锁骨远端向后运动。当放松站立时，锁骨相对于胸部冠状面的起始位置约为后缩 20°[6, 7]。这种后缩可以在体格检查时通过触诊相对于胸锁关节稍后方位置的肩锁关节观察到。锁骨前伸和后缩的总体活动范围在文献中并没有得到特征性描述，但被认为是大约前伸 20° 和从最初的后缩位

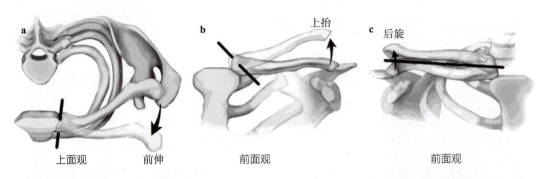

图2.2 胸锁关节的活动:(a)绕垂直轴的前伸和后缩 (b)绕前轴的上抬和下降 (c)绕长轴的前旋和后旋[6]

后缩 30°。

胸锁关节的上抬和下降发生在前后轴上(图2.2b)。上抬是使锁骨远端相对于其休息位向上升高,下降则是使锁骨远端降低。在放松站立位时,锁骨相对于胸部水平面的初始位置通常是轻微抬高的(10°或更小)[6,7]。这种轻微的抬高可以在体格检查时通过触诊相对于胸锁关节稍上方位置的肩锁关节观察到。从轻微抬高的初始位置开始,由于紧邻锁骨下方的胸廓的约束,锁骨只能出现轻度下降(10°~15°)[8]。锁骨上抬的总体活动范围在研究文献中并没有得到确切的定义,但曾被描述为从初始位置抬高45°[8]。稍后将要提到,在功能性手臂抬高时,锁骨上抬角度要小得多。

胸锁关节的前后旋转围绕锁骨的长轴发生(图2.2c)。前旋使锁骨锥状结节向后移动,而后旋使其转向前侧。目前没有解剖学标准来定义锁骨的初始轴向旋转位置,因此,其在放松站立位时通常被认为是0°旋转。由于第1肋的限制,锁骨前旋的总体活动范围是很小的。锁骨后旋的总体活动范围是50°[2],手臂抬高期间胸锁关节的主要运动即对应此旋转[2,6]。

肩锁关节位置和运动

肩锁关节允许锁骨远端和肩胛骨前内侧肩峰之间发生相对运动,并且该关节盘内经常包括一个中间带。这通常被描述为更远端的肩胛骨相对于锁骨移动(图2.3)。与胸锁关节的动作一样,肩锁关节也存在多种动作命名惯例。我们将使用上旋和下旋、内旋和外旋,以及前倾和后倾来描述肩锁关节的三类旋转动作。读者可以参考其他文献[5]对肩锁关节平移和关节运动的描述。

肩锁关节内旋和外旋通常也分别被称为前伸和后缩。然而,我们更喜欢使用内旋和外旋来区分胸锁关节和肩锁关节在水平面的旋转。肩锁关节的内旋和外旋是围绕肩锁关节处的近似垂直轴描述的(图2.3a)。内旋将使关节盂朝向前方,而外旋将使关节盂朝向后方。在放松站立时,观察肩锁关节内旋和外旋初始位置的最好角度是俯视肩胛骨和锁骨的水平面(图2.4)。

参考肩胛轴（沿肩胛冈根部指向肩锁关节后部）相对于锁骨长轴的对线（图2.4），肩锁关节内旋的初始位置略小于60°[6, 9]。肩锁关节的内外旋转活动范围鲜有人研究[8]。由于胸廓的约束，肩锁关节可获得的活动范围取决于胸锁关节的后缩程度。例如，当锁骨处于更加后缩的位置时，肩胛骨和锁骨间水平面的夹角将会减小。随之而来的是，肩胛骨前外侧缘与胸部的接触将会限制肩锁关节内旋，而肩胛骨椎体侧前缘与胸部的接触将会限制肩锁关节外旋。相反，当胸锁关节的后缩减少时，肩胛骨沿着胸廓曲面滑动限制了胸锁关节前伸，肩胛骨和锁骨间水平面的夹角将会增大。当肩胛骨位于胸部更外侧时，由于来自圆形胸部的约束较小，肩锁关节的内旋和外旋活动范围可能更大。

肩锁关节的上旋和下旋是围绕垂直于肩胛骨平面的前后斜轴描述的（图2.3b）。上旋将使关节盂向上，下旋将使关节盂向下（图2.3b）。参考肩胛轴（沿肩胛冈根部指向肩锁关节后部）相对于锁骨长轴的对线，在放松站立时，肩锁关节上旋的初始位置小于5°[6]。最新文献没有描述肩锁关节的总活动范围[8]。然而，在无症状受试者的手臂抬高过程中可测量到20°的上旋[6]，这种运动幅度使上旋成为肩锁关节的主要动作之一。

肩锁关节的前倾和后倾是围绕穿过肩锁关节的斜侧轴描述的（图2.3c）。该动作是相对于肩峰进行定义的，前倾使肩峰前方向下和向前，后倾使肩峰前方向上和向后。值得注意的是，肩胛骨下角在前后倾运动期间的运动呈相反方向（如前倾使肩胛骨下角向后方运动），因此该运动的定义有容易混淆的地方。当放松站立时，肩锁关节前倾的初始位置约为10°或更小[6]。肩锁关节前倾和后倾的总活动范围也没有在

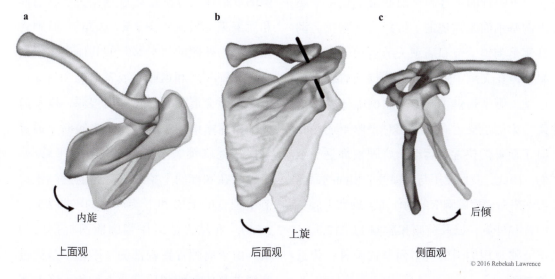

图2.3　肩锁关节的运动：（a）内旋和外旋　（b）上旋和下旋　（c）前倾和后倾（经Rebekah L. Lawrence许可转载）

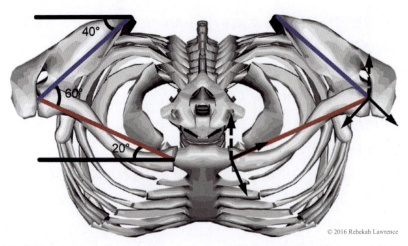

图2.4 肩锁关节和胸锁关节的轴包括肩胛轴（蓝色）、锁骨长轴（红色）和躯干冠状面轴（黑色）。肩胛轴相对于锁骨长轴的倾斜方向定义了胸锁关节运动和肩胛胸壁运动之间的间接耦合关系。在放松站立位，锁骨通常后缩20°，肩胛骨相对于躯干的冠状面内旋约40°。因此，肩锁关节处通常显示肩胛骨相对于锁骨长轴有60°的内旋角（经Rebekah L. Lawrence许可转载）

最近的研究中得出[8]。然而，在无症状受试者的手臂抬高过程中至少可以测到20°的后倾[6]。这种运动幅度使后倾成为肩锁关节除上旋外的主要动作。

肩胛胸壁位置和运动

肩胛骨的位置和运动通常是相对于躯干的基本面来描述的。虽然肩胛胸壁运动其实是胸锁关节和肩锁关节运动的直接结果，但在文献中还是会直接提到肩胛胸壁运动。躯干提供了一个有用的临床参考框架。无论是描述肩胛骨相对于躯干还是相对于锁骨的位置和运动，肩胛轴都是一致的。因此，我们使用与肩锁关节相同的命名习惯来命名肩胛胸壁的动作（上旋和下旋、内旋和外旋，以及前倾和后倾）（图2.3），但要注意用躯干的基本面取代锁骨作为近端参考。

肩胛骨在胸部的运动通常被描述为"平移"。因为肩胛骨不能在胸锁关节或肩锁关节没有运动、甚至两者都没有运动的情况下在胸部单独移动，并且因为这两个关节仅允许非常有限的平移，所以重要的是认识到肩胛骨的"平移"实际上是通过胸锁关节旋转产生的。肩胛骨在胸部内外侧的"平移"分别是通过胸锁关节的前伸和后缩来完成的（图2.5a、2.5b）。肩胛骨在胸部内外侧的"平移"的其他表述包括肩胛胸壁外展和内收，或者前伸和后缩。由于可能会混淆"平移"的根源，以及前伸和后缩术语的重叠，我们更倾向于通过直接描述胸锁关节旋转来描述"平移"。肩胛骨在胸部的上抬和下降是通过胸锁关节中锁骨的上旋和下旋产生的（图2.5c、2.5d），重要的是记住胸廓曲面提供的约束。由于肩胛骨在胸部的"平移"是通过胸锁关节的前伸和后缩或上抬和下降而产生的,因此在肩锁关节处需要调节角度,以使肩胛骨适应弯曲的胸廓表面。

肩胛骨在胸部的整体上旋和下旋是围绕垂直于肩胛骨平面的前后斜轴描述的。在肩锁关节处,上旋将使关节盂向上,下旋使关节盂向下(图2.3b)。参考肩胛轴(沿肩胛冈根部指向肩锁关节后部)相对于躯干水平面的对线,在放松站立时,肩锁关节上旋的初始位置小于5°[6]。胸锁关节和肩锁关节联合运动引起的肩胛骨在胸部的主要运动是上旋,总活动范围常被报道为60°或更大[2]。

重要的是认识到所有关于关节位置和运动的描述,其报道价值取决于为定义旋转轴而选择的解剖标志,以及受试者样本,这对于描述肩胛骨上旋尤其重要。按照从肩胛冈根部到肩锁关节后部的旋转轴的描述,肩胛骨在放松站立时的初始位置通常存在上旋,即使肩胛骨椎体缘处于垂直位置(图2.6)。这是因为肩胛骨椎体缘不与肩胛轴垂直(图2.6)。以肩胛骨椎体缘为轴的肩胛骨上旋值很小,因此通常将放松

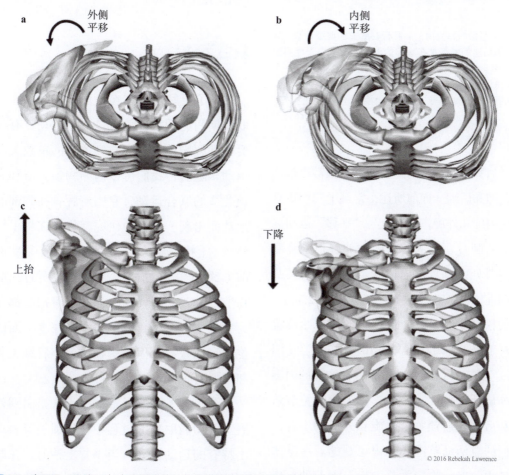

图2.5 肩胛骨"平移":(a)通过胸锁关节前伸产生的肩胛骨在胸部的外侧"平移"或肩胛骨外侧移动 (b)通过胸锁关节后缩产生的肩胛骨内侧"平移"(c)通过胸锁关节上抬产生的肩胛骨上抬或肩胛骨在胸部的上抬运动 (d)通过胸锁关节下降产生的肩胛骨下降(经Rebekah L. Lawrence许可转载)

站立时肩胛骨在胸壁的位置定义为0°[5]。

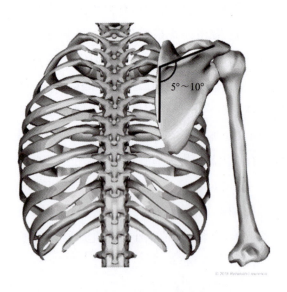

图2.6 当放松站立时，肩胛骨在胸部的典型位置。注意，所描述的肩胛骨在胸部的上旋幅度取决于使用的轴。平行于肩胛骨内侧缘的轴不直接与肩胛轴垂直。两轴夹角为95°~100°。这样，当上肢放松放在体侧时，以肩胛骨内侧缘为轴，肩胛骨上旋0°；以肩胛冈为轴时，肩胛骨上旋5°~10°（经Rebekah L. Lawrence许可转载）

肩胛骨在胸部的内旋和外旋通常也被称为前伸和后缩。如前所述，常规上我们更喜欢用内旋和外旋，并避免与"平移"运动混淆。肩胛骨在胸部的内旋和外旋是围绕肩锁关节处的垂直轴描述的。内旋将使关节盂向前，外旋将使关节盂向后（图2.3a）。在放松站立时，肩胛骨在胸部的初始位置相对于躯干的冠状面向前30°~40°[6,7]（图2.4）。尚未直接研究出肩胛骨在胸部的内旋和外旋活动范围。然而，作为胸锁关节前伸和后缩与肩锁关节内旋和外旋的组合，它们的总活动范围还是很可观的。在身体交叉内收时，胸锁关节发生最大前伸，肩锁关节发生最大内旋，这种状态证明了以

上观点（图2.1b）。

肩胛骨在胸部的前倾和后倾是围绕斜侧轴的。例如在肩锁关节，运动是相对于肩峰进行描述的，如前倾将使肩峰向上、向前，而后倾将使肩峰向下、向后（图2.3c）。在放松站立时，肩胛骨在胸部的初始位置为前倾5°~10°[6]。同样，在研究文献中也没有关于肩胛骨在胸部前倾和后倾的总活动范围的描述。然而，由于在这种肩胛骨复合运动中胸锁关节没有实质性的贡献[6,9]，所以总活动范围应该与肩锁关节的活动范围类似。

复合运动

为了更好地理解在平面上抬和功能性取物期间肩胛骨在胸部的复合运动，有必要先理解胸锁关节和肩锁关节的单独关节运动。随后，我们可以回顾胸锁关节和肩锁关节的联合运动，它因肩胛骨在胸部的运动而出现。大多数研究都集中在将手臂外展（上抬手臂至肩胛骨平面或躯干冠状面前方约40°）或屈曲[6,7]，以及随意过头取物上[10]。我们将任何平面的手臂抬起都视为肱骨上抬。尽管上抬的手臂在水平面的位置存在差异，但是胸锁关节、肩锁关节和肩胛胸壁的运动是一样的。

在任何平面的手臂上抬（从屈曲到外展）及功能取物的过程中，胸锁关节表现出特有的运动模式。当手臂上抬时，在胸锁关节发生的主要运动是后旋[2,6]。手臂在任何平面抬高到120°时，胸锁关节处的锁

骨后旋约30°。为了手臂上抬得更高，锁骨将进一步后旋。随着手臂从屈曲变为外展，这种运动的数量或模式没有实质性变化[6]。

胸锁关节在手臂上抬过程中发生了后缩。在肩胛骨平面外展达到120°时，胸锁关节预期发生约15°的后缩。但是，胸锁关节的后缩程度将直接受到手臂上抬平面的影响。例如，为了使手臂屈曲，肩胛骨（特别是关节盂）需要更向前，以保持与肱骨的一致性。为了使手臂外展，肩胛骨需要更向后，与肱骨一致。为了允许肩胛骨在水平面发生这样的变化，胸锁关节和肩锁关节在水平面的复合位置也必须改变。在屈曲的过程中，胸锁关节仍然会进行整体后缩，但只是从初始的放松站立位稍微后缩一点，并且在手臂上抬的过程中，整体后缩会减少[6]。在冠状面的手臂外展过程正好相反：胸锁关节从初始放松站立位开始，后缩会进一步增加，并在外展的过程中，再稍微后缩一点[6]，以使关节盂与肱骨平面达到最佳对线。由于功能取物发生在肩胛骨平面之前，但又在屈曲平面的后方[10]，因此可以推断，在功能取物的过程中，各个运动平面都会发生胸锁关节后缩。

在任何平面的手臂上抬过程中，胸锁关节的最终旋转结果都是锁骨上抬。然而，在健康的肩运动中，这种旋转角度应该很小。要将手臂上抬至120°，胸锁关节的上抬角度应该低于10°。与上斜方肌过度激活相关的胸锁关节上抬增加，是在患者中常见的运动代偿，将在之后进行讨论。

手臂在任何平面的从屈曲到外展的上抬过程中，以及在功能取物过程中，肩锁关节也展示出特有的运动模式。当手臂上抬时，在肩锁关节发生的主要运动是上旋和后倾[2, 6]。在任何平面将手臂上抬至120°，肩锁关节将发生约15°的上旋和20°的后倾。进一步上抬手臂，肩锁关节将进一步后倾。随着手臂从屈曲变为外展，这些运动的数量或模式只会发生细微的变化[6]。

过去的观点是，在手臂功能性抬高的过程中，肩锁关节并没有发生实质性运动。这样想的原因是我们认为喙锁韧带的张力限制了肩锁关节上旋。然而，我们现在已经知道，在功能运动过程中，肩锁关节的实质性运动是正常存在的。我们现在也知道，喙锁韧带的主要功能可能是将肩胛骨的旋转传递给锁骨，而不仅仅是限制肩锁关节旋转[11]。例如，据我们所知，胸锁关节肌肉组织并不直接有助于锁骨的主要运动——后旋。当肩锁关节通过作用在肩胛骨上的前锯肌产生的扭矩而上旋和后倾时，这些运动很可能主要是由喙锁韧带的张力产生的。

当手臂的上抬发生在如上所述的任何平面时，肩锁关节是内旋状态。在肩胛骨平面外展期间，要将手臂上抬至120°，肩锁关节内旋约10°。类似于胸锁关节水平面的后缩旋转，发生在肩锁关节的内旋程度将直接受到手臂上抬平面的影响。如前所述，为了适应屈曲与外展所需的关节盂朝向，肩锁关节的位置和运动必须改变。在屈曲的过程中，从初始放松站立位开始，肩锁关节内旋将增加，并且在上抬运动期间将有更多的整体内旋。在冠状面的手臂外展过程正好相反。虽然肩锁关节仍将整体内旋，但它将在初始放松站立位以较少的内旋开始，并且在外展运动期间内旋得更少[6]，以使关节盂与肱骨平面达到最佳对线。

胸锁关节和肩锁关节的联合运动

关于肩部的复杂运动，最难理解的概念之一是胸锁关节和肩锁关节单独的旋转是如何组合或耦合产生肩胛胸壁整体的位置和运动的[9]。当从上方观察时，锁骨长轴和肩胛轴（与肩胛冈大致对齐）彼此倾斜（图2.4）。在正常的放松站立位，这两个轴之间的角度（对应上述的肩锁关节内旋）通常约为60°（图2.4）。因此，除了垂直轴，任何特定胸锁关节旋转轴的运动将不对应任何特定肩锁关节旋转轴的运动，反之亦然。然而，无论肩锁关节的内旋角度如何，胸锁关节和肩锁关节的垂直轴是大致对齐的，因此它们各自的水平面运动通常更容易解释[9]。

此外，如前所述，肩锁关节轴与描述肩胛胸壁运动的轴存在同样的定义。接下来，当手臂上抬时，肩锁关节上旋、后倾并内旋，如果不通过胸锁关节的抵消运动，则这些运动将直接耦合到肩胛胸壁运动中。因此，如果肩锁关节是唯一有助于肩胛骨在胸部运动的关节，在正常手臂上抬至肱骨胸壁成120°时，我们会看到肩胛胸壁上旋约15°，后倾约20°，以及内旋约10°。与描述肩锁关节一样，肩胛骨内旋的程度也将取决于上抬平面，手臂在屈曲时内旋更多，而在冠状面外展时内旋较少。假设胸锁关节后缩，在功能取物的过程中，肩锁关节的内旋程度预计会介于屈曲与肩胛骨平面外展之间。

此外，回想一下胸锁关节在手臂上抬过程中发生的3次旋转，主要是后旋、后缩，最后是上抬。因为胸锁关节垂直轴与肩胛胸壁运动的垂直轴大致对齐，如果没有肩锁关节的抵消运动，在手臂上抬过程中，胸锁关节后缩和肩胛胸壁外旋的程度一样。但是，我们知道，在手臂上抬期间，当胸锁关节后缩时，肩锁关节同时内旋[6]。因此，就整体的肩胛胸壁运动而言，胸锁关节和肩锁关节在水平面的旋转倾向于相互抵消。在肩胛骨平面外展的过程中，最终结果是肩胛胸壁的内旋位置发生了非常小的变化。这是因为引起肩胛骨外旋的胸锁关节后缩被肩锁关节内旋所抵消，这将引起极小的肩胛胸壁内旋。在之后的肩胛骨平面外展时，胸锁关节后缩（总体上约15°）大于肩锁关节内旋（总体上约10°）。这样就产生了净肩胛胸壁外旋运动[6]。与之相反，在屈曲期间，胸锁关节后缩减少并且肩锁关节内旋增加，最终结果是发生有限的肩胛胸壁内旋运动[6]。这种肩胛胸壁内旋有助于关节盂向前，与前屈的肱骨对位得更好。在冠状面外展过程中，胸锁关节后缩增加，肩锁关节内旋减少，最终结果是发生有限的肩胛胸壁外旋运动[6]。这种肩胛胸壁外旋有助于关节盂向外，与侧向外展的肱骨对位得更好。

为了将后旋和上抬这两个剩余的胸锁关节单轴旋转直接耦合到肩胛胸壁单轴旋转中，考虑胸锁关节轴与肩胛胸壁轴直接对齐的两种假设情况（图2.7a、2.7b）。如果锁骨长轴与肩胛轴对齐，使肩锁关节内旋角度为0°（图2.7a），胸锁关节后旋将直接与肩胛骨后倾相连，胸锁关节上抬将直接与肩胛胸壁上旋耦合[9]。如果锁骨长轴与肩胛轴垂直对齐，使肩锁关节内旋角度为90°（图2.7b），胸锁关节后旋将直接与肩胛胸壁上旋耦合，胸锁关节上抬将直接与肩胛胸壁前倾相关（前倾不是理想的运动，后面将在肩胛骨运动障碍部分讨论）[9]。我们当然知道这两个假设都不会发生。事实上，肩锁关节的内旋角度约为60°(图2.4)。随后，胸锁关节旋转与肩胛胸壁以复杂的方式耦合。大约2/3的胸锁关节后旋将与肩胛胸壁上旋耦合（90°耦合关系），约1/3的胸锁关节后旋将与肩胛胸壁后旋耦合（0°耦合关系）[9]。同样地，大约2/3的胸锁关节上抬将与肩胛胸壁前倾耦合（90°耦合关系），大约1/3的胸锁关节上抬将与肩胛胸壁上旋耦合（0°耦合关系）[9]。

由于这些复杂的耦合关系很难可视化，一个数值例子可能有助于演示（图2.8）。应该注意的是，为了简化演示，数值经过了四舍五入。在手臂上抬过程中常见的胸锁关节和肩锁关节运动，要么是对整个肩胛胸壁运动的叠加，要么是以相互抵消的方式运动。例如，胸锁关节和肩锁关节的整体旋转对肩胛胸壁上旋（主要的旋转动作）起叠加作用，并且抵消肩胛胸壁的内旋和外旋。在手臂上抬至120°时发生的30°胸锁关节后旋，其中20°（2/3）将与肩胛胸壁上旋耦合。此外，肩锁关节上旋（通常为15°）将直接与肩胛胸壁上旋耦

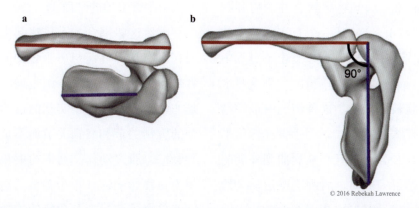

图2.7 锁骨长轴与肩胛轴对齐的两个假设方案，用于了解胸锁关节和肩锁关节单独的旋转是如何耦合产生肩胛胸壁整体的位置和运动的：平行轴（a）的排列将胸锁关节上抬、肩胛胸壁上旋和胸锁关节后旋耦合到肩胛胸壁后倾中。垂直轴（b）的排列将胸锁关节上抬耦合到肩胛胸壁前倾、胸锁关节后旋耦合到肩胛胸壁上旋中（经Rebekah L. Lawrence许可转载）

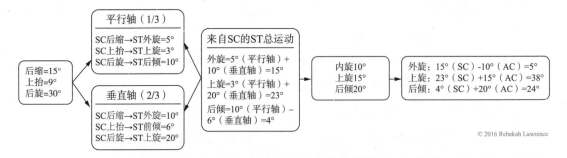

图2.8 数值例子展示了胸锁关节运动如何与肩锁关节运动耦合,从而在手臂上抬到120°时产生了肩胛胸壁运动。左侧方框展示了在肱骨胸壁上抬过程中典型的胸锁关节运动幅度。中间方框量化了胸锁关节运动是如何耦合到肩胛胸壁运动中的,进一步与肩锁关节运动相加,产生最右方框中肩胛胸壁运动的最终结果(经Rebekah L. Lawrence许可转载)

合。在手臂上抬过程中发生的9°胸锁关节上抬,其中3°(1/3)将与肩胛胸壁上旋耦合。在这种情况下,这些旋转组合增加了38°的肩胛胸壁上旋,这就是手臂在肩胛骨平面外展的过程中进行这种运动的真正价值[6, 7]。在这种情况下发生的胸锁关节后旋30°也会导致肩胛胸壁后倾10°(1/3)。然而,胸锁关节也同时上抬9°,其中6°(2/3)将导致肩胛胸壁前倾,从而将整个肩胛胸壁后倾减少至4°。这样的话,加上肩锁关节的20°后倾将导致合并的肩胛胸壁后倾(24°),这又是一个有实际意义的值[6, 7]。如果胸锁关节在此手臂上抬过程中后缩15°,而肩锁关节内旋10°,则这些水平面旋转将彼此抵消。这种情况的最终结果会是肩胛胸壁外旋5°。当手臂在任何平面可抬高到120°,并且在从屈曲到外展的不同范围都可完成时,肩胛胸壁运动大约是上旋40°,后倾20°,以及少量的、不同程度的内旋或外旋,这取决于上抬的平面和角度[6, 7]。

综上所述,在手臂上抬过程中,胸锁关节后旋和肩锁关节上旋相结合,产生了可观察到的绝大多数的整体肩胛胸壁上旋[9]。这些主要运动通过胸锁关节上抬完成有限的补充(<5°)。胸锁关节后旋也有助于肩胛胸壁后倾,但这一贡献在很大限度上被相应的胸锁关节上抬抵消[9]。因此,肩胛胸壁后倾主要是由肩锁关节后旋产生的。最后,胸锁关节后缩和肩锁关节内旋相互抵消,产生有限的内旋或外旋运动,取决于手臂上抬的平面[9]。

虽然这些耦合关系描述起来很复杂,但在对有肩部疼痛与肩胛骨功能失调的患者进行诊断和治疗时,医生理解这些关系是非常重要的。由于实际的运动发生在单个的胸锁关节和肩锁关节而不是复合的肩胛胸壁,肌肉动作、韧带约束和关节反作用力正在影响这些单个关节的运动。考虑这些单个关节运动和功能的诊断和治疗方法,在改善患者护理方面具有很大的潜力。

异常运动（运动障碍）甄别

理解了在手臂上抬过程中胸锁关节和肩锁关节的正常运动及整体肩胛胸壁运动后，一旦这些运动模式有偏离，通常就被认为是不正常的。对于肩胛骨，这些异常通常被称为肩胛骨运动障碍[12]。在许多与各种病理相关的肩痛研究中，研究者发现了各种各样的异常活动[13, 14]。已确定的异常活动包括胸锁关节上抬增加[15-17]和减少[18]、胸锁关节后缩增加[15]、胸锁关节后旋减少[18]、肩锁关节上旋和后倾增加[19]、肩胛胸壁上旋增加[15]和减少[18, 20, 21]、肩胛胸壁后倾增加[15, 16]和减少[21]，以及肩胛胸壁内旋增加[21, 22]。鉴于文献中描述的偏差方向不一致，很难确定观察到的变化是因果关系还是代偿关系[23]。此外，与无症状受试者相比，这些微小的变化引起了一些研究者的疑问：这些变化实际上是异常的？还是仅仅是正常变化的预期范围[24]？

我们认为，各研究缺乏一致的运动偏差，更多地与小样本量和样本大小不同有关[13, 14]，再加上测量技术的精确度有限，以及用于定义同质患者样本的病理解剖学诊断效用有限[25, 26]，并不是患者群体缺乏真实的运动偏差。然而，在得出明确的结论之前，还需要进一步的调查研究。我们认为，当肩胛骨的位置和运动偏差与重复的运动暴露相结合时，可能会导致有害的病理力学。运动偏差的一些常见临床表现如下。

胸锁关节上抬增加的表现通常能在"耸肩"患者试图抬起手臂时观察到（图2.9）。这种偏差是过度使用上斜方肌造成的，这种代偿性模式可能是肩袖撕裂、关节囊粘连限制盂肱关节运动、盂肱关节骨关节炎或其他一些情况导致的[15-17, 27]。由于胸锁关节上抬主要与肩胛胸壁前倾相结合，因此这种运动偏差通常被认为是一种负性的补偿策略，原因在于它可能进一步限制了肩胛胸壁的正常后倾。

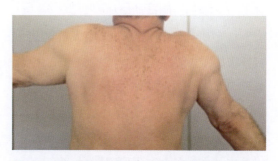

图2.9 患者试图将双臂举过头顶，展示双侧"耸肩"。这种运动是通过增加上斜方肌活动和抬高胸锁关节产生的（经Paula M. Ludewig许可转载）

在一些患者中可以观察到胸锁关节上抬减少[18]。这通常是一种姿势偏差，当手臂在放松站立位放于体侧时，锁骨没有处于典型的轻微抬高位置。这种偏差可能与肩胛胸壁上旋减少和肩胛骨内旋增加有关，它被描述为肩胛骨的"病态"现象[28]。

在患者中，胸锁关节后缩增加也得到了证实[15]。这种偏差与胸锁关节上抬增加相结合，表明上斜方肌活动增加可能是导致这两种偏差的原因。

由于胸锁关节后旋很难通过非侵入性方法准确测量，因此研究者很少对患者的这部分运动进行研究。一项使用骨固定跟踪传感器的研究[18]确定了符合肩部撞击表现的患者其胸锁关节后旋显著减少。由于胸锁关节后旋与肩胛胸壁上旋耦合，因此这一发现被认为与患者肩胛胸壁上旋减少有关。

肩锁关节偏差也很难用非侵入性方法准确测量。一项研究[19]确实发现，肩锁关节炎患者在进行手臂上抬的过程中，肩锁关节上旋和后倾明显增加。另一项单一受试者分析显示，盂肱关节骨关节炎患者的肩锁关节上旋和后倾运动增加[29]。

许多研究已经发现，肩痛人群的肩胛胸壁上旋减少[13, 14, 18, 20, 21, 27, 30, 31]（图2.10）。最常见的是，这些减少发生在手臂抬高的角度较低时[14, 20, 21]。上旋减少经常被认为有助于肩峰下或内部撞击条件的发展[13]，以及向下方或多方向不稳定[30-32]。

另外，研究还发现患者的肩胛胸壁上旋增加[15, 33]。这一看似矛盾的发现可能与肩关节上旋增加是肩痛和病理学的代偿性偏差而非致病性偏差有关。肩袖撕裂患者的肩胛胸壁上旋增加[33]、肩袖撕裂手术后肩胛骨运动学正常化[34]，以及一项表明健康受试者在肩胛上神经阻滞后上旋增加的研究[35]均支持这一假设。肩胛胸壁上旋增加也可能是由于骨关节炎[29, 36]或软组织紧张[36, 37]（图2.11）而导致的盂肱关节运动减少，受试者出现代偿性运动。

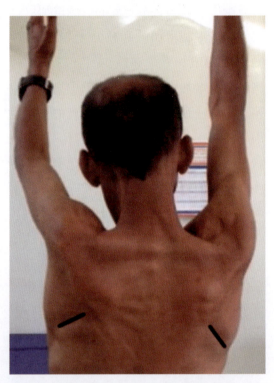

图2.11 患者表现为左肩胛骨上旋增加，继发于盂肱关节软组织僵硬。线条表示肩胛骨内侧缘或椎体缘（经Paula M. Ludewig许可转载）

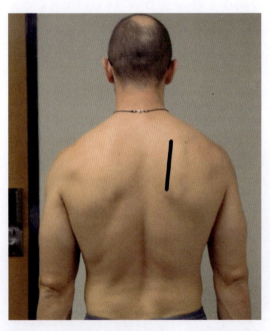

图2.10 患者表现为肩胛骨上旋减少。右肩胛骨内侧缘上的线条描绘了向下的坡度（经Paula M. Ludewig许可转载）

在患者中也观察到肩胛胸壁后倾增加[15, 16]和减少[17, 20, 21, 27]，以及肩胛胸壁内旋（图2.12）增加[21, 22, 30, 38]。这些不同的发现进一步说明了区分与疼痛和功能有关的因果性运动偏差、代偿性运动偏差及非因果性运动偏差的必要性。

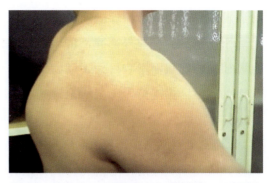

图2.13 患者表现为屈曲时右肩前倾增加，后倾减少（经Paula M. Ludewig许可转载）

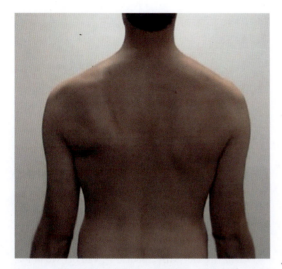

图2.12 患者表现为肩胛骨内旋增加，如图所示，左侧肩胛骨内侧缘或椎体缘突出。据肩胛骨内侧缘的向下坡度显示，肩胛骨上旋减少（经Paula M. Ludewig许可转载）

有趣的是，一些患者后倾减少（甚至前倾增加，图2.13）、内旋增加，或者上旋减少可能与三角肌的反向动作有关。任何肌肉收缩时都会在其近端和远端的附着部位施力。通常情况下，肌肉远端附着在较小质量的节段上，随后该部分向近端附着处移动。然而，在三角肌与肩胛骨相连的情况下，如果肩胛胸壁的肌肉系统未充分激活或不能产生足够的力，较轻的肩胛骨将被拉扯为前倾或下旋。这可能是激活或时相问题，而不是力量问题。另一个临床值得注意的问题是，肩胛骨运动障碍更多的是离心障碍[39]。

肩胛骨异常位置和运动对肩痛和组织病理学的潜在影响

针对肩胛骨位置和运动与肩痛和组织病理学相关性的研究还很有限。因为盂肱关节是大多数疾病的病理学观察点，所以肩胛胸壁偏差的影响力很大限度上取决于盂肱关节是否受到影响。如果发生肩胛骨运动障碍，但肱骨与肩胛骨同步运动，则可能没有负面影响。然而，如果发生肩胛骨运动障碍，使盂肱关节旋转或平移运动增加，则可能会增加盂肱关节结构的应力。

决定肩胛骨运动障碍是否有害的一个关键因素是它是否影响盂肱关节的稳定性。如果关节接触力的净结果指向凹陷中心的关节盂，则盂肱关节是最稳定的[40]。如果肩胛骨位置变化或运动障碍改变了关节合力方向，可能会导致盂肱关节不稳定、半脱位或脱位；也可能出现微不稳定的不典型情况，其中肩胛骨运动障碍可能会导致盂肱关节过度平移。

较多人认为，肩胛骨运动障碍会增加肩峰下压迫和内部或外部撞击的风险。运动障碍的普遍负面影响得到了动物模型的组织病理学证据支持[41]。历史上，一直用测量肩峰肱骨距离的方法来调查异常的肩胛骨运动学是否会对肩袖产生负面影响[42, 43]。然而，最近已经澄清，测量肩峰肱骨距离需要考虑肩袖软组织结构[44, 45]，以便更好地了解肩袖受压的潜在风险。迄今为止，肩峰下肩袖受压和体内特定的肩胛骨运动障碍之间还没有明确的联系[23, 42, 43]。关于内部撞击，Mihata等人在尸体模型中证明了肩胛骨上旋减少和肩胛骨内旋增加的负面影响[46]。还需要进行更多的研究，将肩胛骨位置和运动的变化与肩袖和潜在撞击结构的接近程度联系起来，还有与评估组织应力和变形的有限元模型联系起来。这样的研究可以进一步确定，在患者中发现的肩胛骨位置和运动改变带来的临床后果。

总之，肩胛骨运动障碍不一定是肩胛骨本身的病理状态（如与副神经或胸长神经损伤有关）[47]。然而，肩胛骨运动障碍可能导致异常的关节应力，并最终导致组织病理变化。虽然还需要进一步的研究，但我们认为肩胛骨运动障碍是对最理想运动模式的损害，可能是肩关节组织病理学的危险因素。有危险因素的人不一定会发展成病理学改变。在肩关节病变的案例中，决定组织病变继续发展的，很可能是多个危险因素。这些因素可能包括个人的基础解剖结构、肩部运动概况、组织对重复性应力（血液和炎症反应）的恢复能力、遗传因素，以及肩部位置和运动变化造成的风险。为了全面了解这些危险因素及其影响，需要持续进行调查。

（何红晨）

参考文献

1. Dvir Z, Berme N. The shoulder complex in elevation of the arm: a mechanism approach. J Biomech, 1978, 11(5): 219–225.

2. Inman VT, Saunders JB, Abbott LC. Observations of the function of the shoulder joint. Clin Orthop Relat Res, 1944, 26(1): 1–30.

3. Dempster WT. Mechanisms of shoulder movement. Arch Phys Med Rehabil, 1965, 46: 49–70.

4. Klein Breteler MD, Spoor CW, van der Helm FC. Measuring muscle and joint geometry parameters of a shoulder for modeling purposes. J Biomech, 1999, 32(11): 1191–1197.

5. Ludewig PM, Borstad JD. Joint structure and function: a comprehensive analysis. 5th ed. Philadelphia: FA Davis Company, 2011.

6. Ludewig PM, Phadke V, Braman JP, et al. Motion of the shoulder complex during multiplanar humeral elevation. J Bone Joint Surg, 2009, 91(2): 378–389.

7. McClure PW, Michener LA, Sennett BJ, et al. Direct 3-dimensional measurement of scapular kinematics during dynamic movements in vivo. J Shoulder Elbow Surg, 2001, 10(3): 269–277.

8. Conway AM. Movements at the sternoclavicular and acromioclavicular joints. Phys Ther Rev, 1961, 41: 421–432.

9. Teece RM, Lunden JB, Lloyd AS, et al. Three-dimensional acromioclavicular joint motions during elevation of the arm. J Orthop Sports Phys Ther, 2008, 38(4): 181–190.

10. Braman JP, Engel SC, RF LP, et al. In vivo assessment of scapulohumeral rhythm during unconstrained overhead reaching in asymptomatic subjects. J Shoulder Elbow Surg, 2009, 18(6): 960–967.

11. van der Helm FCT, Pronk GM. Three-dimensional recording and description of motions of the shoulder mechanism. J Biomech Eng, 1995, 117(1): 27–40.

12. Kibler WB, Ludewig PM, McClure PW, et al. Clinical implication of scapular dyskinesis in shoulder injury: the 2013 consensus statement from the "scapular summit". Br J Sports Med, 2013, 47: 877–885.

13. Ludewig PM, Reynolds J. The association of scapular kinematics and glenohumeral joint pathologies. J Orthop Sports Phys Ther, 2009, 39(2): 90–104.

14. Timmons MK, Thigpen CA, Seitz AL, et al. Scapular kinematics and subacromialimpingement syndrome: a meta analysis. J Sport Rehabil, 2012, 21(4): 354–370.

15. McClure PW, Michener LA, Karduna AR. Shoulder function and 3-dimensional scapular kinematics in people with and without shoulder impingement syndrome. Phys Ther, 2006, 86(8): 1075–1090.

16. Laudner KG, Myers JB, Pasquale MR, et al. Scapular dysfunction in throwers with pathologic internal impingement. J Orthop Sports Phys Ther, 2006, 36(7): 485–494.

17. Lukasiewicz AC, McClure P, Michener LA, et al. Comparison of 3-dimensional scapular position and orientation between subjects with and without shoulder impingement. J Orthop Sports Phys Ther, 1999, 29(10): 574–583.

18. Lawrence RL, Braman JP, LaPrade RF, et al. Comparison of 3-dimensional shoulder complex kinematics in individuals with and without shoulder pain. J Orthop Sports Phys Ther, 2014, 44(9): 636–645.

19. Sousa CO, Camargo PR, Ribeiro IL, et al. Motion of the shoulder complex in individuals with isolated acromioclavicular osteoarthritis and associated with rotator cuff dysfunction. J Electromyogr Kinesiol, 2014, 24(4): 520–530.

20. Endo K, Ikata T, Katoh S, et al. Radiographic assessment of scapular rotational tilt in chronic shoulder impingement syndrome. J Orthop Sci, 2001, 6(1): 3–10.

21. Ludewig PM, Cook TM. Alterations in shoulder kinematics and associated muscle activity in people with symptoms of shoulder impingement. Phys Ther, 2000, 80(3): 276–291.

22. Lopes AD, Timmons MK, Grover M, et al. Visual scapular dyskinesis: kinematics and muscle activity alterations in patients with subacromial impingement syndrome. Arch Phys Med Rehabil, 2015, 96(2): 298–306.

23. Karduna AR, Kerner PJ, Lazarus MD. Contact forces in the subacromial space: effects of scapular orientation. J Shoulder Elbow Surg, 2005, 14(4): 393–399.

24. McQuade KJ, Borstad J, de Oliveira AS. Critical and theoretical perspective on scapular stabilization: What does it really mean, and are we on the right track? Phys Ther, 2016, 96(8): 1162–1169.

25. Braman JP, Zhao KD, Lawrence RL, et al. Shoulder impingement revisited: evolution of diagnostic understanding in orthopaedic surgery and physical therapy. Med Biol Eng Comput, 2014, 52(3): 211–219.

26. Ludewig PM, Lawrence RL, Braman JP. What's in a name? Using movement system diagnoses versus pathoanatomic diagnoses. J Orthop Sports Phys Ther, 2013, 43(5): 280–283.

27. Lin JJ, Hanten WP, Olson SL, et al. Functional activity characteristics of individuals with shoulder dysfunctions. J Electromyogr Kinesiol, 2005, 15: 576–586.
28. Burkhart SS, Morgan CD, Kibler WB. The disabled throwing shoulder: spectrum of pathology. Arthroscopy, 2003, 19(6): 641–661.
29. Braman JP, Thomas BM, LaPrade RF, et al. Three-dimensional in vivo kinematics of an osteoarthritic shoulder before and after total shoulder arthroplasty. Knee Surg Sports Traumatol Arthrosc, 2010, 18(12): 1774–1778.
30. Ogston JB, Ludewig PM. Differences in 3-dimensional shoulder kinematics between persons with multidirectional instability and asymptomatic controls. Am J Sports Med, 2007, 35(8): 1361–1370.
31. Ozaki J. Glenohumeral movements of the involuntary inferior and multidirectional instability. Clin Orthop Relat Res, 1989, 238: 107–111.
32. Illyes A, Kiss RM. Kinematic and muscle activity characteristics of multidirectional shoulder joint instability during elevation. Knee Surg Sports Traumatol Arthrosc, 2006, 14(7): 673–685.
33. Mell AG, LaScalza S, Guffey P, et al. Effect of rotator cuff pathology on shoulder rhythm. J Shoulder Elbow Surg, 2005, 14(1 Suppl S): 58S–64S.
34. Kolk A, de Witte PB, Henseler JF, et al. Three-dimensional shoulder kinematics normalize after rotator cuff repair. J Shoulder Elbow Surg, 2016, 25(6): 881–889.
35. McCully SP, Suprak DN, Kosek P, et al. Suprascapular nerve block disrupts the normal pattern of scapular kinematics. Clin Biomech, 2006, 21(6): 545–553.
36. Fayad F, RobyBrami A, Yazbek C, et al. Three-dimensional scapular kinematics and scapulohumeral rhythm in patients with glenohumeral osteoarthritis or frozen shoulder. J Biomech, 2008, 41(2): 326–332.
37. Vermeulen HM, Stokdijk M, Eilers PH, et al. Measurement of three dimensional shoulder movement patterns with an electromagnetic tracking device in patients with a frozen shoulder. Ann Rheum Dis, 2002, 61(2): 115–120.
38. von Eisenhart-Rothe R, Matsen FA 3rd, Eckstein F, et al. Pathomechanics in atraumatic shoulder instability: scapular positioning correlates with humeral head centering. Clin Orthop Relat Res, 2005, 433: 82–89.
39. Borstad JD, Ludewig PM. Comparison of scapular kinematics between elevation and lowering of the arm in the scapular plane. Clin Biomech, 2002, 17(9–10): 650–659.
40. Marchi J, Blana D, Chadwick EK. Glenohumeral stability during a handpositioning task in previously injured shoulders. Med Biol Eng Comput, 2014, 52(3): 251–256.
41. Reuther KE, Thomas SJ, Tucker JJ, et al. Scapular dyskinesis is detrimental to shoulder tendon properties and joint mechanics in a rat model. J Orthop Res, 2014, 32(11): 1436–1443.
42. Silva RT, Hartmann LG, Laurino CF, et al. Clinical and ultrasonographic correlation between scapular dyskinesia and subacromial space measurement among junior elite tennis players. Br J Sports Med, 2010, 44(6): 407–410.
43. Seitz AL, McClure PW, Lynch SS, et al. Effects of scapular dyskinesis and scapular assistance test on subacromial space during static arm elevation. J Shoulder Elbow Surg, 2012, 21(5): 631–640.
44. Bey MJ, Brock SK, Beierwaltes WN, et al. Invivo measurement of subacromial space width during shoulder elevation: technique and preliminary results in patients following unilateral rotator cuff repair. Clin Biomech, 2007, 7: 767–773.
45. Giphart JE, van der Meijden OA, Millett PJ. The

effects of arm elevation on the three-dimensional acromiohumeral distance: a biplane fluoroscopy study with normative data. J Shoulder Elbow Surg, 2012, 21(11): 1593–1600.

46. Mihata T, Jun BJ, Bui CNH, et al. Effect of scapular orientation on shoulder internal impingement in a cadaveric model of the cocking phase of throwing. J Bone Joint Surg, 2012, 94(17): 1576–1583.

47. Roren A, Fayad F, Poiraudeau S, et al. Specific scapular kinematic patterns to differentiate two forms of dynamic scapular winging. Clin Biomech, 2013, 28(8): 941–947.

第3章　与肩胛骨功能和功能障碍相关的肌肉激活

David Ebaugh, Margaret Finley

本章将讨论在肩胛胸壁运动和盂肱关节运动产生和控制的过程中肌肉是如何参与的，重点讨论肩胛胸壁运动和盂肱关节运动的原动肌群和力偶；还会讨论肌肉活动改变和肌肉灵活性不足对肩胛胸壁运动的影响，以及它们在康复治疗中的意义。

正常肩胛带活动是建立在肩胛胸壁和盂肱关节协调的交互运动上的。例如，在盂肱关节外展（冠状面抬起）过程中，典型的肩胛胸壁运动模式包括上抬、后缩、上旋、后倾和外旋[1]。这些肩胛胸壁运动是保持肱骨头和盂窝的最佳对线、保持肩峰下的最佳空间、保持肩袖理想的长度－张力关系和保持全范围的手臂上抬所必需的。

肩胛骨上附着有17块肌肉。5块肌肉主要负责产生和控制肩胛胸壁运动，包括斜方肌（上中下三部分）、肩胛提肌、菱形肌、前锯肌和胸小肌。冈上肌、冈下肌、肩胛下肌、小圆肌和三角肌主要负责产生盂肱关节运动。几乎没有文献研究其他的肩胛骨周围肌肉（背阔肌、胸大肌、肱三头肌长头、肱二头肌长头和短头、喙肱肌和肩胛舌骨肌）在产生和控制肩胛胸壁运动中的作用。接下来我们会讨论产生肩胛胸壁运动和盂肱关节运动的原动肌，以及这些肌肉是如何一起工作使手臂抬起的。

肩胛骨在胸壁上的平移运动（上抬、下降、前伸和后缩）可以不伴有盂肱关节的运动。肩胛骨上抬（耸肩）动作是由上斜方肌、肩胛提肌和菱形肌收缩产生的[2, 3]（图3.1a）。上斜方肌附着在锁骨的外侧，使肩胛骨在上抬的同时产生上旋，而肩胛提肌和菱形肌附着的位置使肩胛骨在上抬的过程中产生下旋。上斜方肌、肩胛提肌和菱形肌的收缩比例不同，使肩胛骨在上抬的过程中可以伴有上旋或下旋，或者使肩胛骨保持便于上旋或下旋的中立位置。

下斜方肌、胸小肌、背阔肌和胸大肌下部收缩使肩胛骨产生有力的下降，并伴有肩胛骨的下旋[4, 5]（图3.1b）。在肩胛骨下降的过程中，前方肌群（胸大肌和胸小肌）和后方肌群（斜方肌和背阔肌）的收缩比例决定肩胛骨是前伸、后缩还是保持中立位。

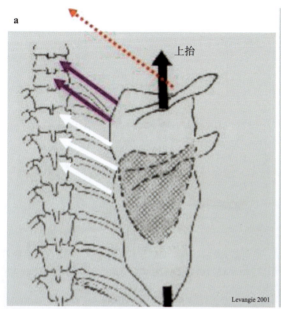 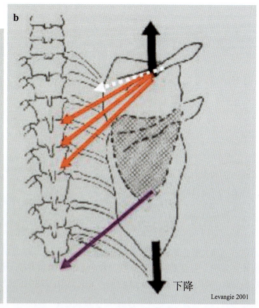

图3.1 （a）产生肩胛骨上抬的肌肉：红色虚线＝上斜方肌，紫色实线＝肩胛提肌，白色实线＝菱形肌 （b）产生肩胛骨下降的肌肉：白色虚线＝胸大肌和胸小肌，红色实线＝下斜方肌，紫色实线＝背阔肌（引自 Pamela K. Levangie, Cynthia C. Norkin. Joint Structure and Function： A Comprehensive Analysis, 3rd. ISBN 9780803607101）

　　肩胛骨前伸是由胸小肌、前锯肌和胸大肌收缩产生的[6, 7]（图3.2a）。在肩胛骨前伸的过程中，这些肌肉的收缩比例决定伴随肩胛骨前伸的其他动作（上旋和下旋、内旋和外旋、前倾和后倾）。例如，如果胸小肌和胸大肌在运动中占主导地位，基于它们的附着位置，肩胛骨在前伸的过程中会伴有下旋、内旋和前倾。与之相反，如果前锯肌在运动中占主导位置，肩胛骨在前伸的过程中会伴有上旋、外旋和后倾。

　　肩胛骨后缩是由斜方肌、菱形肌和背阔肌收缩产生的[2, 3]（图3.2b）。菱形肌和背阔肌使肩胛骨在后缩的同时产生下旋，斜方肌使肩胛骨在后缩的同时产生上旋，并抵消了下旋，这样肩胛骨在后缩的过程中保持了便于上旋和下旋的中立位。

　　三角肌（前部、中部和后部）和肩袖（肩胛下肌、冈上肌、冈下肌和小圆肌）是产生盂肱关节运动、提供盂肱关节稳定的原动肌。在冈下肌、冈上肌和肩胛下肌[11-13]为盂肱关节提供稳定的基础上，三角肌前部和中部[8-10]肌肉收缩产生矢状面的肩关节上抬（屈曲）。在冈下肌和肩胛下肌[11-13, 16-18]提供稳定的基础上，三角肌前部、中部[10, 14, 15]和冈上肌[9, 11, 16]是盂肱关节冠状面上抬（外展）的原动肌。

　　在手臂的不同抬起角度，产生盂肱关节内旋和外旋的原动肌是不同的。冈下肌在中立位（手臂抬起0°）和抬起90°位时主要负责外旋[10, 18]，冈上肌[19]、小圆肌和三角肌后部辅助冈下肌[8]。同样地，当手臂在体侧时，肩胛骨下角使盂肱关节产生内

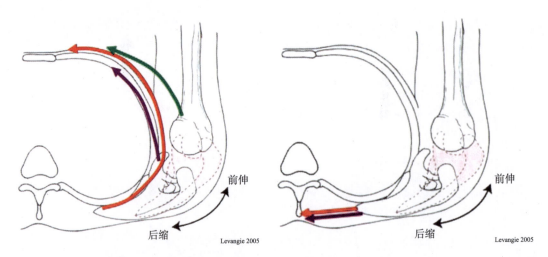

图3.2 （a）产生肩胛骨前伸的肌肉：绿色箭头=胸大肌，红色箭头=前锯肌，紫色箭头=胸小肌 （b）产生肩胛骨后缩的肌肉：红色箭头=菱形肌，紫色箭头=中斜方肌（引自Pamela K. Levangie, Cynthia C. Norkin. Joint Structure and Function: A Comprehensive Analysis, 4th. ISBN 9780803611917）

旋；当手臂抬高90°的时候，则需要来自冈上肌[11]、三角肌中部[11]和胸大肌[8]的额外辅助，使盂肱关节产生内旋。

三角肌前部、胸大肌和肩胛下肌共同收缩产生盂肱关节的水平内收[18, 20]。三角肌后部和冈下肌收缩产生盂肱关节的水平外展[18, 20, 21]。

手臂可以在很多平面上抬，包括冠状面、矢状面和肩胛骨平面。Poppen和Walker[22]建议将肩胛骨平面上抬，位于冠状面前方30°~45°，这个平面的盂肱关节处于最佳对位，增强了关节稳定性，也保持了盂肱关节肌肉系统理想的长度-张力关系。因此，大部分过头运动都发生在肩胛骨平面，需要肩胛胸壁运动和盂肱关节运动协调、平衡[22, 23]。这些运动包括肩胛胸壁上旋、外旋和后倾，盂肱关节上抬和外旋[2, 24-27]。

当手臂抬举到过头的位置时，肩胛胸壁的主要运动是上旋。传统上认为上斜方肌、下斜方肌和前锯肌是产生这个动作的力偶。与之不同，Johnson等人[3]声称中斜方肌与前锯肌是产生肩胛骨上旋的一对力偶。通过尸体解剖，作者提出，一旦前锯肌启动上旋运动，中斜方肌便位于最佳对线来辅助该运动[3]。前锯肌和中斜方肌持续收缩，形成一对力偶，在手臂上抬过头的过程中使肩胛骨上旋（图3.3）。下斜方肌被认为是通过抵消上斜方肌和前锯肌产生的肩胛骨上抬和前伸来稳定肩胛骨的，上斜方肌被认为是参与锁骨和肩胛骨上抬和后缩的肌肉之一[3]。

在肩胛骨平面手臂上抬的末端范围，肩胛骨后倾、外旋[27]。前锯肌、菱形肌和斜方肌作为力偶共同收缩产生这些运动[14, 26, 28, 29]。在肩胛骨下角的广泛附着使前锯肌下部处在理想的位置，从而产生肩胛骨后倾。下斜方肌起自胸椎下段棘突，止于肩胛冈的三角肌粗隆，能够与前锯肌下部共同产生肩胛骨后倾（图3.4）。前锯肌和菱形肌形成的力偶可以产生肩胛骨外旋。这两块肌肉附着在肩胛骨的椎侧缘，力线产生肩胛骨外旋（图3.5）。

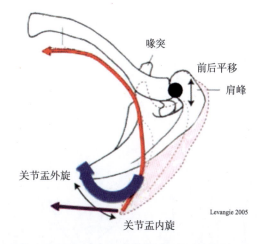

图3.5 产生肩胛骨外旋的肌肉：黑点＝旋转轴，蓝色箭头＝外旋运动，红色箭头＝前锯肌，紫色箭头＝菱形肌（引自 Pamela K. Levangie, Cynthia C. Norkin. Joint Structure and Function: A Comprehensive Analysis, 4th. ISBN 9780803611917）

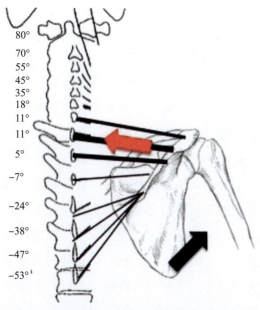

图3.3 产生肩胛骨上旋的肌肉：红色箭头＝中斜方肌，黑色箭头＝前锯肌下部[3]

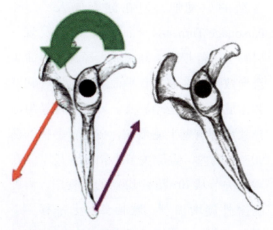

图3.4 产生肩胛骨后倾的肌肉：黑点＝旋转轴，绿色箭头＝后倾运动，紫色箭头＝前锯肌，红色箭头＝下斜方肌

在手臂过头运动中，盂肱关节的灵活性和稳定性需要达到平衡。盂肱关节的稳定性主要是靠凹侧应力机制[30]维持的。凹侧应力机制是指凹陷的盂窝和肩袖的应力对肱骨头平移的稳定作用。引发这一机制的其他因素包括关节盂软骨的厚度和盂唇[30]。

随着手臂抬起，三角肌和肩袖构成的力偶完成过头时的盂肱关节上抬（图3.6）。在盂肱关节上抬的最初阶段，三角肌提起肱骨，肩袖通过将肱骨头压向盂窝来稳定盂肱关节[15, 16, 31, 32]。另外，冈上肌辅助三角肌产生手臂上抬，冈下肌和小圆肌朝着手臂上抬的终点方向产生肱骨外旋。

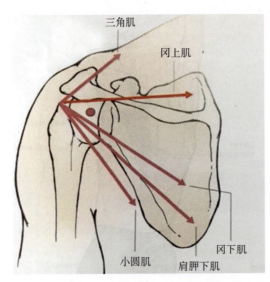

图3.6 盂肱关节上抬过程中三角肌和肩袖构成的力偶（引自 Carol A. Oatis. Kinesiology: The Mechanics and Pathomechanics of Human Movement, 3rd. ISBN 9781451191561）

异常的肌肉激活及产生的运动

在手臂上抬的过程中，适当的肌肉活动是产生协调的肩胛胸壁运动和盂肱关节运动所必需的。神经损伤（如神经卡压、神经炎）会导致肌肉激活异常，从而产生异常运动。具体而言，已有报道显示胸长神经（前锯肌）[33]、副神经（斜方肌）[33]、肩胛背神经（菱形肌）[34, 35]和肩胛上神经（冈上肌、冈下肌）[36, 37]的病变会导致肩胛胸壁和盂肱关节的运动异常。

Roren等人[33]研究了胸长神经麻痹（LTNP）患者（n=5）和副神经麻痹（SANP）患者（n=4）的手臂上抬过程。LTNP患者的手臂在矢状面（屈曲）和冠状面（外展）上抬过程中，肩胛胸壁上旋减少了3.4°~13°，后倾减少了3.6°~8.8°，内旋少量减少（<3.5°）。SANP患者的手臂在两个平面上抬过程中，肩胛胸壁上旋减少了9.2°~28.6°，内旋增加了18.5°~20.3°。手臂在冠状面上抬过程中，肩胛胸壁后倾减少了2.4°~8.9°；但是在休息位或矢状面上抬的初始位置，后倾增加了2.6°~5.6°，上抬90°以上的活动范围减少了2.1°。此类异常的运动模式在临床上通常被描述为动态翼状肩胛。

经肌电诊断确诊肩胛背神经损伤的患者，其表现为肩胛骨静态位置和运动模式均异常[34, 35]。视诊肩胛骨休息位，肩胛骨内侧缘和下角是突出的，患侧肩胛骨在胸壁上的位置也更靠外侧。手臂在冠状面和矢状面上抬的过程中，翼状肩胛更加明显（肩胛骨内侧缘抬离后侧胸壁，导致肩胛胸壁内旋并向内、向上平移）。这些研究结果支持菱形肌在辅助肩胛胸壁后缩和外旋过程中起重要作用的结论。

尽管冈上肌和冈下肌都不是肩胛骨运动的原动肌，但在健康成人[36, 37]和Parsonage-Turner综合征[38]患者中发现，肩胛上神经损伤（健康成人经神经阻滞）会导致手臂在肩胛骨平面上抬时肩胛胸壁和盂肱关节的运动异常。肩胛上神经阻滞导致肩胛胸壁上旋增加，在手臂上抬的前90°范围内，盂肱关节上抬减少[36, 37]。在盂肱关节从70°抬到120°的过程中，肩胛胸壁外旋增加[36]，肱骨头向上平移[37]。Camargo等人[38]记录了肩胛上神经病变的病例，患者肩胛胸壁的上旋和内旋增加，后倾减少，手臂上抬的活动范围并没有减小。这些研究结果支持冈上肌和冈下肌的激活缺失会导致肩胛骨运动代偿性改变的说法，冈上肌和冈下肌被认为是在手臂上举时肩峰上抬的重要因素。

软组织柔韧性

有人提出，与肩胛带相关的软组织柔韧性不良会影响肩胛骨的位置和运动[39]。近期的研究聚焦在胸小肌、肩袖后方肌肉或盂肱关节后方关节囊上，我们将在此讨论这些内容。

胸小肌长度影响肩胛骨在胸壁上的静态位置及运动[39, 40]。在健康年轻人中开展了这项研究[41-43]。当自然放松站立的时候，静态下胸小肌较短的人比胸小肌较长的人表现出更多的肩胛骨内旋[41]；而且在手臂上举的过程中，静态下胸小肌较短的人还会表现出肩胛骨上旋和后倾减少[43]。这项研究的意义在于，这种运动模式与继发于肩峰下撞击、肩袖病变及盂肱关节不稳定的肩痛患者的表现类似[28, 44]。

值得注意的是，虽然研究发现胸小肌静态长度与肩胛骨位置、肩痛、肩胛胸壁运动有关，但是胸小肌长度是在受试者呈站立位或仰卧位，手臂放在体侧的时候测量的[43, 45, 46]。虽然这个位置可以测出胸小肌静态长度，但是，不能明确肌肉是紧张的还是短缩的。胸小肌静态长度对肩胛骨位置和肩胛胸壁运动有意义。确定胸小肌是紧张的还是短缩的，能为临床决策提供其他有价值的信息。在手臂过头运动时，紧张或短缩的胸小肌会影响肌肉的正常延展。一项建模研究结果显示，在充分的过头运动中，胸小肌长度较其静态长度延长67%[14]。需要进一步研究，明确胸小肌紧张或短缩是什么原因造成的，以及胸小肌紧张或短缩对肩胛胸壁运动和肩关节功能有什么影响。

通过测量过头类项目运动员的盂肱关节内旋角度和水平内收角度，以及超声测量盂肱关节后方关节囊的厚度来理解肩关节后方软组织柔韧性不良对肩胛骨位置和肩胛胸壁运动的影响[47-50]。存在盂肱关节水平内收受限的运动员，与水平内收活动范围更大的人相比，他们在站立位的肩胛骨位置更加靠前（前伸和前倾）[48]。盂肱关节内旋不足（GIRD）的运动员在保持肩关节上抬90°时，从最大外旋位向最大内旋位运动，肩胛胸壁前倾的角度增加[47]。肩关节后方软组织柔韧性不良对肩胛胸壁上旋的影响存在矛盾的研究结果。Thomas等人[50]测量GIRD显示，GIRD大于15°的运动员在手臂上举60°、90°和120°时，肩胛胸壁上旋较少。但是在他们2011年的研究中，Thomas等人[49]报告，盂肱关节后方关节囊较厚（超声测量）的运动员在手臂上举60°、90°和120°时，肩胛胸壁上旋更多。这些差异，从一定程度上可以用对肩关节后方软组织的测量方法不同来解释。因为测量盂肱关节内旋角度可能会受到肱骨后倾的影响，所以直接超声测量盂肱关节后方关节囊厚度可能是评价组织柔韧性更好的方法。这些研究共同证实，肩关节后方软组织柔韧性不良会影响肩胛骨位置和肩胛胸壁运动，这将是未来研究的基础。

康复指南的临床意义

正常肩胛带运动依赖于肩胛胸壁和盂肱关节肌群的协调收缩，以此产生和控制肩胛胸壁运动和盂肱关节运动。从临床角度来说，当检查肩痛和有活动障碍的患者时，应考虑该情况。理解正常情况下肩胛带肌肉是如何一起工作来产生和控制肩胛胸壁运动和盂肱关节运动的，以及这些肌肉出现功能障碍的时候会有什么表现，能为临床人员评价和治疗肩痛和功能障碍、制订康复干预计划提供强有力的支持。

（马钊）

参考文献

1. Ludewig PM, Phadke V, Braman JP, et al. Motion of the shoulder complex during multiplanar humeral elevation. J Bone Joint Surg Am, 2009, 91(2): 378–389.
2. Ebaugh DD, McClure PW, Karduna AR. Three-dimensional scapulothoracic motion during active and passive arm elevation. Clin Biomech, 2005, 20(7): 700–709.
3. Johnson G, Bogduk N, Nowitzke A, et al. Anatomy and actions of the trapezius muscle. Clin Biomech, 1994, 9(1): 44–50.
4. Paine RM, Voight M. The role of the scapula. J Orthop Sports Phys Ther, 1993, 18(1): 386–391.
5. Perry J. Normal upper extremity kinesiology. Phys Ther, 1978, 58(3): 265–278.
6. Bertelli JA, Ghizoni MF. Long thoracic nerve: anatomy and functional assessment. J Bone Joint Surg Am, 2005, 87(5): 993–998.
7. Culham E, Peat M. Functional anatomy of the shoulder complex. J Orthop Sports Phys Ther, 1993, 18(1): 342–350.
8. Kuechle DK, Newman SR, Itoi E, et al. The relevance of the moment arm of shoulder muscles with respect to axial rotation of the glenohumeral joint in four positions. Clin Biomech, 2000, 15(5): 322–329.
9. Liu J, Hughes RE, Smutz WP, et al. Roles of deltoid and rotator cuff muscles in shoulder elevation. Clin Biomech, 1997, 12(1): 32–38.
10. Arwert HJ, de Groot J, van Woensel WW, et al. Electromyography of shoulder muscles in relation to force direction. J Shoulder Elbow Surg, 1997, 6(4): 360–370.
11. Kronberg M, Nemeth G, Brostrom LA. Muscle activity and coordination in the normal shoulder. An electromyographic study. Clin Orthop Relat Res, 1990, 257: 76–85.
12. Kadaba MP, Cole A, Wootten ME, et al. Intramuscular wire electromyography of the subscapularis. J Orthop Res, 1992, 10(3): 394–397.
13. Sarrafian SK. Gross and functional anatomy of the shoulder. Clin Orthop Relat Res, 1983, 173: 11–19.
14. van der Helm FC. A finite element musculoskeletal model of the shoulder mechanism. J Biomech, 1994, 27(5): 551–569.
15. Yanagawa T, Goodwin CJ, Shelburne KB, et al. Contributions of the individual muscles of the shoulder to glenohumeral joint stability during abduction. J Biomech Eng, 2008, 130(2): 21–24.
16. Otis JC, Jiang CC, Wickiewicz TL, et al. Changes in the moment arms of the rotator cuff and deltoid muscles with abduction and rotation. J Bone Joint Surg Am, 1994, 76(5): 667–676.

17. Hughes RE, Niebur G, Liu J, et al. Comparison of two methods for computing abduction moment arms of the rotator cuff. J Biomech, 1998, 31(2): 157–160.
18. Kuechle DK, Newman SR, Itoi E, et al. Shoulder muscle moment arms during horizontal flexion and elevation. J Shoulder Elbow Surg, 1997, 6(5): 429–439.
19. Reinold MM, Wilk KE, Fleisig GS, et al. Electromyographic analysis of the rotator cuff and deltoid musculature during common shoulder external rotation exercises. J Orthop Sports Phys Ther, 2004, 34(7): 385–394.
20. Basmajian JV, de Luca C. Muscles alive: their functions revealed by electromyography. Baltimore:Williams & Wilkins,1985.
21. Brandell B, Wilkinson D. An electromyographic study of manual testing procedures for the trapezius and deltoid muscles. Physiother Can, 1991, 43(3): 33–39.
22. Poppen NK, Walker PS. Forces at the glenohumeral joint in abduction. Clin Orthop Relat Res, 1978, 135: 165–170.
23. Johnston T. The movements of the shoulder-joint a plea for the use of the plane of the scapula's the plane of reference for movements occurring at the humeroscapular joint. Br J Surg, 1937, 25(98): 252–260.
24. Karduna AR, Kerner PJ, Lazarus MD. Contact forces in the subacromial space: effects of scapular orientation. J Shoulder Elbow Surg, 2005, 14(4): 393–399.
25. Ludewig PM, Behrens SA, Meyer SM, et al. Three-dimensional clavicular motion during arm elevation: reliability and descriptive data. J Orthop Sports Phys Ther, 2004, 34(3): 140–149.
26. Ludewig PM, Cook TM, Nawoczenski DA. Three-dimensional scapular orientation and muscle activity at selected positions of humeral elevation. J Orthop Sports Phys Ther, 1996, 24(2): 57–65.
27. McClure PW, Michener LA, Sennett BJ, et al. Direct 3-dimensional measurement of scapular kinematics during dynamic movements in vivo. J Shoulder Elbow Surg, 2001, 10(3): 269–277.
28. Ludewig PM, Cook TM. Alterations in shoulder kinematics and associated muscle activity in people with symptoms of shoulder impingement. Phys Ther, 2000, 80(3): 276–291.
29. Freedman L, Munro RR. Abduction of the arm in the scapular plane: scapular and glenohumeral movements. J Bone Joint Surg Am, 1966, 48(8): 1503–1510.
30. Lippitt S, Matsen F. Mechanisms of glenohumeral joint stability. Clin Orthop Relat Res, 1993, 291: 20–28.
31. Inman VT, Saunders JB, Abbott LC. Observations on the function of the shoulder joint. J Bone Joint Surg, 1944, 26(1): 1–30.
32. Payne L, Deng X, Craig E, et al. The combined dynamic and static contributions to subacromial impingement. Am J Sports Med, 1997, 25(6): 801–808.
33. Roren A, Fayad F, Poiraudeau S, et al. Specific scapular kinematic patterns to differentiate two forms of dynamic scapular winging. Clin Biomech, 2013, 28(8): 941–947.
34. Akgun K, Aktas I, Terzi Y. Winged scapula caused by a dorsal scapular nerve lesion: a case report. Arch Phys Med Rehabil, 2008, 89(10): 2017–2020.
35. Sultan HE, Younis El-Tantawi GA. Role of dorsal scapular nerve entrapment in unilateral interscapular pain. Arch Phys Med Rehabil, 2013, 94(6): 1118–1125.
36. McCully SP, Suprak DN, Kosek P, et al. Supras-

capular nerve block disrupts the normal pattern of scapular kinematics. Clin Biomech, 2006, 21(6): 545–553.

37. San Juan JG, Kosek P, Karduna AR. Humeral head translation after a suprascapular nerve block. J Appl Biomech, 2013, 29(4): 371–379.

38. Camargo PR, Zanca GG, Okino PS, et al. Scapular kinematics and muscle performance in a single case of parsonage-turner. Man Ther, 2014, 19(1): 77–81.

39. Kibler WB, McMullen J. Scapular dyskinesis and its relation to shoulder pain. J Am Acad Orthop Surg, 2003, 11(2): 142–151.

40. Sahrman S. Diagnosis and treatment of movement impairment syndromes. St Louis: Mosby, 2002.

41. Borstad JD. Resting position variables at the shoulder: evidence to support a posture-impairment association. Phys Ther, 2006, 86(4): 549–557.

42. Borstad JD. Measurement of pectoralis minor muscle length: validation and clinical application. J Orthop Sports Phys Ther, 2008, 38(4): 169–174.

43. Borstad JD, Ludewig PM. The effect of long versus short pectoralis minor resting length on scapular kinematics in healthy individuals. J Orthop Sports Phys Ther, 2005, 35(4): 227–238.

44. Kibler WB, Ludewig PM, McClure P, et al. Scapular summit 2009. J Orthop Sports Phys Ther, 2009, 39(11): A1–A13.

45. Struyf F, Meeus M, Fransen E, et al. Interrater and intrarater reliability of the pectoralis minor muscle length measurement in subjects with and without shoulder impingement symptoms. Man Ther, 2014, 19(4): 294–298.

46. Yesilaprak S, Yuksel E, KalKan S. Influence of pectoralis minor and upper trapezius lengths on observable scapular dyskinesis. Phys Ther Sport, 2016, 19: 7–13.

47. Borich MR, Bright JM, Lorello DJ, et al. Scapular angular positioning at end range internal rotation in cases of glenohumeral internal rotation deficit. J Orthop Sports Phys Ther, 2006, 36(12): 926–934.

48. Laudner KG, Moline MT, Meister K. The relationship between forward scapular posture and posterior shoulder tightness among baseball players. Am J Sports Med, 2010, 38(10): 2106–2112.

49. Thomas SJ, Higginson JS, Kaminski TW, et al. A bilateral comparison of posterior capsule thickness and its correlation with glenohumeral range of motion and scapular upward rotation in collegiate baseball players. J Shoulder Elbow Surg, 2011, 20(5): 708–716.

50. Thomas SJ, Swanik KA, Swanik CB, et al. Internal rotation deficits affect scapular positioning in baseball players. Clin Orthop Relat Res, 2010, 468(6): 1551–1557.

第4章 肩胛骨检查

Phil McClure, Aaron D. Sciascia, Tim L. Uhl

肩胛骨运动与病理

因为认识到肩胛骨在正常肩关节功能中的生物力学作用，一些临床研究试图找出肩胛骨的异常运动即所谓的肩胛骨运动障碍与肩关节的病理变化如肩关节撞击综合征[1-6]或不稳定[6]的联系。这些研究通过莫尔云纹法、机电数字化、X线摄影、磁共振成像、电磁追踪等技术来捕捉肩胛骨的运动轨迹。在三维空间内这些评估肩胛骨病理运动的研究结果并不一致。例如已经发现肩关节撞击综合征患者表现出肩胛骨后倾增加[7, 8]、后倾减少[1, 3, 4]、上旋增加[2, 8]、上旋减少[1, 3]、上移增加[4, 8]和内旋增加[3, 6]等变化。这些研究结果的差异使人困惑，因为健康肩关节与病变肩关节的活动度差异值通常很小（3°~5°）。尽管在一些研究中观察到有统计学意义，但这些差异是否具有临床意义尚不清楚。此外，最近的前瞻性研究发现，肩胛骨运动障碍与过头类项目运动员具有的症状之间的关系存在互相矛盾的结果。两项研究发现，在高中棒球运动员[9]与大学水球运动员[10]中，肩胛骨运动障碍与肩部症状并无关联。Clarsen等人[11]发现，挪威精英手球运动员的肩胛骨运动障碍与一个赛季后肩部症状的发展确实存在着正相关关系。尽管有些研究者称肩胛骨的异常运动模式与肩关节的病理变化之间存在很强的关联[12-14]，但支持这一观点的实际研究证据是有限的。其他基于肩胛骨手法复位改变症状的临床试验有望明确哪些患者确实存在肩胛骨功能障碍驱动症状的情况[15-17]。

检查

肩胛骨检查应当和肩关节检查一同进行。这是为了确定潜在的肩关节功能障碍是否与肩胛骨的异常位置及运动障碍有关[18-20]。肩胛骨运动障碍通常在无症状的个体中也会出现，因此将其与肩关节功能障碍患者的症状相联系是存在一定风险的。肩胛骨是在皮肤及其他软组织覆盖下运动的，这对肩胛骨运动障碍的评估也是一个挑战；同时它在三维空间内的运动取决于上抬的平面及所做的运动，这也给测试者带来挑战。鉴别肩胛骨运动障碍的方法已经被认为具有足够的信度，但是有效性尚且存疑，因为它们与症状之间缺乏直接的联系[18]。本章将为大家勾勒出一个检查肩胛骨的体系，它包括以下三个主要部分：① 对具有症状的患者进行视觉观察以确定其是否存在肩胛骨运动障碍；② 手法矫正肩胛骨的位置和运动，看是否对症状有改善；③ 评估可能导致肩胛骨及肩关节功能障碍的周围组织[18]。

本章将详细介绍这三个部分的整体情况，图4.1为检查流程总结。

视诊

在检查时需要直接观察肩胛骨。一个比较常见的评估错误就是没有从后方直观地观察肩胛骨的静态位置（图4.2），但这是全面评估一位肩关节疼痛患者时必不可少的手段。作为经典的姿势评估步骤，视诊静

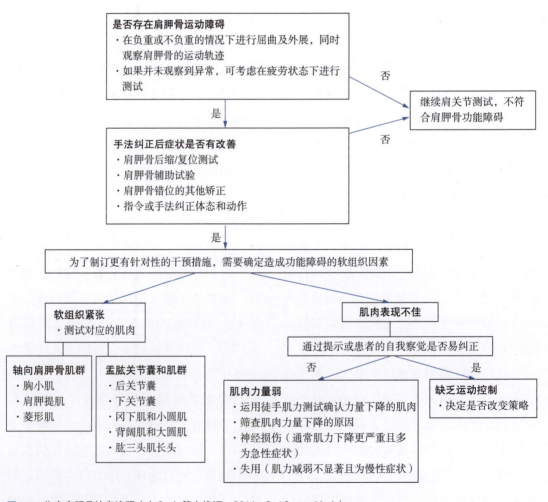

图4.1 临床肩胛骨检查流程（由Cools等人修订，2014，Br J Sports Med）

态位的肩胛骨时还应该考虑颅骨与脊柱的对线问题。在初次视诊时，观察脊柱侧弯和脊柱后凸也应按常规进行，因为它们可能是导致肩胛骨力学改变及产生肩胛骨运动障碍的潜在的生物力学因素[21, 22]。

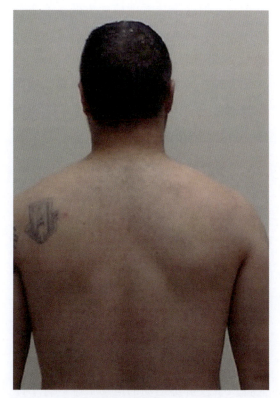

图 4.2　从后方对肩胛骨进行视诊

很多研究者提到头前伸及胸椎后凸增加都可能对肩胛骨前伸有影响，它们会进一步导致前侧的姿势肌适应性短缩或肌肉力量失衡[23-26]。肩胛骨前伸的体态常与肩峰下空间狭窄[27, 28]、胸椎屈曲增加有关。肩胛骨位置朝前还会改变肩胛骨的运动，从而导致上抬的力量输出减少[23, 29]（图 4.3）。

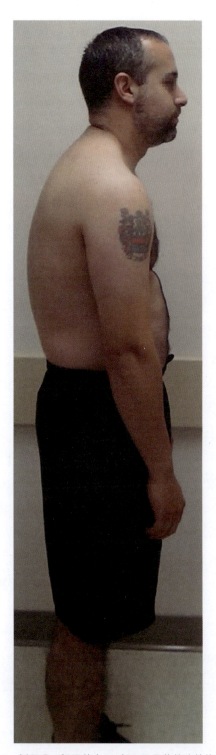

图 4.3　侧面观：躯干的上 1/4 部可见显著的头前伸及圆肩姿势

不论受试者的肩关节是否存在病变，静态评估都提示肩胛骨错位[6]。Warner分别对肩袖撞击、肩关节不稳定人群及健康人使用了莫尔云纹法，通过增强视觉观察后发现：在29名肩关节病变患者中，有30%~50%在屈肘90°并手持4.5kg重物时存在静态肩胛骨错位问题[6]。值得注意的是，在对照组（22名肩关节未损伤的健康人）中，有3名（14%）存在双侧肩胛骨不对称。很重要的是，发现肩胛骨位置不对称，并不意味着发生了病变。

肩胛骨外侧滑动测试是指静态测量两侧肩胛骨下角至相邻棘突之间的距离，得出差值[30]。在双手臂置于体侧、双手叉腰及手臂在最大内旋位外展90°这三个不同的姿态下分别进行测试。如果双侧差距大于1.5 cm，应当考虑存在病理变化。这个测试在临床上很容易应用，信度中等[30, 31]，但效度还有一定的争议。因为有研究发现，肩关节有症状与无症状的个体在用这个方法进行测试时都会出现不对称[32, 33]，而且病理性运动障碍也可能会在双侧对称时出现，所以只与对侧进行比较的话其效度是有问题的。此外，这是一个静态、二维平面的测试，它并不能全面地评估伴随肩胛骨运动发生的动态三维运动[10, 32, 34]。临床检查时，考虑测试结果的效度问题，这个测试需要与其他测试配合进行。

用线性或静态评估方法来对肩胛骨运动障碍进行分类的视诊评估方案已发展出来[15, 34, 35]。这些方法涉及将肩胛骨运动归为异常和正常情况，在临床应用中更具有功能性和全面性，并且能在三维模式下判断肩胛骨运动。Kibler等人[15]首先描述了一种基于视诊、将肩胛骨功能障碍划分为四类的方法，其中三类属于异常，一类属于正常。但这个体系的信度太低，不适合临床应用，研究者改进出一种更简便的分类方法[35]。

肩胛骨运动障碍测试也是一种以视诊为基础、用于评估肩胛骨运动障碍的方法，它要求受试者负重进行肩前屈及肩外展，观察受试者肩胛骨的表现[34]。这个测试将特征性肩胛骨运动障碍分为存在或不存在两类，肩胛骨的每一侧都单独评分。运动障碍意味着要么存在翼状肩胛（肩胛骨内侧缘的任何部分突起或肩胛骨下角抬离胸壁），要么存在肩肱节律紊乱（在手臂上抬或放下时肩胛骨运动出现提前、过度或卡顿）（图4.4）。这项测试的信度比之前提到的其他视诊分类体系要好，效度也在大批从事投掷类运动的运动员中进行了评估。结果显示，被这项测试判断为异常的人，在三维动作捕捉追踪时表现出肩胛骨上旋减少、锁骨上抬减少及锁骨后缩减少[10]。与冠状面的肩外展相比，肩前屈出现异常的情况更为普遍。这些结果表明，用这个测试判断出的肩胛骨运动障碍会引起肩胛骨三维运动的明显改变，尤其是在肩前屈时。然而，即使在视诊中观察到运动障碍导致了肩胛骨三维运动出现改变，受试者也不一定会报告有症状[10]。

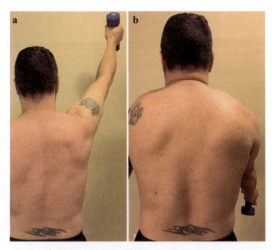

图4.4 肩胛骨运动障碍测试的后面观：在手臂上抬或放下时伴随着右侧肩胛骨内缘的突起

Uhl等人[35]使用了本质上相同的一套评判标准（翼状肩胛或肩肱节律紊乱），只是他们将肩胛骨运动异常归为"是"，运动正常归为"否"。他们研究了分成有或无各种软组织病变症状的两组患者，当将通过三维动作捕捉技术发现的不对称性作为金标准时，这个测试表现出了更高的信度、特异性及敏感性[35]。还有一项重要的发现与以往的研究结论一致[10]：在肩前屈时，有症状个体（54%）相比无症状个体（14%）出现肩胛骨运动障碍的频率更高，但是在肩胛骨平面上抬时两组患者并无太大差异。

手法矫正

由于肩胛骨运动障碍在无症状个体中也常发现，因此评估时要判断肩胛骨运动障碍是否是症状持续的一个重要异常因素。肩胛骨运动改变可能是一种代偿策略，以避免对疼痛、敏感的组织产生应力。症状改变测试用来推断症状是否是肩胛骨位置异常导致的，通过测试者在激惹试验中徒手对受试者的肩胛骨活动重新定向来判断。如果肩胛骨的位置改变后症状即刻改善，就直接说明该患者的肩胛骨运动障碍是导致肩部症状的一个因素。两种主要的症状改变测试包括肩胛骨辅助试验[16, 30]和肩胛骨后缩/复位测试[17, 36]。

肩胛骨辅助试验就是在患者肩关节上抬时手法辅助肩胛骨上旋，同时评估该动作对疼痛的影响[37]（图4.5）。随后Rabin对这项测试进行了改良，加入了肩胛骨后倾[16]（图4.6）。测试阳性结果是指在辅助操控时随着手臂上抬，肩关节疼痛减轻或消失。这项测试显示出可接受的信度水平[16]，肩峰下空间增加，肩胛骨上旋及后倾增加[38]。

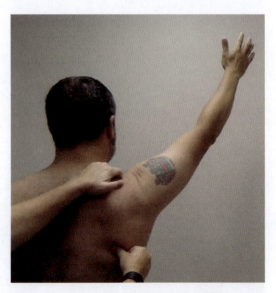

图4.5 测试者的拇指在受试者的肩胛骨下角施加一个向前外侧的力

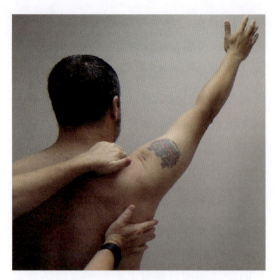

图4.6 整个手对受试者的肩胛骨下角施加向前外侧的力

肩胛骨后缩测试是指通过手法定位并固定肩胛骨的整个内侧缘,使肩胛骨保持在胸壁的后缩位置[37]。这项测试可用于鉴别那些由于肩胛骨近端不稳定而致肩部上抬的肌力缺失患者。在进行测试时,要求受试者主动后缩双侧肩胛骨,同时测试者用前臂固定受试者的肩胛骨内侧缘(图4.7)。测试阳性结果是指受试者在肩胛骨稳定的情况下,在肩胛骨平面上抬手臂达到90°时进行静力收缩,表现出肩关节疼痛减轻或力量上升[19, 37]。Kibler等人[36]研究了此测试在有症状和无症状受试者中的应用情况,结果表明受试者的疼痛等级并未改变,但不论症状如何,他们的力量输出都得到了改善。

肩胛骨复位测试是对肩胛骨后缩测试的改进,更强调肩胛骨后倾和外旋,并避免完全的肩胛骨后缩[17](图4.8)。此调整是因为以往有研究发现,当肩胛骨达到最大主动后缩位时肩部上抬的力量会减弱[29]。在对一大组投掷类项目运动员进行测试时,该测试表现出可靠的信度;大约有一半在撞击测试中伴随疼痛的运动员(46/98)疼痛减轻,还有26%的运动员等

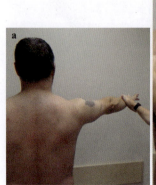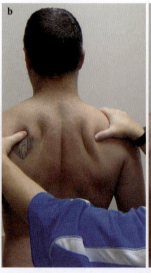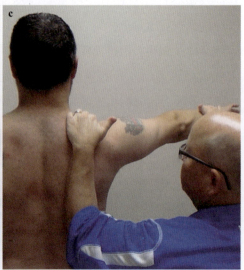

图4.7 肩胛骨后缩测试由三个部分组成:(a)在没有肩胛骨固定或后缩的情况下测试者测试受试者手臂的力量 (b)嘱咐受试者主动后缩肩胛骨 (c)测试者以一侧前臂稳定受试者的肩胛骨内侧缘,另一只手在受试者外展的手臂上施加向下的力

长上抬力量显著提高。因此这项测试可能有助于筛选出能受益于旨在改善肩胛骨肌群功能的干预措施的有肩关节病变的患者。

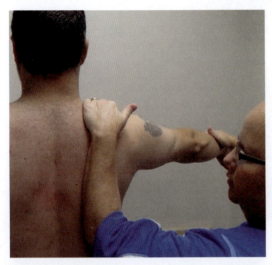

图4.8 除了不要求受试者主动后缩肩胛骨，肩胛骨复位测试类似于肩胛骨后缩测试。测试者用一侧前臂稳定受试者的肩胛骨内侧缘，另一只手在受试者外展的手臂上施加向下的力

周围组织评估

一旦测试者判断受试者存在肩胛骨运动障碍，同时认为肩胛骨运动障碍与整个肩部病变有关时，就需要对肩关节周围组织进行评估，以确定是什么因素导致了肩胛骨的运动轨迹出现变化。肌肉力量不足？肩胛骨稳定肌群对肩部的运动控制不佳[17, 18, 30, 39]？姿势异常[23, 26, 40]？柔韧性受损[13, 41]？这些因素都与肩胛骨运动障碍密切相关。因此设计一套针对这些因素的检查是很有必要的（图4.1）。

涉及肩胛骨稳定机制的主要肌肉的力量可以通过Kendall等人[42]提出的标准姿势与标准步骤进行评估。这个测试主要针对连接躯干与肩胛骨的肌肉[43]。神经损伤如胸长神经、副神经、肩胛背神经等损伤也应该被考虑为是肩胛骨运动障碍的潜在因素。由胸长神经支配的前锯肌对肩胛骨上旋、前伸和锁骨前伸有重要作用。评估肩胛骨围绕胸壁做前伸及对抗后缩阻力的能力是确定前锯肌功能正常的必要条件。上抬手臂过头顶（尤其是在矢状面检查中）且能对抗后缩阻力，使肩胛骨沿着胸壁前伸，提示前锯肌功能正常（图4.9）。

在矢状面手臂上抬时出现翼状肩胛或不能保持肩胛骨内侧缘下段紧贴胸壁，提示前锯肌功能不良。这可能是运动控制不佳的问题，也可能是肌肉失用，或者是神经损伤导致的肌力问题。它们的干预策略截然不同。如果是由于运动控制不佳导致的翼状肩胛，那么在恰当的提示下受试者的问题可以很快得到纠正，同时他在进行徒手肌力测试时的表现也可能是正常的。但如果是很难矫正的翼状肩胛或单独进行徒手肌力测试时一直有力弱的表现，那么往往提示胸长神经存在病变或损伤[44]。

除前锯肌外，上斜方肌和下斜方肌也形成了一对使肩胛骨上旋的力偶。在冠状面手臂外展时，斜方肌是最主要的稳定肌[19, 39, 45-47]。测试斜方肌的一个关键点是即使阻力是通过受试者的手臂施加的，我们也应该通过观察肩胛骨在测试中的位置是否改变来判断是否存在力弱，而非观察手臂的位置。在实施这项测试时，需要为肩袖或三角肌无力者的手臂提供支撑，同时直接对肩胛骨施加阻力，这样才能准确

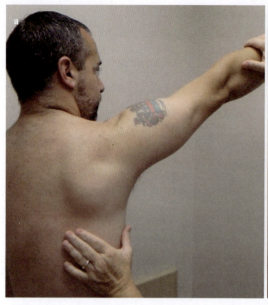
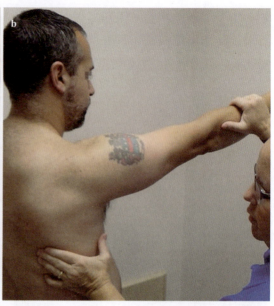

图4.9 前锯肌的徒手肌力测试用于评估肩胛骨紧贴胸壁，在受到向后下方的阻力时能否保持稳定（a），出现翼状肩胛或肩胛骨离开胸壁提示前锯肌无力（b）

测出肩胛骨周围肌力的强弱。在肩胛骨的不同方向施加阻力评估肌力的方式应该更具针对性。以肩胛骨上抬或耸肩为例，它们主要是上斜方肌起作用，但上斜方肌在徒手肌力测试中大多又是正常的。在对下斜方肌进行测试时，受试者取俯卧位，手臂外展135°，同时抬离地面（这里的地面指治疗床床面）（图4.10）。沿着下斜方肌的走向在肩峰后外侧施加一个向前（指向地面）的力，促进下斜方肌激活[48]。

在评估菱形肌（由肩胛背神经支配）与中斜方肌时，受试者取俯卧位，在肩峰后外侧施加向前的力，同时嘱咐受试者主动后缩肩胛骨（图4.11）。目前为止还没有人能用复合测试体位来区分这两块肌肉[48, 49]。在进行测试时，关键是要将受试者的肩胛骨放在正确的后缩位，以便更好地募集肩胛骨后缩肌群。

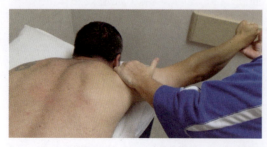

图4.10 对下斜方肌进行徒手肌力测试时，受试者取俯卧位，测试者在肩峰后外侧施加向前的力，这些力直接作用于肩袖和三角肌

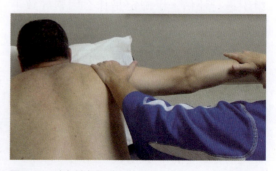

图4.11 对中斜方肌进行徒手肌力测试时，受试者取俯卧位，测试者在肩峰后外侧施加向前的力，使力通过肩袖和三角肌更好地向肩胛骨肌肉组织传递。如果受试者的力臂太长，那么测试者需要密切关注受试者先启动的是肩胛骨后缩还是手臂水平外展

评估肩关节周围肌肉的柔韧性及肩关节的活动度，是完整地评估肩胛骨运动障碍的关键。胸小肌适应性短缩已经被发现与肩胛骨运动学异常有关，它有可能是导致肩关节撞击综合征的原因之一[41, 50]。Sahrmann[50] 提出了一种测量胸小肌长度的方法，用直尺测量受试者在仰卧位时肩峰后侧到治疗床的距离，如果＞2.54 cm 则认为胸小肌短缩（图4.12）。

紧张导致肩前伸的个体。这个方法不能确定某一块肌肉的紧张度，但显示出对前倾姿势的敏感性[26, 55]。

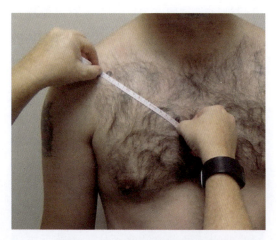

图4.13　测量第4肋到喙突的距离即得到胸小肌的长度

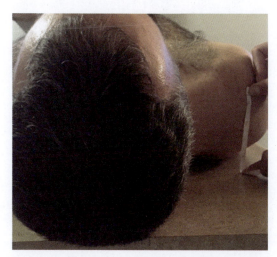

图4.12　Sahrmann 提出的测量胸小肌长度的方法：受试者在仰卧位，测量肩峰后侧到治疗床的距离

虽然这项测试的信度很高，但是有人质疑它的效度，因为它并不能鉴别肩关节疼痛[51]。而另一种通过皮尺或卷尺测量胸小肌起点与止点之间直线距离的测试，被发现具有良好的效度（同类相关系数=0.82～0.87）与信度[52]（图4.13）。这个测试要求仔细地触诊，它在具有和不具有撞击症状的受试者之间并没有表现出差异[53]。

还有一种评估肩前伸的方法——测量受试者在靠墙直立时肩峰前侧到墙壁的距离[54]（图4.14）。它用于筛查由于前侧结构

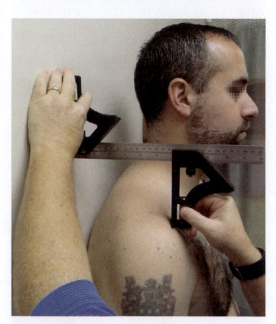

图4.14　采用双平法评估肩前伸的体态

传统肩关节内外旋的关节活动范围测量是在肩胛骨保持稳定、肩关节外展90°的情况下进行的。确定盂肱关节的活动度是评估肩胛骨运动障碍成因的重要内容。盂肱关节受限可能是肩胛骨运动异常的一个

原因，这个问题亟待在肩关节病变的评估和治疗中得到解决。

肩关节后方紧张（关节囊或肩袖）与肩胛骨过度前伸有关[56]，它也有可能导致肩胛骨运动障碍[13]。有两种方法可评估肩关节后方的紧张度，一是在肩外展90°时内旋[57, 58]（图4.15）；二是观察手伸背后时所能达到的脊柱平面[59, 60]。这两个方法在临床应用中都表现出了可靠的信度。Gerber等人[61]提出：与肩外展90°位相比，当手臂置于体侧时，关节囊的各部分会限制肩关节内旋。因此有研究者建议临床工作者同时使用这两种方法来评估肩关节后方紧张度[62]。肩关节内旋角度的大小还受肱骨及关节盂的个体差异的影响，因此很难区分到底是软组织紧张还是骨性结构改变导致了内旋角度变小。为了解决这一问题，Laudner等人[63]提出了一种方法：固定肩胛骨后将上臂抬高90°，在水平内收后测量，它的信度令人满意（图4.16）。

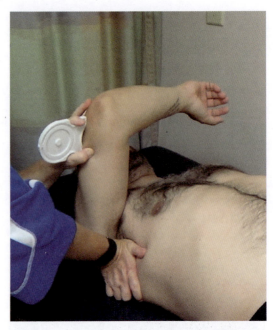

图4.16　肩关节后方紧张度的测试要求在固定肩胛骨的同时进行水平内收。这个测试的0°位为肱骨与躯干垂直时的位置；水平内收方向的运动被记录为正值，水平外展方向的运动则为负值

任何测试的最终目的都是更好地进行诊断，确定合适的干预措施以解决在检查时发现的损伤或功能障碍。肩胛骨检查是为了确定是否存在潜在的肩胛骨功能障碍而使患者产生肩部疼痛。肩胛骨检查的三个要素有助于进一步确定是肩关节周围组织的柔韧性有问题还是运动控制有问题。为了顺利实施干预（在第15章和16章将详细说明），应将患者组织激惹度纳入检查，以便确定适宜的干预水平。在进行合适的干预时，也需要考虑组织激惹度的3个阶段[64]。在高激惹度状态下（第1阶段），患者表现为因剧烈疼痛引起的运动障碍、失能，以及在主动活动肩关节时采取过度的自我保护措施。干预这类患者，需要采用最小的组织负荷，同时采取一些止痛措

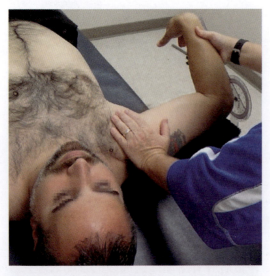

图4.15　在固定肩胛骨时测量盂肱关节在肩胛骨平面的内旋角度大小

施。然而，对于同样有肩胛骨周围肌群运动控制障碍但激惹度较低的患者，我们可以直接去解决他们的肌肉功能障碍问题。有经验的临床工作者能够将肩胛骨检查与激惹度的3个阶段进行统筹，这样他们能准确地诊断患者的病情并为其制订阶段性的干预措施。

（孙扬）

参考文献

1. Endo K, Ikata T, Katoh S, et al. Radiographic assessment of scapular rotational tilt in chronic shoulder impingement syndrome. J Orthop Sci, 2001, 6(1): 3–10.
2. Graichen H, Stammberger T, Bonel H, et al. Three-dimensional analysis of shoulder girdle and supraspinatus motion patterns in patients with impingement syndrome. J Orthop Res, 2001, 19(6): 1192–1198.
3. Ludewig PM, Cook TM. Alterations in shoulder kinematics and associated muscle activity in people with symptoms of shoulder impingement. PhysTher, 2000, 80(3): 276–291.
4. Lukasiewicz AC, McClure P, Michener LA, et al. Comparison of 3-dimensional scapular position and orientation between subjects with and without shoulder impingement. J Orthop Sports Phys Ther, 1999, 29(10): 574–586.
5. McClure PW, Bialker J, Neff N, et al. Shoulder function and 3-dimensional kinematics in people with shoulder impingement syndrome before and after a 6-week exercise program. Phys Ther, 2004, 84(9): 832–848.
6. Warner JJ, Micheli LJ, Arslanian LE, et al. Scapulothoracic motion in normal shoulders and shoulders with glenohumeral instability and impingement syndrome. Clin Orthop Relat Res, 1992, 285: 191–199.
7. Laudner KG, Myers JB, Pasquale MR, et al. Scapular dysfunction in throwers with pathologic internal impingement. J Orthop Sports Phys Ther, 2006, 36(7): 485–494.
8. McClure PW, Michener LA, Karduna AR. Shoulder function and 3-dimensional scapular kinematics in people with and without shoulder impingement syndrome. Phys Ther, 2006, 86(8): 1075–1090.
9. Myers JB, Oyama S, Hibberd EE. Scapular dysfunction in high school baseball players sustaining throwing-related upper extremity injury: a prospective study. J Shoulder Elbow Surg, 2013, 22(9): 1154–1159.
10. Tate AR, McClure PW, Kareha S, et al. A clinical method for identifying scapular dyskinesis. J Athl Train, 2009, 44: 165–173.
11. Clarsen B, Bahr R, Andersson SH, et al. Reduced glenohumeral rotation, external rotation weakness and scapular dyskinesis are risk factors for shoulder injuries among elite male handball players: a prospective cohort study. Br J Sports Med, 2014, 48(17): 1327–1333.
12. Burkhart SS, Morgan CD, Kibler WB. The disabled throwing shoulder: spectrum of pathology. Arthroscopy, 2003, 19(4): 404–420.
13. Burkhart SS, Morgan CD, Kibler WB. The disabled throwing shoulder: spectrum of pathology. Arthroscopy, 2003, 19(6): 641–661.
14. Kibler WB, McMullen J. Scapular dyskinesis and its relation to shoulder pain. J Am Acad Orthop Surg, 2003, 11: 142–151.
15. Kibler WB, Uhl TL, Maddux JQ, et al. Qualitative clinical evaluation of scapular dysfunction: A reliability study. J Shoulder Elbow Surg, 2002, 11(6):

550–556.

16. Rabin A, Irrgang JJ, Fitzgerald GK, et al. The intertester reliability of the scapular assistance test. J Orthop Sports Phys Ther, 2006, 36(9): 653–660.

17. Tate AR, McClure PW, Kareha S, et al. Effect of the scapula reposition test on shoulder impingement symptoms and elevation strength in overhead athletes. J Orthop Sports Phys Ther, 2008, 38(1): 4–11.

18. Kibler WB, Ludewig PM, McClure PW, et al. Scapular summit 2009. J Orthop Sports Phys Ther, 2009, 39(11): A1–A13.

19. Kibler WB, Sciascia AD. Current concepts: scapular dyskinesis. Br J Sports Med, 2010, 44(5): 300–305.

20. Tate AR, McClure PW. Rehabilitation of the hand and upper extremity. Philadelphia: Mosby/Elsevier, 2010.

21. Otoshi K, Takegami M, Sekiguchi M, et al. Association between kyphosis and subacromial impingement syndrome: LOHAS study. J Shoulder Elbow Surg, 2014, 23(12): e300–e307.

22. Yang S, Feuchtbaum E, Werner BC, et al. Does anterior shoulder balance in ado-lescent idiopathic scoliosis correlate with posterior shoulder balance clinically and radiographically? Eur Spine J, 2012: 21(10): 1978–1983.

23. Kebaetse M, McClure P, Pratt N. Thoracic position effect on shoulder range of motion, strength, and three-dimensional scapular kinetics. Arch Phys Med Rehabil, 1999, 80: 945–950.

24. Lewis JS, Green A, Wright C. Subacromial impingement syndrome: the role of posture and muscle imbalance. J Shoulder Elbow Surg, 2005, 14(4): 385–392.

25. Lewis JS, Valentine RE. Clinical measurement of the thoracic kyphosis □ A study of the intra-rater reliability in subjects with and without shoulder pain. BMC Musculoskelet Disord, 2010, 11: 39.

26. Lynch SS, Thigpen CA, Mihalik JP, et al. The effects of an exercise intervention on forward head and rounded shoulder postures in elite swimmers. Br J Sports Med, 2010, 44(5): 376–381.

27. Seitz AL, McClure PW, Finucane S, et al. Mechanisms of rotator cuff tendinopathy: intrinsic, extrinsic, or both? Clin Biomech, 2011, 26(1): 1–12.

28. Solem-Bertoft E, Thuomas KA, Westerberg CE. The influence of scapular retraction and protraction on the width of the subacromial space. An MRI study. Clin Orthop Relat Res, 1993, (296): 99–103.

29. Smith J, Kotajarvi BR, Padgett DJ, et al. Effect of scapular protraction and retraction on isometric shoulder elevation strength. Arch Phys Med Rehabil, 2002, 83: 367–370.

30. Kibler WB. The role of the scapula in athletic shoulder function. Am J Sports Med, 1998, 26(2): 325–337.

31. Odom CJ, Taylor AB, Hurd CE, et al. Measurement of scapular asymmetry and assessment of shoulder dysfunction using the lateral scapular slide test: a reliability and validity study. Phys Ther, 2001, 81(2): 799–809.

32. Koslow PA, Prosser LA, Strony GA, et al. Specificity of the lateral scapular slide test in asymptomatic competitive athletes. J Orthop Sports Phys Ther, 2003, 33(6): 331–336.

33. Nijs J, Roussel N, Vermeulen K, et al. Scapular positioning in patients with shoulder pain: a study examining the reliability and clinical importance of 3 clinical tests. Arch Phys Med Rehabil, 2005, 86(7): 1349–1355.

34. McClure PW, Tate AR, Kareha S, et al. A clinical method for identifying scapular dyskinesis. J Athl Train, 2009, 44: 4.

35. Uhl TL, Kibler WB, Gecewich B, et al. Evaluation

of clinical assessment methods for scapular dyskinesis. Arthroscopy, 2009, 25(11): 1240–1248.
36. Kibler WB, Sciascia AD, Dome D. Evaluation of apparent and absolute supraspinatus strength in patients with shoulder injury using the scapular retraction test. Am J Sports Med, 2006, 34(10): 1643–1647.
37. Burkhart SS, Morgan CD, Kibler WB. Shoulder injuries in overhead athletes, the "dead arm" revisited. Clin Sports Med, 2000, 19(1): 125–158.
38. Seitz AL, McClure PW, Finucane S, et al. The scapular assistance test results in changes in scapular position and subacromial space but not rotator cuff strength in subacromial impingement. J Orthop Sports Phys Ther, 2012, 42(5): 400–412.
39. Ludewig PM, Hoff MS, Osowski EE, et al. Relative balance of serratus anterior and upper trapezius muscle activity during push-up exercises. Am J Sports Med, 2004, 32(2): 484–493.
40. Thigpen CA, Padua DA, Michener LA, et al. Head and shoulder posture affect scapular mechanics and muscle activity in overhead tasks. J Electromyogr Kinesiol, 2010, 20(4): 701–709.
41. Borstad JD, Ludewig PM. The effect of long versus short pectoralis minor resting length on scapular kinematics in healthy individuals. J Orthop Sports Phys Ther, 2005, 35(4): 227–238.
42. Kendall FP, EK MC, Provance PG, et al. Muscles testing and function. Baltimore: Williams & Wilkins, 1993.
43. Inman VT, Saunders JB, Abbott LC. Observations of the function of the shoulder joint. Clin Orthop Relat Res, 1996, (330): 3–12.
44. Watson CJ, Schenkman M. Physical therapy management of isolated serratus anterior muscle paralysis. Phys Ther, 1995, 75(3): 194–202.
45. Cools AM, Dewitte V, Lanszweert F, et al. Rehabilitation of scapular muscle balance: which exercises to prescribe? Am J Sports Med, 2007, 35(10): 1744–1751.
46. Cools AM, Witvrouw EE, Declercq GA, et al. Scapular muscle recruitment patterns: trapezius muscle latency with and without impingement symptoms. Am J Sports Med, 2003, 31(4): 542–549.
47. Johnson G, Bogduk N, Nowitzke A, et al. Anatomy and actions of the trapezius muscle. Clin Biomech, 1994, 9: 44–50.
48. Michener LA, Boardman ND, Pidcoe PE, et al. Scapular muscle tests in subjects with shoulder pain and functional loss: reliability and construct validity. Phys Ther, 2005, 85(11): 1128–1138.
49. Smith J, Padgett DJ, Kaufman KR, et al. Rhomboid muscle electromyography activity during 3 different manual muscle tests. Arch Phys Med Rehabil, 2004, 85: 987–992.
50. Sahrmann SA. Diagnosis and treatment of movement impairment syndromes. St. Louis: Mosby, 2002.
51. Lewis JS, Valentine RE. The pectoralis minor length test: a study of the intra-rater reliability and diagnostic accuracy in subjects with and without shoulder symptoms. BMC Musculoskelet Disord, 2007, 8: 64.
52. Borstad JD. Measurement of pectoralis minor muscle length: validation and clinical application. J Orthop Sports Phys Ther, 2008, 38(4): 169–174.
53. Rosa DP, Borstad JD, Pires ED, et al. Reliability of measuring pectoralis minor muscle resting length in subjects with and without signs of shoulder impingement. Braz J Phys Ther, 2016, 20(2): 176–183.
54. Peterson DE, Blankenship KR, Robb JB, et al. Investigation of the validity and reliability of four objective techniques for measuring forward shoulder posture. J Orthop Sports Phys Ther, 1997,

25(1): 34–42.
55. Kluemper M, Uhl TL, Hazelrigg H. Effect of stretching and strengthening shoulder muscles on forward shoulder posture in competitive swimmers. J Sport Rehabil, 2006, 15(1): 58–70.
56. Laudner KG, Moline MT, Meister K. The relationship between forward scapular posture and posterior shoulder tightness among baseball players. Am J Sports Med, 2010, 38(10): 2106–2112.
57. Awan R, Smith J, Boon AJ. Measuring shoulder internal rotation range of motion: a comparison of 3 techniques. Arch Phys Med Rehabil, 2002, 83: 1229-1234.
58. Ellenbecker TS, Roetert EP, Piorkowski PA, et al. Glenohumeral joint internal and external rotation range of motion in elite junior tennis players. J Orthop Sports Phys Ther, 1996, 24(6): 336–341.
59. Edwards TB, Bostick RD, Greene CC, et al. Interobserver and intraobserver reliability of the measurement of shoulder internal rotation by vertebral level. J Shoulder Elbow Surg, 2002, 11(1): 40–42.
60. Hayes K, Walton JR, Szomor ZR, et al. Reliability of five methods for assessing shoulder range of motion. Aust J Physiother, 2001, 47(4): 289–294.
61. Gerber C, Werner CM, Macy JC, et al. Effect of selective capsulorrhaphy on the passive range of motion of the glenohumeral joint. J Bone Joint Surg Am, 2003, 85(1): 48–55.
62. McClure P, Balaicuis J, Heiland D, et al. A randomized controlled comparison of stretching procedures for posterior shoulder tightness. J Orthop Sports Phys Ther, 2007, 37(3): 108–114.
63. Laudner KG, Stanek JM, Meister K. Assessing posterior shoulder contracture: the reliability and validity of measuring glenohumeral joint horizontal adduction. J Athl Train, 2006, 41(4): 375–380.
64. McClure PW, Michener LA. Staged approach for rehabilitation classification: shoulder disorders (STAR-Shoulder). Phys Ther, 2015, 95(5): 791–800.

第二部分

肩胛骨和肩部病变

第5章 撞击综合征和肩袖疾病

Katherine E. Reuther, Brent J. Morris, John E. Kuhn

背景

肩胛骨运动障碍存在于大多数肩部损伤中（68%~100%）[1]。我们对肩胛骨运动障碍的理解已经取得了重大进展。目前，世界各地都确认肩胛骨运动障碍存在，且其影响力是广泛的。我们现在对肩胛骨的理解已经远远超出了我们对翼状肩胛和神经系统状况的基本认识，并且开始探索肩胛骨对其他病况的影响，还探索其中更多的因果关系。肩胛骨为肩袖的有效功能发挥和肩关节的正常运动建立了一个平台。肩胛骨运动的改变可能与多种病理状况有关，包括肩袖无力和肩袖病理改变[2]。临床研究和实验模型系统（包括尸体和动物）也被开发出来评估肩胛骨在撞击综合征和肩袖疾病中的作用。目前，已经存在有限的证据来指导我们治疗或预防继发于肩胛骨运动障碍的肩袖损伤。更好地了解肩胛骨在肩袖病变中的角色，将有助于优化临床治疗。

本章将重点介绍目前如何通过临床研究和实验模型系统对肩胛骨在撞击综合征和肩袖疾病中的角色进行评估。以这些研究为框架，我们将强调肩胛骨在这些疾病发展中的作用。最后，我们将讨论肩胛骨在肩袖病变治疗中的重要性。

评估肩胛骨在撞击综合征和肩袖疾病中的角色

早期识别肩胛骨运动障碍是基于临床观察，现在则可以通过一项有效的观察测试，得到可靠的肩胛骨运动障碍特征[3]。肩胛骨运动障碍测试是一种诊断肩胛骨运动障碍的动态观察测试。矫正性体格检查操作可以引起症状改变和肩袖力量改善，从而对肩胛骨运动障碍的临床观察和诊断起到补充作用。肩胛骨辅助试验和肩胛骨后缩测试是可以改变损伤症状的矫正性体格检查[1, 4, 5]。这些矫正性体格检查操作证实了肩胛骨运动障碍在肩袖病变中的作用，因为在它们纠正了异常的肩胛骨位置后，症状和肩袖力量即改善。

临床观察和矫正性体格检查有助于更好地确定肩胛骨运动障碍及其与肩袖疾病

的关系，现在流行病学研究也强调了这种关系。特定的体型和姿势与肩胛骨运动障碍、肩袖撕裂也存在关系。错误的姿势，尤其是胸椎过度后凸，已经被证明与肩胛骨运动障碍有关[6]。一项针对单个山村379名参与者的超声研究表明，姿势异常是肩袖撕裂的独立预测因素，肩袖撕裂在胸椎过度后凸和腰椎过度前凸患者中患病率最高[7]。姿势异常被证明会改变肩胛骨运动，而这又被认为会引起肩袖机械磨损。

伴前伸、后倾和上旋的肩胛骨运动障碍可能是肩袖疾病发生的原因，肩峰下空间减少、肩袖间隙减小，导致肩袖机械磨损[6]。肩胛骨运动障碍也可能是肩袖损伤的负代偿，并可能导致进一步的肩关节功能障碍。

不幸的是，临床研究无法解决发生撞击综合征和肩袖疾病的根本原因。在对肩袖疾病的特征进行描述和理解的过程中，以及检查肩胛骨静态和动态的变化后寻求治疗方法时，尸体和动物等实验模型系统起到了关键作用。这些模型系统有其优点与局限性，在评价和解释结果时应予以考虑。

尸体研究

人类尸体研究有几个优点，包括解剖评估和肩胛骨的控制性生物力学评估。关于肩峰类型和关节盂定向等静态解剖变异及它们与肩袖疾病的关系已有研究[8-11]。在控制肩胛骨方向和改变应力和/或模拟撕裂的情况下，研究者进行了生物力学测试[12,13]。不幸的是，尸体研究的作用是有限的，因为它们不能解释发生损伤的根本原因，也无法评估随着时间的推移损伤发展的过程。此外，大多数肩部生物力学研究的重点只是盂肱关节的驱动，并不包括肩胛胸壁运动，或只考虑改变肩胛骨位置，而忽视在活体中观察到的动态的、复杂的三维运动[14,15]。

动物模型

以往认定，老鼠的肩关节模型在解剖学方面和功能方面都与人的肩关节相似[16]。更确切地说，老鼠和人类有着相似的骨骼结构和软组织解剖结构，包括存在喙肩弓，以及在向前运动的过程中从其下方通过的冈上肌腱（图5.1）。Reuther等人[17,18]最近将老鼠的肩关节模型扩展，通过引起副神经和胸长神经的急性损伤造成鼠肩胛骨运动障碍。使用动物模型进行肩部研究，与临床研究相比有几个优点，包括可以重复实验、控制研究参数，以及可以检查行为表现、功能和肌腱性能的纵向变化并阐明这些变化的发生机制。不过，也应该承认鼠模型具有局限性，如使用四足动物并不能准确复制人类的情况，急性神经损伤造成的肩胛骨运动障碍仅代表很少的一部分临床患者。然而，鼠模型与人类在解剖学上相似，可控制、可重复，便于研究人员评估异常肩胛骨运动与肩袖病理学之间的因果关系。

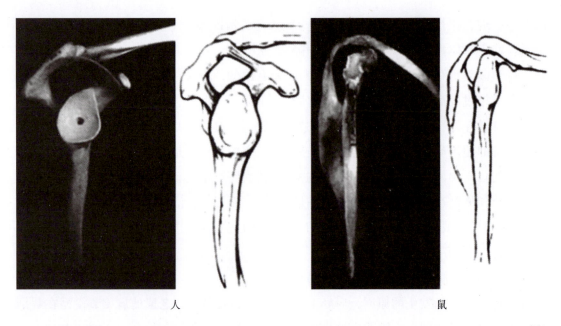

图5.1 人体肩部解剖与鼠肩部解剖的比较。这一视图表明在人和鼠的肩部都存在喙肩弓,在其下方有冈上肌腱通过[16]

肩袖疾病、撞击综合征形成

肩袖撕裂是非常常见的。据报道,普通人群中多达20%的人存在肩袖撕裂,在60岁和70岁的人群中发生率超过50%[19]。肩袖撕裂患者存在高比例的肩胛骨运动障碍[20]。在这项前瞻性多中心研究中,28%的有症状但无创伤的肩袖撕裂患者存在肩胛骨运动障碍。肩胛骨运动障碍与治疗前肩功能评分较差有关。

除了临床观察到的相关因素,实验模型系统还发现肩胛骨的静态和动态变异可能导致肩袖疾病或撞击综合征形成。

静态解剖变异

肩胛骨的静态解剖变异包括肩峰和关节盂的解剖变异,它们与肩袖疾病的关系在尸体实验模型中早已被研究过。Bigliani等人[21]开发了一个肩峰形状的分类系统,包括扁平(1型)、弯曲(2型)和钩状(3型)(图5.2)。3型肩峰与尸体肩部存在肩袖撕裂的相关性。为了支持这项工作,Flatow等人[22]进行了另一项尸体研究,通过生物力学测试、立体摄影测量和X线评估肩关节下的肩袖偏移,作者发现3型肩峰的肩峰下接触增加。与肩袖疾病有关的肩峰其他特征包括肩峰前倾[23]、肩峰侧向延伸[24]、肩峰侧向倾斜[25],以及存在肩峰骨[26]。与肩峰形态相关的是发现冈上肌出口狭窄与肩袖撕裂有关[27]。

尸体研究还表明,关节盂方向在肩袖疾病中也起着重要作用。在伴随或不伴随肩袖撕裂的尸体肩部进行关节盂倾角的检查,即在肩胛骨平面测量关节盂角度,观

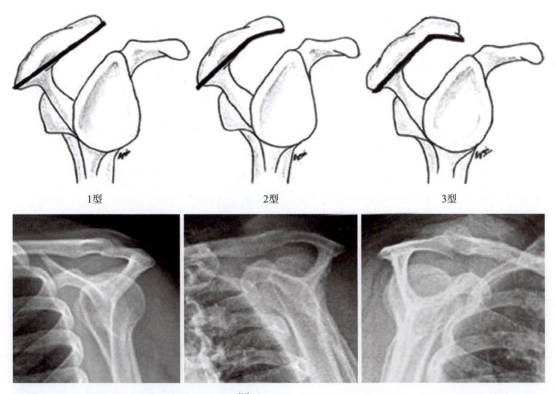

图5.2 Bigliani的肩峰分类法显示及相应的X线片[29]

察到有肩袖撕裂的肩部存在更大的关节盂倾角,即关节盂更加向上[28]。另一项尸体研究发现,具有较大关节盂倾角的肱骨头,其上移的风险会增加,这表明更向上的关节盂可能会引发肩袖疾病和撞击综合征[11, 28]。与此相反,Kandemir等人[9]发现,对比肩袖完好的尸体和肩袖撕裂的尸体,关节盂的样式或倾角并没有差别。最后,肩峰的侧向延伸与关节盂倾角之间存在关系,两者产生"临界肩角",此角度较大则与肩袖撕裂有关,角度较小则与盂肱关节骨关节炎有关[10]。

肩胛骨运动学及其动态影响

研究人员对尸体肩部进行了生物力学评估,已经深入了解了肩胛骨在盂肱关节中的力学和病理学作用,又在尸体实验模型中对撞击综合征(包括内型、外型和肩峰下型)进行了研究。Karduna等人[12]改变了肩胛骨的方向(包括后倾、上旋和外旋),并评估了肩峰下空间。结果表明,肩胛骨上旋增加,肩峰下空间减少。这与预期相反,因为临床数据表明,肩峰下撞击综合征伴随上旋减少,提示关节运动学的代偿性改变[30]。

内型撞击综合征的特点是肩袖后侧的下表面与肱骨、上盂唇和盂边缘存在接触。肩胛骨位置在内型撞击综合征中的作用已通过生物力学评估进行了研究。Mihata等人[13]改变肩胛骨的方向来评估盂肱关节的位置和接触压力,发现减少上旋和增加内旋会增加尸体肩关节的接触压力和撞击面积。这与Karduna等人的肩峰下撞击综合征研究相反,表明肩胛骨位置在两种撞击综合征中的作用仍有争议。

尽管我们通过临床观察和尸体评估对肩胛骨在肩袖疾病和撞击综合征中的作用有了更好的认识,但肩胛骨运动障碍与肩袖疾病之间关系的证据仍然是复杂、混乱的。最近,为了从基础科学的角度更好地理解这种关系,研究者开发了一个新的肩胛骨运动障碍鼠模型[17, 18]。鼠模型允许可控制和可重复地诱导肩胛骨运动障碍,并有机会对随后的关节功能(包括空间、时间、动力学参数和被动关节力学)和冈上肌腱特性(包括力学、结构学和组织学)进行定性和定量评估,以对应肩胛骨运动中的既定改变。

鼠模型研究的目的是探讨肩胛骨运动障碍对盂肱关节功能和肩袖肌腱特性的影响。在肩胛骨运动障碍组,研究者对鼠进行了副神经和胸长神经的手术横切,在运动过程中可以观察到鼠的整个肩胛骨内侧突出,显示这些动物的肩胛骨和肩峰定位不正常。肩胛骨运动障碍组还有关节功能改变,表现为推进力增加、垂直力减少和内旋活动范围增加。推进力是大鼠前进运动所需要的,而这一参数的增加可能表明关节需要承受更大的应力。垂直力减少提示功能缺陷及疼痛的可能。内旋活动范围增加表明肩后部结构的松动对不稳定的肩胛骨有影响。肩胛骨运动障碍组还存在肌腱特性改变(图5.3)。这些改变有两种可能的力学机制:①肩峰位置改变和肩峰下空间减少导致肌腱机械磨蚀和磨损。②在肩胛骨运动障碍组,需要肩袖更加用力,才能试图恢复关节的动态稳定性。此研究首次直接地将肩胛骨运动障碍确定为盂肱关节功能和肩袖肌腱特性改变的发病机制。

Reuther等人的后续研究考察了肩胛骨运动障碍对过度使用人群的影响[17, 18]。与预期一致,过度使用和肩胛骨运动障碍的

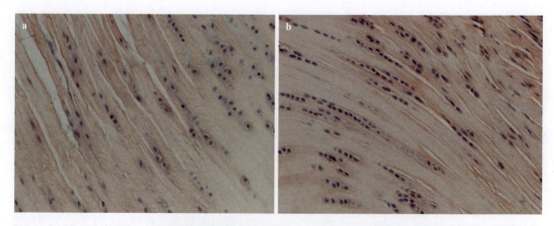

图5.3 与对照组(a)相比,在有肩胛骨运动障碍(b)的情况下,鼠冈上肌腱组织学图像显示细胞密度增加[17,18]

结合对肩袖肌腱特性的影响大于仅有肩胛骨运动障碍。该研究表明，肩胛骨运动障碍患者肩关节损伤的风险在经常进行过头运动的个体中较高。

不仅有大量的生物力学研究和动物模型研究评估肩胛骨运动障碍与肩袖疾病之间的关系，临床研究的证据也是十分充裕可靠的。Warner等人[31]利用莫尔云纹法发现，撞击综合征患者在休息位下肩胛骨位置不正常。有症状表现的肩袖疾病患者会出现肩胛骨运动异常，肌肉活动比例与无症状的该疾病患者和正常人相比也存在异常[32-36]。游泳者中与撞击综合征有关的肩痛和前锯肌、下斜方肌的异常募集相关联[37]，与肩袖撕裂相关的疼痛和肩胛骨运动障碍之间存在线性关系[38]。

肩胛骨康复可能有助于治疗与肩袖相关的疼痛和疲劳[39]。最近有两篇系统文献综述得出结论：以肩胛骨为中心的治疗方法在早期改善患者的功能障碍[40]和肩胛骨力量[41]方面有显著的作用，但对于疼痛或活动范围的影响似乎没有那么显著。由于文献中的试验次数有限（7次），我们很难得出明确的结论。

总之，临床研究和尸体及动物实验模型系统证据都表明肩胛骨的静态和动态变异可能引起肩袖疾病。肩胛骨的异常位置和运动会增加肩袖的应力，导致撞击综合征。在临床上处理这类情况时，应仔细考虑这些研究发现。

肩胛骨在治疗肩袖疾病时的重要作用

肩胛骨运动障碍已被确定是治疗肩袖撕裂的一个非手术的可改变因素[20]。在一项前瞻性多中心研究中，物理治疗作为一种可行的治疗方案，用于治疗有症状的非创伤性全层肩袖撕裂患者[42]。针对肩胛骨的物理治疗对75%的患者有长达2年的疗效。

临床研究和体外及体内实验模型系统都表明肩胛骨的静态、动态变异与肩袖疾病和撞击综合征有明显的联系。因此，在治疗时应考虑这些变异。已经有研究开始检查肩胛骨在肩袖修补术后的作用。Reuther等人[43]利用鼠模型评估肩胛骨运动障碍是如何在修补术后影响肌腱修复的。结果表明，与正常肩胛骨运动组的肌腱相比，肩胛骨运动障碍组的肌腱力学性能表现不足。这是第一个表明肩胛骨运动障碍可能减少肩袖修补后愈合的研究。临床可能需要成功的术前肩胛骨康复，才能在术后取得成功的结局；然而，由于缺乏长期的临床数据评价，这个问题值得进一步研究。

实验模型系统也被用来评估肩峰在肩袖病理和治疗中的作用。肩峰成形术（切除肩峰下表面）或肩峰下减压术（切除肩峰下空间内的组织）常与肩袖修复联合进行，为肩峰下肩袖提供更大的间隙，减轻疼痛。尸体生物力学评估结果已经表明对这种技术的支持，数据显示肩峰下减压降低了肩袖的峰值压力[44]。与之类似，鼠模型中的体内实验数据表明，缩小肩峰下空间，随后肩峰下外部撞击结合过度使用对肩袖肌腱造成的损害大于单纯的过度使用[45]。

总结

总而言之，临床研究和实验模型系统证据表明，异常的肩胛骨位置和运动会导致撞击综合征，增加肩袖的应力，如果不治疗就会进一步导致肌腱损伤。对异常肩胛骨运动进行评估和康复，有助于预防肌腱损伤，改善修复术后的肌腱愈合。

（何红晨）

参考文献

1. Kibler WB. The role of the scapula in athletic shoulder function. Am J Sports Med, 1998, 26: 325–337.
2. Lintner D, Noonan TJ, Kibler WB. Injury patterns and biomechanics of the athlete's shoulder. Clin Sports Med, 2008, 27: 527–551.
3. McClure P, Tate AR, Kareha S, et al. A clinical method for identifying scapular dyskinesis. J Athl Train, 2009, 44: 160–164.
4. Merolla G, de Santis E, Campi F, et al. Infraspinatus scapular retraction test: a reliable and practical method to assess infraspinatus strength in overhead athletes with scapular dyskinesis. J Orthop Traumatol, 2010, 11(2): 105–110.
5. Rabin A, Irrgang JJ, Fitzgerald GK, et al. The intertester reliability of the scapular assistance test. J Orthop Sports Phys Ther, 2006, 36: 653–660.
6. Kibler WB, Ludewig PM, McClure PW, et al. Clinical implications of scapular dyskinesis in shoulder injury: the 2013 consensus statement from the "Scapular Summit". Br J Sports Med, 2013, 47: 877–885.
7. Yamamoto A, Takagishi K, Kobayashi T, et al. The impact of faulty posture on rotator cuff tears with and without symptoms. J Shoulder Elbow Surg, 2015, 24: 446–452.
8. Halder A, Zobitz ME, Schultz F, et al. Mechanical properties of the posterior rotator cuff. Clin Biomech, 2000, 15: 456–462.
9. Kandemir U, Allaire RB, Jolly JT, et al. The relationship between the orientation of the glenoid and tears of the rotator cuff. J Bone Joint Surg, 2006, 88: 1105–1109.
10. Moor BK, Bouaicha S, Rothenfluh DA, et al. Is there an association between the individual anatomy of the scapula and the development of rotator cuff tears or osteoarthritis of the glenohumeral joint? a radiological study of the critical shoulder angle. Bone Joint J, 2013, 95(7): 935–941.
11. Wong AS, Gallo L, Kuhn JE, et al. The effect of glenoid inclination on superior humeral head migration. J Shoulder Elbow Surg, 2003, 12: 360–364.
12. Karduna AR, Kerner PJ, Lazarus MD. Contact forces in the subacromial space: effects of scapular orientation. J Shoulder Elbow Surg, 2005, 14: 393–399.
13. Mihata T, Jun BJ, Bui CN, et al. Effect of scapular orientation on shoulder internal impingement in a cadaveric model of the cocking phase of throwing. J Bone Joint Surg Am, 2012, 94: 1576–1583.
14. Labriola JE, Lee TQ, Debski RE, et al. Stability and instability of the glenohumeral joint: the role of shoulder muscles. J Shoulder Elbow Surg, 2005, 14(1 Suppl S): 32S–38S.
15. Thompson WO, Debski RE, Boardman ND 3rd,

et al. A biomechanical analysis of rotator cuff deficiency in a cadaveric model. Am J Sports Med, 1996, 24: 286–292.

16. Soslowsky LJ, Carpenter JE, DeBano CM, et al. Development and use of an animal model for investigations on rotator cuff disease. J Shoulder Elbow Surg, 1996, 5: 383–392.

17. Reuther KE, Thomas SJ, Tucker JJ, et al. Scapular dyskinesis is detrimental to shoulder tendon properties and joint mechanics in a rat model. J Orthop Res, 2014, 32: 1436–1443.

18. Reuther KE, Thomas SJ, Tucker JJ, et al. Overuse activity in the presence of scapular dyskinesis leads to shoulder tendon damage in a rat model. Ann Biomed Eng, 2015, 43(4): 917–928.

19. Yamamoto A, Takagishi K, Osawa T, et al. Prevalence and risk factors of a rotator cuff tear in the general population. J Shoulder Elbow Surg, 2010, 19: 116–120.

20. Harris JD, Pedroza A, Jones GL, et al. Predictors of pain and function in patients with symptomatic, atraumatic full-thickness rotator cuff tears: a time- zero analysis of a prospective patient cohort enrolled in a structured physical therapy program. Am J Sports Med, 2012, 40: 359–366.

21. Bigliani LU, Morrison DS, April EW. The morphology of the acromion and its relationship to rotator cuff tears. Orthop Trans, 1986, 10: 216.

22. Flatow EL, Soslowsky LJ, Ticker JB, et al. Excursion of the rotator cuff under the acromion. Patterns of subacromial contact. Am J Sports Med, 1994, 22: 779–788.

23. Prato N, Peloso D, Franconeri A, et al. The anterior tilt of the acromion: radiographic evaluation and correlation with shoulder diseases. Eur Radiol, 1998, 8(9): 1639–1646.

24. Nyffeler RW, Werner CM, Sukthankar A, et al. Association of a large lateral extension of the acromion with rotator cuff tears. J Bone Joint Surg Am, 2006, 88(4): 800–805.

25. Banas MP, Miller RJ, Totterman S. Relationship between the lateral acromion angle and rotator cuff disease. J Shoulder Elbow Surg, 1995, 4(6): 454–461.

26. Boehm TD, Rolf O, Martetschlaeger F, et al. Rotator cuff tears associated with os acromiale. Acta Orthop, 2005, 76(2): 241–244.

27. Ogata S, Uhthoff HK. Acromial enthesopathy and rotator cuff tear. A radiologic and histologic postmortem investigation of the coracoacromial arch. Clin Orthop Relat Res, 1990, 254: 39–48.

28. Hughes RE, Bryant CR, Hall JM, et al. Glenoid inclination is associated with full-thickness rotator cuff tears. Clin Orthop Relat Res, 2003, 407: 86–91.

29. Pandey V, Jaap Willems W. Rotator cuff tear: a detailed update. Asia Pac J Sports Med Arthroscopy Rehabil Technol, 2015, 2(1): 1–14.

30. Ludewig PM, Reynolds JF. The association of scapular kinematics and glenohumeral joint pathologies. J Orthop Sports Phys Ther, 2009, 39: 90–104.

31. Warner JJ, Micheli LJ, Arslanian LE, et al. Scapulothoracic motion in normal shoulders and shoulders with glenohumeral instability and impingement syndrome: A study using Moiré topographic analysis. Clin Orthop Relat Res, 1992, 285: 191–199.

32. Kijima T, Matsuki K, Ochiai N, et al. In vivo 3-dimensional analysis of scapular and glenohumeral kinematics: comparison of symptomatic or asymptomatic shoulders with rotator cuff tears and healthy shoulders. J Shoulder Elbow Surg, 2015, 24(11): 1817–1826.

33. Leong HT, Tsui SS, Ng GY, et al. Reduction of the subacromial space in athletes with and without

rotator cuff tendinopathy and its association with the strength of scapular muscles. J Sci Med Sport, 2016, 19(12): 970–974.

34. Lopes AD, Timmons MK, Grover M, et al. Visual scapular dyskinesis: kinematics and muscle activity alterations in patients with subacromial impingement syndrome. Arch Phys Med Rehabil, 2015, 96(2): 298–306.

35. Michener LA, Sharma S, Cools AM, et al. Relative scapular muscle activity ratios are altered in subacromial pain syndrome. J Shoulder Elbow Surg, 2016, 25(11): 1861–1867.

36. Struyf F, Cagnie B, Cools AM, et al. Scapulothoracic muscle activity and recruitment timing in patients with shoulder impingement symptoms and glenohumeral instability. J Electromyogr Kinesiol, 2014, 24(2): 277–284.

37. Wadsworth DJ, Bullock-Saxton JE. Recruitment patterns of the scapular rotator muscles in freestyle swimmers with subacromial impingement. In J Sports Med, 1997, 18: 618–624.

38. Scibek JS, Carpenter JE, Hughes RE. Rotator cuff tear pain and tear size and scapulohumeral rhythm. J Athl Train, 2009, 44(2): 148–159.

39. van de Velde A, de Mey K, Maenhout A, et al. Scapular-muscle performance: two training programs in adolescent swimmers. J Athl Train, 2011, 46(2): 160–167.

40. Bury J, West M, Chamorro-Moriana G, et al. Effectiveness of scapula-focused approaches in patients with rotator cuff related shoulder pain: a systematic review and meta-analysis. Man Ther, 2016, 25: 35–42.

41. Reijneveld EA, Noten S, Michener LA, et al. Clinical outcomes of a scapular-focused treatment in patients with subacromial pain syndrome: a systematic review. Br J Sports Med, 2017, 51(5): 436–441.

42. Kuhn JE, Dunn WR, Sanders R, et al. Effectiveness of physical therapy in treating atraumatic full-thickness rotator cuff tears: a multicenter prospective cohort study. J Shoulder Elbow Surg, 2013, 22: 1371–1379.

43. Reuther KE, Tucker JJ, Thomas SJ, et al. Effect of scapular dyskinesis on supraspinatus repair healing in a rat model. J Shoulder Elbow Surg, 2015, 24: 1235–1242.

44. Denard PJ, Bahney TJ, Kirby SB, et al. Contact pressure and glenohumeral ranslation following subacromial decompression: how much is enough? Orthopedics, 2010, 33: 805.

45. Soslowsky LJ, Thomopoulos S, Esmail A, et al. Rotator cuff tendinosis in an animal model: role of extrinsic and overuse factors. Ann Biomed Eng, 2002, 30: 1057–1063.

第6章 投掷类、过头类项目运动员的肩胛骨

Stephen J.Thomas, John D. Kelly 4th

引言

投掷类动作是一种非常独特和复杂的行为,通常在人2岁时就已经开始出现。这个阶段的孩子们正在发育协调、有效的投掷所需的神经肌肉系统。类似于其他任务的发育,如走路或跑步,神经肌肉系统需要经过大量的重复才能变得高效。刚开始,动作会非常不协调,特别是上下肢的动作,但随着重复次数的增加,神经肌肉系统变得更加高效,动作更加流畅[1]。随着神经肌肉系统的不断发育和骨骼的生长,运动会增加。此时,身体的力量和承受的应力增加,尤其是上肢[2,3]。随着肩部肌肉和肩胛骨的应力增加,组织的适应性也会增强。起初,适应性对于增强力量和稳定性非常重要。然而,要使适应性继续朝着积极的方向发展,必须考虑两个因素。首先要考虑的是施加应力的频率,必须在应力和应用频率之间保持平衡。随着应力的增加,施加应力的频率必须相应地降低。由于没有办法持续监测应力,因此常常难以实现临床管理。许多像少年棒球联盟一样的组织尝试把投球计数合并,作为一个限制频率的方法[4]。然而,当选手参与多个联赛和选秀时,这很难监控。此外,这些指南都是普适性的,并没有考虑每个球员的个体应力。第二个必须考虑的因素是恢复。虽然管理应力频率很重要,但允许适当的恢复可以将有害的适应(比如高频拳击比赛后的慢性疲劳和肌肉萎缩)降到最低。肩胛骨后部稳定肌由于肌肉的离心收缩而承受着很高的应力。在投掷类动作的减速阶段,肩胛骨稳定肌既要为肩袖提供稳定,使其正常发挥作用,又要绕着胸廓前伸,使应力消散[5-8]。由于高应力和高频率,这些肌肉会同时出现急性和慢性疲劳。

肩胛骨稳定肌发生的急性和慢性疲劳通常会影响肩胛骨的位置和运动[5,6]。静态位置的改变通常由软组织结构紧张引起,肩胛骨运动的改变通常由神经肌肉控制模式改变外加软组织紧张引起。这些适应将极大地影响肩胛骨的正常功能。肩胛骨功能不正常,往往会对远端节段产生更大的应力(如肩关节和肘关节)。远端节段上有额外的应力可导致稳定结构的组织退化,

导致诸如盂唇和尺侧副韧带撕裂之类的损伤。本章将深入探讨过头类项目运动员的肩胛骨正常和异常功能及它们的临床表现。此外，还将讨论肩胛骨异常功能的临床意义。

肩胛骨正常功能

静态姿势

要了解如何评估和治疗过头类项目运动员的肩胛骨问题，首先必须了解什么是正常的肩胛骨。在临床上，评估肩胛骨的第一件事是观察运动员的休息姿势。由于投掷侧手臂需承受应力，即使是健康的运动员也经常会出现左右不对称的情况。一个常见的不对称现象是优势侧肩胛骨的上旋角度增加[9-12]。这通常被认为是一个积极的适应，因为上旋角度增加理论上会增加肩峰下的空间，并将发生肩峰下撞击综合征的风险降到最低。然而，当检查过头类项目运动员的肩峰下空间时，结果是不一致的。Thomas等人[13]发现肩峰下空间在盂肱关节外展0°和90°时两侧并无差异。检查90°位是因为90°位是投掷动作的功能位，也是最常见的重现肩峰下撞击症状的体位。然而，Maenhout等人[14]发现，优势侧的肩峰下空间在盂肱关节外展0°、45°和60°时会增大。最近的研究表明，冈上肌止点位于肩峰内侧，而且一旦盂肱关节外展超过60°就不会受到撞击[15]，因此研究者对这些位置进行了检查。这两项研究的结果结合，可能表明肩峰下撞击综合征在较低的外展位置时即已形成。然而，一旦冈上肌腱退变，患者可能在肩外展90°时出现症状，因为冈上肌腱受到较大的内在应力或张力。

位置、比赛水平和年龄也可能影响过头类项目运动员的肩胛骨上旋角度。首先，Laudner等人[16]发现投手的上旋角度比防守球员小。其次，Thomas等人[17]发现大学棒球运动员的肩胛骨上旋角度比高中棒球运动员小。最后，Cools等人[18]发现，年龄较大（>16岁）的网球运动员的肩胛骨上旋角度比年龄较小（<14岁）的网球运动员小。将这三项研究的结果结合起来，可能得出结论：使用量对肩胛骨上旋有不利影响。事实上，额外的研究发现，高中和大学的球员们在赛季过程中都损失了肩胛骨上旋[19, 20]。这可能表明，即使是健康的无症状运动员，其参与肩胛骨上旋的肌肉（上斜方肌、下斜方肌和前锯肌）也产生了慢性疲劳。维持适当的肩胛骨上旋，对维持盂肱关节的最佳功能和使因过度使用造成损伤的风险（如肩峰下撞击综合征）最小化是非常重要的[5, 8]。

运动学

过头类投掷运动是人体最快的运动之一，可在盂肱关节处产生每秒7000°的速度[21]。由于此极端速度，肩胛骨也必须高速工作，以保持适当的盂肱关节力量和稳定性。肩胛骨以前被描述成一只用鼻子顶着球保持平衡的海狮[22, 23]。海狮（肩胛骨）必须移动以保持球（肱骨头）的平衡和稳定。由于在活体内评估肩胛骨的高速运动比较困难，目前仅有两项研究对投掷过程中肩胛骨的运动进行了研究[24, 25]。为了简化运动学研究，研究人员仅在投掷运动的特定部分（跨步足接触、最大外旋和最大内旋）评估了肩胛骨。在跨步足接触时，研究人员发现肩胛骨处在后缩、微上旋、前倾的位置。从该位置移动到最大外旋处，肩胛骨进一步后缩和上旋，同时也变为外旋和后倾。这已提示，在投掷运动的最大外旋角度时，肩胛骨的作用类似于漏斗，将能量从下肢和躯干传递到手臂[7, 8]。充分的肩胛骨后缩将最大限度地将能量转移到肩关节，同时肩胛骨上旋、外旋和后倾，提供最大的冈上肌腱空间。最大内旋发生在球释放之后，需要消散大量在加速阶段产生的能量。肩胛骨处于前伸、内旋和前倾的位置。与最大外旋相比，这些位置是可活动范围的另一个极端。为了有效地消散能量，关节会产生大范围的活动。在较大范围内消散的能量会降低周围软组织结构（关节囊、韧带、肌腱和肌肉）上的应力峰值。理论上，这将保护这些结构，避免其被过度使用、退化和损伤。虽然通过投掷了解肩胛骨正常的高速运动方式是很重要的，但在临床评估时是不可能达成的。因此，测试者经常让受试者缓慢而有控制力地抬高肩部，以观察其肩胛骨的运动。与非优势侧相比，在上抬过程中优势侧的肩胛骨表现出更多的上旋、后倾和内旋[12]。此外，与非投掷类项目运动员相比，投掷类项目运动员通常有更多的肩胛骨上旋、内旋和后缩[9]。因此，投掷类项目运动员不太可能有完美的肩胛骨对称性，两侧肩胛骨通常存在着细微的差异。临床评估过头类项目运动员时，这些差异是需要重点记录的。

动力学

在投掷过程中，需要力来产生速度和加速度，从而与运动学相联系。没有动力学，就不会发生正常的运动。在正常投掷过程中有时会产生极端的力量，导致创伤性损伤，不过动力是亚极量，不会导致急性组织破坏[26]。而且，力学刺激会使组织适应[27]。一般来说，这种适应将使组织更强，能够承受更大的力量。然而，如果负荷过大或频率过高，则会导致组织退化[28, 29]。投掷是一种高速运动，研究已证明其将在整个上肢产生很大的力量和扭矩[26, 30-32]。投掷产生最大力量的两个主要阶段是加速阶段和减速阶段。在加速阶段，肩关节处产生很大的向前（300 N）和向上（400 N）的力[26]。研究者认为这些力量被肩袖和肱二头肌腱收缩所产生的力量抵消，以保持盂肱关节的稳定。投掷减速阶段产生的压缩力大于1000 N，相当于1.5倍体重[26]。这是加速阶段产生的力量的两倍多。这种力是由后部肩袖和肩胛骨稳定肌的离心收缩产生的，以帮助消散能量[5, 6]。如前所述，从最大外旋到最大内旋，肩胛骨的活动范围很大。大范围的运动减少了周围关节结构上的峰值力，并在离心收缩期间最大限度地减少了肌肉损伤，并有可能加速恢复。

力量

肌肉力量对过头类项目运动员来说是非常重要的。由于投掷有很大的动力和重复性，肩胛骨肌肉必须适应并且变得更强。事实上，已有几项研究探讨了过头类项目运动员优势侧手臂肌肉力量的不对称性。在临床检查时，上、中、下斜方肌的肌肉力量都有所增强[11, 33, 34]。此外，检查也发现前锯肌在优势侧更加强壮[11]。这些特殊的肌肉对肩胛骨的正常功能至关重要，尤其是在肩胛骨上旋时。随着运动员的成长，上肢的肌肉力量、速度和加速度通常都会增加。肩胛骨稳定肌产生的离心收缩力也会增加，以达到减速作用，并使传递到盂肱关节和肘关节的应力最小化。因此，过头类项目运动员在整个职业生涯中维持肩胛骨的力量，对于减少肩关节和肘关节损伤是至关重要的。

肌肉活动

肌肉的激活常常独立于神经肌肉系统，与力量不同，它常常是神经肌肉和机械元素（肌动蛋白和肌球蛋白）的组合。因此，对过头类项目运动员的肩胛骨稳定肌的肌肉活动进行检查，将有助于更全面地了解肩胛骨肌肉在执行这类任务时发挥的功能。在检查中，我们发现上斜方肌和前锯肌在过头类投掷动作的最大外旋和最大内旋之间活动最强[35]。在模拟投掷动作的减速阶段，优势侧前锯肌活动也会增加[36]。

这些结果与前面讨论的运动学结果一致。在投掷阶段，肩胛骨保持上旋并前伸以吸收能量。上斜方肌将帮助保持上旋，前锯肌将使肩胛骨运动到前伸位。有趣的是，研究也发现肩胛骨肌肉的活化与对侧臀中肌的活化有关[35]。这表明过头类项目运动员优势侧肩胛骨和对侧髋关节之间有神经肌肉联系。另一个需要检查的肌肉活动的重要方面是时序。潜伏期或恰当时机激活的肌肉应该发生于正常的功能中，从而产生正常的运动。一项研究发现，优势侧上斜方肌和中斜方肌的潜伏期有所增加[37]。与中斜方肌和前锯肌相比，上斜方肌的潜伏期也有所增加。为了使肩胛骨功能正常化，必须先激活前锯肌和下斜方肌。若上斜方肌的激活优先于下斜方肌和前锯肌，将导致肩胛骨上提而不是上旋，有造成肩袖撞击的隐患。事实上，这种异常运动常见于肩袖撕裂患者[38]。

综上所述，由于投掷时上肢反复承受应力，肩胛骨常呈现正常的不对称。如果不了解这些正常的不对称，测试者可能会将其识别为异常，受试者将被错误地诊断。因此，了解肩胛骨和周围肌肉的正常功能对评估过头类项目运动员至关重要。临床人员具备适当的知识，不仅可以充分地评估受伤运动员，而且可以帮运动员制订预防计划。

应力适应

肩胛骨运动障碍

肩胛骨运动障碍被定义为一种可观察

到的肩胛骨位置或运动的改变[8, 39]。它并不是一个诊断或一种疾病，虽然它经常被认为是。它是影响最佳肩胛骨运动的缺陷，并且可能是肩部和肘部损伤的危险因素。据报道，健康且无症状的过头类项目运动员，其有肩胛骨运动障碍的概率为61%，而非过头类项目运动员为33%[40]。因此，在损伤之前，运动障碍可能已经存在，并发展为功能障碍。有趣的是，大鼠模型研究检验了肩胛骨运动障碍的影响，证明它会导致冈上肌腱和肱二头肌腱退化[41]。这表明，如果过头类项目运动员存在运动障碍，应对其采取矫正治疗，尽量减少受伤的风险。据报道，94%有肩部或肘部损伤的过头类项目运动员有肩胛骨运动障碍[5]。这是将肩胛骨运动障碍与肩部和肘部损伤联系起来的证据。从临床角度来看，患者通常可以单纯通过有针对性的肩胛骨锻炼来改善肩部和肘部症状。重建正常的肩胛骨功能可以最大限度地减少盂肱关节和肘关节周围结构的应力，从而减轻或消除症状。关于过头类项目运动员的肩胛骨功能改变与特定适应性，下文将做详细讨论。

肌肉疲劳

过头类项目运动员通常经历的第一个适应是肌肉疲劳。一般而言，疲劳可以被认为是有两个成分在同时作用：神经和机械[42]。神经疲劳会导致非最佳的放电模式和神经脉冲振幅减少。取代以非常复杂的放电模式产生最佳的肌肉激活的方式，改为不复杂的肌肉内大量运动单元同时放电的模式[43, 44]。这是一种为了弥补神经脉冲振幅减少的尝试。这种补偿模式导致肩胛骨运动不协调，盂肱关节后侧关节囊和肩袖在后续减慢手臂速度的过程中将承受更多的力。

机械疲劳通常由离心收缩期间肌球蛋白和肌动蛋白的细微损伤引起[45]。随着肩胛骨稳定肌内受损的肌球蛋白和肌动蛋白数量的增加，肩胛骨机械地产生力和吸收能量的能力会降低。这会产生负反馈回路，进入神经部分产生非最佳神经放电[44]。因此，确定投掷类项目运动员所需的最佳恢复时间将使急性和慢性疲劳造成的不利影响最小化，并使肩胛骨稳定肌能够在投掷过程中改善吸收离心能量的能力。

在过头类项目运动员中，我们可以查出急性和慢性的肌肉疲劳。急性疲劳通常在一场比赛中或训练期间发生，而慢性疲劳通常在赛季期间发生。一项研究比较了一组游泳运动员的训练前后，通过视觉观察发现了肩胛骨运动障碍的存在[46]。在训练开始之前，没有游泳运动员被鉴定为有肩胛骨运动障碍。然而，训练后立即发现，存在肩胛骨运动障碍的人增加至82%。另一项研究检查了业余的过头类项目运动员在肩部疲劳前后的肩胛骨运动学和肩峰下空间[47]。研究人员发现，在肩部疲劳后，当肩关节外展45°和60°时，肩胛骨处于更大的上旋、外旋和后倾角度。与之相一致，肩峰下空间也增加了。另一项研究还发现，肩部疲劳后肩胛骨的上旋角度增加；然而，下斜方肌的肌肉活动减少[48]。这些结果令人惊讶，因为这种变化被认为是有利的（更多的上旋、外旋和后倾）。由于受试者是业余运动员，他们可能在疲劳期间进行代偿，以使受伤的风险最小化。最近有一项针对一组大学网球运动员在网球发球前后检查肩胛骨上旋角度的研究，发现疲劳后立即出现肩胛骨上旋角度减小，但在24小时后恢复到基准线[49]。该结果与先前的假设一致，即疲劳会减少上旋角度，从而减少肩峰下空间并压迫冈上肌腱。

在赛季中检查过头类项目运动员的慢性疲劳也很重要。先前的研究发现，在赛季结束后，高中和大学棒球运动员在各个盂肱关节外展位（60°、90°和120°）的肩胛骨上旋都有显著减少[10,19,20]。此外，另一项研究发现投手的肩胛骨上旋减少，而防守球员在一个赛季中其肩胛骨上旋有所增加[50]。这表明与防守球员相比，由于投手较大力量和重复使用的累积，其负责肩胛骨上旋的肌肉（上、下斜方肌和前锯肌）出现慢性疲劳。如前所述，肩胛骨稳定肌产生高重复的离心收缩力能使手臂减速并维持盂肱关节的稳定性，但该力量可能在比赛期间引起显著的急性疲劳，如果没有适当的恢复将导致慢性疲劳。由于肩胛骨功能不正常，盂肱关节肌肉（肩袖）将不得不进行代偿。这将加速肩袖微小损伤和疲劳的发生，从而使代偿向远端进展至肘部[51]。

软组织紧张

除了肌肉疲劳，过头类项目运动员经常会有多种软组织结构（包括肌肉、肌腱和关节囊）紧张。由于肩胛骨是多达18块肌肉和肌腱的附着部位，因此这些结构紧张会影响肩胛骨的位置和运动，从而导致长期的功能改变。在本节中，我们将讨论常见的易紧张的结构及其对肩胛骨功能的影响。

胸小肌

胸小肌起于肩胛骨喙突并止于第3~5肋。胸小肌的正常功能是使肩胛骨前伸和下降。如前所述，肩胛骨前伸对投掷期间的手臂适当减速非常重要。然而，由于长期的过头运动和正常肩胛骨功能的重复使用，这块肌肉经常发生过度紧张。研究已发现，胸小肌长度与临床确定的肩部向前姿势直接相关[52]。更具体地说，胸小肌紧张的运动员的肩胛骨前倾和内旋增加[53]。这些位置的变化使肩峰下空间减少[54]，并与肩胛骨不稳定相关[5]。有趣的是，牵伸胸小肌确实增加了肌肉的长度，但没有重建正常的肩胛骨运动学[55]。这可能表明长期紧张会改变神经肌肉控制的方式和肩胛骨稳定肌的力量。因此，单独牵伸仅能解决一种有害的适应，最佳治疗方案可能包括肌肉再教育和肩胛骨稳定肌肌力训练。

后侧肩紧张

众所周知，过头类项目运动员会出现后侧肩紧张。与非优势侧相比，优势侧手臂在临床上表现为肩内旋缺失。因此，它被称为盂肱关节内旋不足（GIRD）。GIRD

已被证实会影响肩胛骨的位置和运动。一项研究发现，与盂肱关节内旋减少14°或以下的球员相比，减少15°或以上的棒球运动员的肩胛骨上旋减少，而肩胛骨前伸增加[56]。同样，另一项研究发现后侧肩紧张与肩部向前姿势相关[57]。另一项研究发现，平均减少24°的GIRD患者肩峰下空间较小，而在牵伸后侧肩部肌肉6周后，不仅GIRD好转，并且肩峰下空间也增加了[58]。这表明过度的GIRD会对肩胛骨稳定肌产生不必要的应力，从而导致神经肌肉控制障碍，并使肩袖处于受伤的风险中，还表明单纯牵伸后侧肩部肌肉可以增加肩峰下空间。

要考虑GIRD包含三种组织的适应性。首先，肱骨后倾是一种发生在骨骼成熟之前的骨骼适应[59-61]。在出生时，肱骨处于过度的后倾位（更多的盂肱关节外旋和更少的内旋）。在正常发育的过程中，肱骨转变至前倾位置[61]。然而，如果肱骨在年幼时就暴露在投掷的应力下，其将停留在后倾位。因此，与非优势侧手臂相比，这种适应性会在优势侧手臂产生较少的内旋[62]。由于能在不牵伸或不损伤软组织结构的情况下获得额外的外旋角度，因此后倾通常被认为是一个积极的适应。接下来的两种是软组织适应，如果存在可导致肩胛骨改变。后侧肩袖紧张也被认为可导致GIRD。在比赛后立即对GIRD进行检测，发现GIRD立即增加，并能持续多达3天[63]。由于内旋的突然缺失，后侧肩袖的离心损伤导致GIRD增加。然而，单独直接测量后侧肩袖的紧张度是不可能的，因此目前无法证明其与肩胛骨功能改变有直接关系。后侧关节囊紧张或肥厚也被证明可在过头类项目运动员中发现，并且有GIRD的临床表现[60,64,65]。已发现大学棒球运动员优势侧手臂的后侧关节囊更厚[64]、更硬[65]，并且与盂肱关节内旋角度呈负相关[64]。这表明后侧关节囊越厚，内旋角度越小。有趣的是，也发现后侧关节囊厚度与肩胛骨上旋角度之间存在正相关[64]。这表明关节囊越厚，上旋角度越大。当后侧关节囊紧张或肥厚时，其组织硬度增加[65]，这将减少肩胛骨原来可获得的运动，并因此将肩胛骨拉向更大的肩胛骨上旋位置。这种上旋角度的增加并不是有益的，因为对尸体进行的研究已经证明，后侧关节囊紧张将导致肱骨头在关节盂表面向后上移动[66,67]，肩峰下空间减少，并导致肩峰下撞击或内部撞击。

大圆肌

最近的研究发现，过头类项目运动员的优势侧手臂可能会外旋缺失（多<5°）[68]。由于存在肱骨后倾，临床上真正的外旋缺失通常是很难测量的。然而，利用肱骨后倾来纠正盂肱关节的活动度，可帮助临床人员鉴别是否存在外旋缺失。专业运动员的外旋缺失被认为能使肩部受伤后变残疾的风险增加2倍、肩部手术概率增加4倍[68]。虽然研究尚未确定外旋缺失的原因，但据推测是由大圆肌紧张引起的。大圆肌是唯一的起于肩胛骨外侧缘下段、止于肱骨小结节嵴的肌肉。与其他的肩部肌肉类似，

它作为内旋肌，处于长期过度使用的状态。在临床检查中，大圆肌紧张将在肩胛骨稳定时限制肩外旋。然而，在过头运动期间，大圆肌紧张可以将肩胛骨拉向更大角度的上旋和后倾。实际上，在过头类项目运动员的优势侧可观察到更多的肩胛骨上旋和后倾[9, 12]。这种强力运动可能会给肩胛骨稳定肌带来更大的应力，并加速肌肉疲劳。但是，这需要研究来证实。

肱三头肌长头

肱三头肌长头是一种双关节肌肉，起于盂下结节、止于尺骨鹰嘴。在过头运动期间，肱三头肌负责肩部和肘部的减速动作。在随球动作的过程中，肱三头肌产生很大的离心收缩力来控制两个关节，可能导致明显的肌肉微损伤[69]。这种重复的微损伤可导致肌肉与肌腱慢性紧张。事实上，过头类项目运动员经常出现由于优势侧手臂肩胛骨不稳定而产生的盂肱关节前屈角度缺失[68]。研究也表明，优势侧前屈缺失≥5°，肘关节损伤的风险增加2.8倍[68]。另一种可能导致前屈角度缺失的结构是背阔肌。然而，背阔肌并没有附着在肩胛骨上，因此它只能限制肩胛骨前屈。由于肱三头肌长头附着在肩胛骨上，在肩前屈或外展时，紧绷的肌肉可能会强制肩胛骨上旋。另外，由于它是双关节肌肉，在过头运动中身体可通过改变肘关节的运动来代偿肌肉紧张。例如，如果在投掷动作的加速阶段出现肱三头肌过度紧张，则运动员可能会做更多的肘关节伸直来减小张力。

在加速阶段肘关节伸直增加，会给尺侧副韧带带来过大的外翻应力[26]，久而久之，会对肘关节的稳定性造成不利影响。

疼痛影响

有很多东西可以改变正常的关节运动学、动力学和肌肉功能。如上所述，肌肉疲劳和软组织紧张在过头类项目运动员中是非常普遍的。然而，还有一样东西尚未被讨论过，而且在过头类项目运动员中极其普遍，这就是疼痛。过头类项目运动员疼痛的患病率也非常高，即使在青少年运动员中也是如此。大约16%的青少年棒球运动员经历过肩痛，而29%的人经历过肘部疼痛[70]。同样，据报道，精英游泳运动员在运动期间患肩痛的概率也高达91%[71]。由于大量的过头类项目运动员经常有疼痛表现，因此了解疼痛对肩胛骨功能的影响是很重要的。疼痛是身体结构传递的神经信号，身体感受到异常的应力并由大脑解读出来。为了保护自己，身体会以代偿的方式避免疼痛。这种代偿通常会导致其他结构的暂时性应力增加。过头类项目运动员经常会在引臂后期位置（肩关节90°外展、肘关节屈曲伴最大外旋）或加速阶段出现疼痛，因为在此位置，肩部和肘部受到巨大的关节应力和扭矩[26]。在这些位置时，身体会试图改变动作以减轻疼痛。研究发现，伴有疼痛的过头类项目运动员在盂肱关节外展45°和90°时，肩胛骨上旋减少[72, 73]。这可能通过撞击机制进一步压迫冈上肌。此外，临床报道，伴随疼痛的运动员SICK肩胛骨评分和核心不稳定性均增加[74]。虽然人们常常认为疼痛会导致运动学改变，但运动学改变是否先于疼痛出现仍有待确认。之前的研究已经确定了健康无症状的过头类项目运动员的几种肩胛骨适应性。然而，未来需要前瞻性研究来证实导致疼痛的一系列事件。

综上所述，过头类项目运动员是非常独特的。了解正常的肩胛骨功能和发生在这一人群中的常见适应性将提高临床医生评估、预防和治疗肩损伤的能力。下一节将指导临床医生如何针对这一人群进行全面的临床检查和治疗。

肩胛骨运动障碍的临床意义

如前所述，肩胛骨运动障碍对肩关节功能有多种影响。在临床上，存在肩胛骨运动障碍的过头类项目运动员常伴有肩部其他软组织结构的损伤。本节将重点讨论这些损伤的临床意义和以循证为依据的综合检查方法。

肩袖

肩袖起于肩胛骨。因此，稳定的肩胛骨是肩袖能发挥其最佳功能所必需的。肩胛骨后缩测试说明了这一原则：当有运动障碍的肩胛骨被"减少"运动或被手法固定时，可测量到前屈的阻力增加[75]（图6.1）。正确的肩胛骨位置是优化肩袖的长度-张力关系的必要条件。例如，前伸的肩胛骨不能为冈上肌活动提供适当的张力，因为肌肉、肌腱单元的起点（肩胛骨）和止点（大结节）之间的距离明显缩短。肩袖薄弱的后果包括凹陷压迫功能丧失，从而导致固有肩稳定性丧失[76]。肩袖是盂肱关节重要的动态稳定结构，静态稳定结构（盂唇和关节囊）的张力也将随之变化。此外，薄弱的肌肉与肌腱单位不太能承受肩关节运动时的离心负荷。例如，在投掷的随球阶段，后侧肩袖减速时会产生较大的张力[77]。冈下肌在力学上处于不利位置，它不仅会很快疲劳，将增加的负荷转移到后侧关节囊，而且它在较低的离心负荷下也会

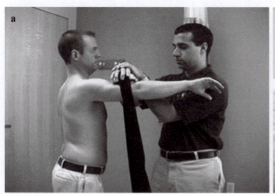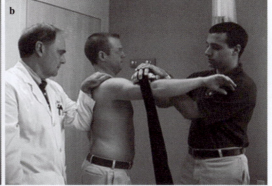

图6.1　空罐试验的检查位置（a）与肩胛骨后缩测试的检查位置（b）。受试者手臂处于倒空罐的位置，测试者将前臂压力作用于受试者的肩胛骨内侧缘，使其肩胛骨保持轻微后缩，同时受试者使用最大的力量来抵抗手持测力计[4]

出问题。换句话说，在非最佳长度-张力关系下的肌肉与肌腱单元，即使在较低的应力水平下也会出问题。因此，约1/3的盂唇撕裂患者同时出现肩袖撕裂也就不足为奇了[78]。此外，随着冈上肌腱前缘负荷的增加，受损冈下肌在减速过程中抑制前侧剪切力的效果也会下降。此外，冈下肌利用其后侧力量来保护盂肱关节，使其免受过度的前移应力，尤其是在外展外旋位[79-81]。因此，冈下肌的应力保护前侧关节囊和盂唇免受磨损。后侧关节囊的张力增加与GIRD有关，而冈上肌前缘的下表面损伤被认为是在随球过程中离心负荷增加所致。肩胛骨前伸使肩胛骨能吸收减速应力的平移区域减小，因此，后侧肩袖和关节囊的张力将会增加。Kibler等人[7]描述了引臂后期的"满罐能量"位置依赖于足够的肩胛骨后缩。如果肩胛骨后缩不足，肱骨的完全外旋被阻止，投掷速度也会降低。肩袖和肘部也因为试图代偿减少的能量而导致应力增加。

过度扭转

GIRD患者的肩胛骨后撤、前侧关节囊松弛增加，以及前侧关节囊假性松弛，使投掷者获得了更多的外旋角度[5,6]。肱骨的过度旋转在肩袖中产生了过度的剪切力，这可能表现为肩袖层间撕裂。Conway[82]描述，冈上肌和冈下肌的上、下薄层可以分离，并形成部分关节撕裂伴腱内延展（PAINT病变）。这种剪切力会因肩胛骨功能障碍而加剧。例如，如果肩胛骨在最大外旋时没有出现后倾，肩袖将经历额外的扭转，从而增加PAINT病变的可能性。

内部撞击

在投掷的引臂后期，过度的肩胛骨前伸和前倾会缩短关节盂和大结节之间的距离。肩胛骨后缩的减少也会导致投掷者的水平外展增加，在肩胛骨平面投出，会导致后上盂唇和大结节之间的接触增加。冈上肌的"挤压"可能导致后续肩袖肌腱纤维的损伤。这种内部撞击[83]表现为冈上肌与冈下肌交界处的下表面撕裂（图6.2）。假以时日，盂唇"挤压"可能导致后上盂唇磨损（图6.3）。肩胛骨前伸和GIRD是密不可分的。Kibler等人[84]描述，内旋丢失将导致肩胛骨翘起，此时肩胛骨将移动到前伸位以提供内旋。如果投掷者被紧张的后侧关节囊限制，肩胛骨会在胸部向上、向周围移动，以使手臂朝向本垒板。静态和动态的限制力薄弱将使肩胛骨处于内旋（肩胛骨前伸）位。此外，后侧关节囊挛缩将导致肱骨头在引臂后期相对地向后、向上移动，进一步增加后上盂唇的"剥离"应力，并可能加剧2型盂唇损伤[85]。在这种情况下，复位测试将是阳性的，因为肩胛骨被手动放置于最佳位置时，施加于肱骨上部的后侧压力将减少结节和盂唇的接触。

外部撞击

肩胛骨前伸使肱骨头和肩峰之间的空间减小。肩胛骨沿着肋骨轮廓前伸并前倾，在肩前屈时，肩峰与大结节的接触增

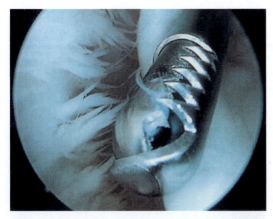

图6.2 关节镜下显示冈上肌与冈下肌交界处的肩袖底面撕裂

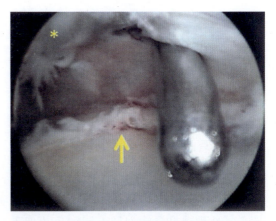

图6.3 关节镜下显示后上盂唇磨损（箭头所指）及并发的肩袖后上底面撕裂（星号所示）

加。外展动作的疼痛弧可由肩胛骨辅助试验缓解，这可能证实了存在有症状的功能性撞击。事实上，Muraki等人[86]表明，在投掷的随球阶段，后下关节囊紧张，增加了肱骨头和喙突肩峰的接触压力。

肩胛骨和肘关节

投手肘部损伤的发生率急剧上升[87]。当然，投球数量增加是造成这种流行病的原因之一。然而，肩胛骨在肘部损伤中扮演重要角色，尤其是尺侧副韧带（UCL）损伤。GIRD[88]、全范围关节活动度受限[88-90]与UCL损伤之间的关系早已经确定。内旋角度丢失本质上减少了上臂的长轴旋转。近端节段损伤可预见远端（肘关节）的负荷将增加，以实现将棒球推向本垒板所必需的内旋。事实上，Suzuki等人[91]已经证明肩胛骨疲劳会导致肘部的代偿性运动。有UCL损伤的投掷类项目运动员，其肱骨外旋的丢失可能是一种保护机制[89]，通过这种保护机制，运动员可避免由于肱骨极度外旋引起的肘外翻力矩失调。肩胛骨前伸可能使肩胛骨跑出肩胛骨平面，如相对地肱骨水平外展，这将增加投掷期间施加在肘关节处的外翻应力负荷的持续时间。上臂在胸部后面的时间越长，肘部就越容易出现外翻。另外，在某些搬运过程中出现的肘部下垂会增加从身体旋转轴中心到力臂（手）末端的距离。该长度的增加仅仅增加了作用在肘部的向心力。投掷时肘部下垂的原因有很多，包括核心肌力薄弱、后侧关节囊紧张、肩胛骨前伸和肩袖薄弱。

检查

肩袖

如前所述，投掷者的肩袖损伤主要发生在三个部位：冈上肌前缘（由于无法承受离心负荷）、冈上肌和冈下肌层间（由于过度扭转）、冈上肌和冈下肌交界处（由于内部撞击）。有效的检查应该划定一个相当精确的受伤区域。

冈上肌

Savoie等人[92]所描述的Whipple测试（图6.4）可检测冈上肌前缘是否薄弱。该测试要求患者将手臂置于前屈和极度内收位。前屈抗阻时出现疼痛和/或无力代表阳性。虽然满罐和空罐对冈上肌的负荷似乎是相等的，但满罐可能是一个更优秀的测试，因为它通常较少诱发疼痛[93]。在正常的满罐试验中，Whipple测试阳性所显示的薄弱提示冈上肌前壁部分增厚。

发生在引臂后期或外展外旋位。复位测试（图6.5）是检测这种现象的极好方法。在外展外旋位，在肱骨近端施加向后的力，如果疼痛得到缓解就被认为是内部撞击的阳性指征。如前所述，在肱骨上施加向后的力，能够增加后上盂唇和大结节之间的距离，减轻撞击。

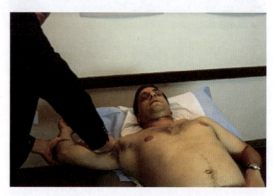

图6.5 复位测试是使受试者仰卧于检查床上，外展90°，肩外旋90°。在这个位置，测试者在肱骨近端前侧施加一个向后的力，从而减轻潜在的内部撞击症状

盂唇撕裂

虽然许多盂唇损伤的检查展示了不一致的结果[94]，但Kibler等人[95]表示动态盂唇剪切（DLS）试验具备良好的敏感性、特异性和准确性。在这个测试中，外展的手臂被带到外旋和水平外展的最大角度；然后手臂被动放下，从而后侧肩袖相对于后上盂唇形成剪切力（图6.6）。Kibler等人[95]也指出，虽然O'Brien试验（前屈、内收和内旋手臂，以此抵抗向下的压力）在盂唇撕裂检测方面不如DLS试验敏感，但这两种试验结合后的预测，与关节镜下发现的盂唇损伤最一致。

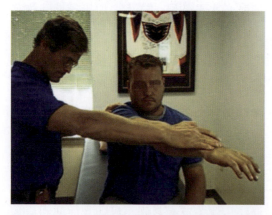

图6.4 Whipple测试是将受试者手臂摆在肩前屈90°和最大水平内收位置。然后测试者对其前臂远端施加一个直接向下的力，受试者保持这个姿势。阳性指征为肌力弱或疼痛

当肩胛骨处于收缩状态（肩胛骨后缩测试）时，Whipple测试阳性确实表示薄弱，因为肩胛骨前伸（基底不稳定）会损害冈上肌功能[75]。

内部撞击

后上盂唇和大结节之间的冈上肌受压

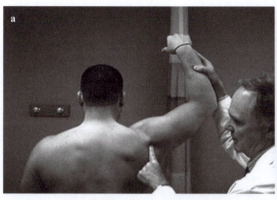 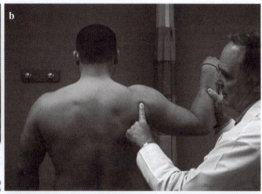

图6.6 （a）受试者站立位，受试侧肘部弯曲90°，手臂在肩胛骨平面外展至120°以上，并且外旋至组织紧绷，然后引导它进入最大水平外展 （b）测试者通过维持外旋和水平外展，对关节施加剪切力，将手臂从外展120°降至外展60°。阳性指征是出现疼痛和/或在外展期间沿着后侧关节线发生疼痛的咔嗒声或卡住[1]

投掷者肩部的影像学表现

先进的成像方法，特别是MRI，可以极大地帮助诊断肩袖和盂唇损伤。将染料注入肩关节囊的MRI关节造影提高了肩袖和盂唇损伤的检出率[96]（图6.7）。然而，必须注意的是，高灵敏度的新一代MRI可能会检测到许多"无关紧要"的盂唇撕裂[97]。事实上，一些盂唇牵拉可能是自适应的，使投掷者表现出"沟槽"（slot）。因此，所有影像学发现必须支持检查结果。对于肩袖下表面撕裂，研究已显示MRI外展外旋视图（在外展外旋位时摄取的轴向图像）可提高对部分关节侧边损伤的检测敏感性[98]。此外，外展外旋视图被认为可以增加对内部撞击和盂唇撕裂的检测效果[99, 100]（图6.8）。正如在内部撞击时所见，冈上肌下表面的轻微撕裂，可能表现为肱骨头后侧冈上肌和冈下肌交界处附近的小囊性改变（图6.9）。

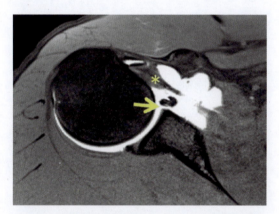

图6.7 MRI关节造影显示可见度增强的条索状盂肱中韧带（星号所示）和Buford复合体——解剖变异，类似于盂唇撕裂（箭头所指）

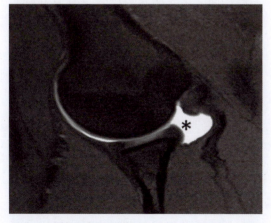

图6.8 外展外旋位MRI关节造影。后上方关节盂、肩袖和盂唇很容易鉴定（星号所示）

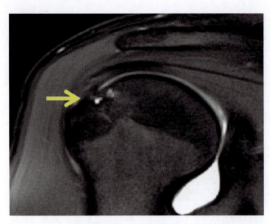

图6.9 MRI显示冈上肌止点位置（箭头所指）因慢性内部撞击而发生囊性改变

治疗

关键康复原则

与肩胛骨相关的投掷性损伤主要以保守治疗为主，以恢复肩部稳态为目标，对有症状的肩胛骨位置不正进行复位。Tate等人[101]发现，并非所有的肩胛骨不对称都伴有症状。事实上，如果肩胛骨复位（后缩测试或肩胛骨辅助试验）可减轻肩袖或盂唇疼痛，这表明是肩胛骨位置有问题。肩胛骨复位可通过增强肩胛骨后缩肌肉和牵拉使肩胛骨前伸的紧张结构来实现。许多从事举重训练的运动员几乎完全专注于前伸运动（卧推），而忽略了重要的肩胛骨后缩训练，如肩胛骨夹紧（scapular pinches），并臂握划船（close-grip rows）和俯卧水平外展伴外旋[102]，而这些训练对维持肩部稳态是必要的。低位划船运动是选择性激活前锯肌和菱形肌的理想方式。

Blackburn练习[103]在训练肩胛骨后缩肌肉方面也很出色。Kibler等人[104]推广的割草机训练引入了更多的核心激活，同时也训练了肩胛骨后缩。综合动力链评估对考量投掷者是否能完全重返投掷运动是最重要的。过头类项目运动员可能存在站立腿外展力弱，导致髋内旋缺失、股四头肌紧张和站立腿踝关节背屈角度缺失。后侧关节囊和肩袖的紧张必须通过侧卧位牵伸和跨身体中线的内收牵伸来解决，以防止肩胛骨"翘起"复发[84]。

手术指征

至少3个月高品质物理治疗无效，并且关节镜评估发现盂唇撕裂的阳性结果。此外，存在明显的机械症状，如锁住、卡住和持续的手臂麻木感，这些都是关节镜干预的指征。如上所述，我们必须注意并非所有的盂唇分离都是病理性的，实际上有一些盂唇牵拉可能是自适应的。

手术拾珍

侧卧位能很好地暴露肩部，特别是后凹处和下凹处，是手术的首选体位。首先建立一个标准的后侧视野入口，大约在肩峰角内侧2 cm和远端2 cm处。接下来建立两个前侧入口，一个位于肩峰的前外角（AL入口），另一个位于喙突尖端外侧2 cm（AP入口）。当从AL入口观察时，使用一种释放型器械将盂唇从关节盂中释放出来。磨损的盂唇伸长不能修复。完整的盂唇分离并伴有关节盂和/或盂唇表面裂痕，通常表明盂唇损伤。动态"剥离"（peel-back）测试是将手臂移开牵引位并放置成外展外旋位，这样做不仅可以发现明显的盂唇分离，还可以增加肱骨后上方的移位和其与冈上肌纤维的接触（内部撞击）。

肩袖失效的体征，不论是在内部撞击中所见的冈上肌和冈下肌交界处磨损，还是由于离心负荷引起肩袖失效而导致的冈上肌下表面纤维断裂，都进一步证明盂唇损伤可能会产生不良后果。在 AL 视图中，通过 Wilmington 口实现经皮锚点入口插入[78]。缝线通过一个 Neviaser 入口来回穿梭，并且只有非常小心才能"捕获"盂唇组织。过度约束任何后侧关节囊的组织，对运动员可能是灾难性的。由于上盂唇的内在弹性，作者更倾向于使用不太柔顺的缝合材料。目前可用的一些较新的缝合材料都非常坚硬，无法承受投掷动作所必需的盂唇偏移。出于两个原因，作者更倾向于采用水平褥式打结结构（图 6.10）。第一，水平缝合模式将盂唇高度恢复到其固有状态[105]。如 Yoo 等人[106]所示，术后肩部功能与盂唇高度有关。无结缝合结构"推动"盂唇向关节盂，并且使关节表面的盂唇不卷起。第二，水平褥式结构使缝合材料移位能较好地远离关节表面。在一些病例中，作者观察到突出的缝合材料造成了相当大的缝合磨损（图 6.11）。如果选择简单的缝合结构，则建议使用可吸收的缝合材料，如 PDS（图 6.12）。

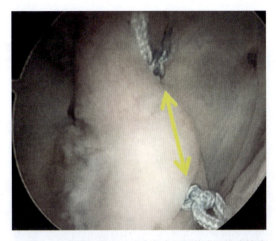

图 6.10 关节镜视窗显示用来固定盂唇的水平褥式缝线结（suture knot）（双箭头所指）

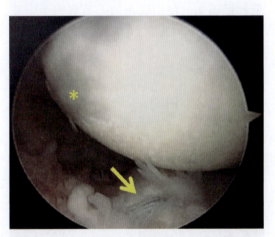

图 6.11 关节镜视窗显示肱骨头软骨软化症（星号所示），原因是突出的缝合材料磨损（箭头所指）

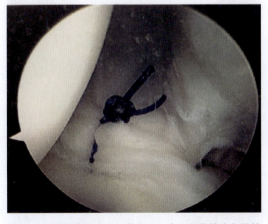

图 6.12 关节镜视窗显示使用 PDS（可吸收缝线）的简单缝合结构

后侧关节囊松解

作者中只有少数做过后侧关节囊松解。它的适应证包括真正的牵伸无反应，只有在肩部治疗师的帮助下才会罕见地遇到此类患者[6]。此外，关节囊必须被证明变得更厚且更坚固。如果遇到变薄的后侧关节囊，则松解术是禁忌。牵伸无反应者往往是更成熟的投掷者（大学后期或专业人员），这些人是有症状的内旋角度缺失至少25°或总运动弧度丢失至少5°。为了避免腋神经损伤，使用成角的关节囊槽子，在切割时向"上"提（图6.13）。

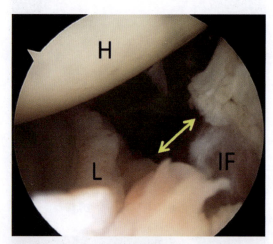

图6.13 关节镜视窗下的肩关节后下方、肱骨头（H）和盂唇（L）。后侧关节囊松解（双箭头所指）可由冈下肌的能见度来确定（IF）

预防

与投掷相关的大部分肩部和肘部损伤确实是可以预防的。对青少年过头类项目运动员进行全面的动力链评估，是避免肩袖和盂唇损伤非常重要的手段。动力链的主要组成部分是肩胛骨。肩胛骨不对称最初可能是投掷者的微小适应性改变，但是随着时间的推移，肩胛骨位置不正的不良机械作用将导致肌肉被抑制，有时候还会伴随肩袖和盂唇组织被破坏。投掷类项目运动员的有症状的肩胛骨不对称如果在早期得到识别和纠正，则可以避免盂唇和肩袖损伤。

（苟艳芸）

参考文献

1. Kibler WB, Sciascia AD, Hester PW, et al. Clinical utility of traditional and new tests in the diagnosis of biceps tendon injuries and superior labrum anterior and posterior lesions in the shoulder. Am J Sports Med, 2009, 37(9): 1840–1847.

2. Blackburn TA, McLeod W, White B, et al. EMG analysis of posterior rotator cuff exercises. J Athl Train, 1990, 25: 40–45.

3. Borstad JD, Ludewig PM. The effect of long versus short pectoralis minor resting length on scapular kinematics in healthy individuals. J Orthop Sports Phys Ther, 2005, 35(4): 227–238.

4. Brindle TJ, Nyland JA, Nitz AJ, et al. Scapulothoracic latent muscle reaction timing comparison between trained overhead throwers and untrained control subjects. Scand J Med Sci Sports, 2007, 17(3): 252–259.

5. Burkhart SS, Morgan CD. The peel-back mechanism: its role in producing and extending posterior type II SLAP lesions and its effect on SLAP repair rehabilitation. Arthroscopy, 1998, 14(6): 637–640.

6. Burkhart SS, Morgan CD, Kibler WB. The disabled throwing shoulder: spectrum of pathology. Arthroscopy, 2003, 19(4): 404–420.

7. Burkhart SS, Morgan CD, Kibler WB. The dis-

abled throwing shoulder: spectrum of pathology. Arthroscopy, 2003, 19(6): 641–661.

8. Burn MB, McCulloch PC, Lintner DM, et al. Prevalence of scapular dyskinesis in overhead and nonoverhead athletes: a systematic review. Orthop J Sports Med, 2016, 4(2): 2325967115627608.

9. Cain PR, Mutschler TA, Fu FH, et al. Anterior stability of the glenohumeral joint. A dynamic model. Am J Sports Med, 1987, 15(2): 144–148.

10. Clabbers KM, Kelly JD 4th, Bader D, et al. Effect of posterior capsule tightness on glenohumeral translation in the late-cocking phase of pitching. J Sport Rehabil, 2007, 16: 41–49.

11. Conte SA, Fleisig GS, Dines JS, et al. Prevalence of ulnar collateral ligament surgery in professional baseball players. Am J Sports Med, 2015, 43(7): 1764–1769.

12. Conway JE. Arthroscopic repair of partial-thickness rotator cuff tears and SLAP lesions in professional baseball players. Orthop Clin North Am, 2001, 32(3): 443–456.

13. Conwit RA, Stashuk D, Suzuki H, et al. Fatigue effects on motor unit activity during submaximal contractions. Arch Phys Med Rehabil, 2000, 81(9): 1211–1216.

14. Cools AM, Dewitte V, Lanszweert F, et al. Rehabilitation of scapular muscle balance: which exercises to prescribe? Am J Sports Med, 2007, 35(10): 1744–1751.

15. Cools AM, Johansson FR, Cambier DC, et al. Descriptive profile of scapulothoracic position, strength and flexibility variables in adolescent elite tennis players. Br J Sports Med, 2010, 44(9): 678–684.

16. Cools AM, Palmans T, Johansson FR. Age-related, sport-specific adaptions of the shoulder girdle in elite adolescent tennis players. J Athl Train, 2014, 49(5): 647–653.

17. Crockett HC, Gross LB, Wilk KE, et al. Osseous adaptation and range of motion at the glenohumeral joint in professional baseball pitchers. Am J Sports Med, 2002, 30(1): 20–26.

18. Cvitanic O, Tirman PF, Feller JF, et al. Using abduction and external rotation of the shoulder to increase the sensitivity of MR arthrography in revealing tears of the anterior glenoid labrum. Am J Roentgenol, 1997, 169(3): 837–844.

19. Dines JS, Frank JB, Akerman M, et al. Glenohumeral internal rotation deficits in baseball players with ulnar collateral ligament insufficiency. Am J Sports Med, 2009, 37(3): 566–570.

20. Donatelli R, Ellenbecker TS, Ekedahl SR, et al. Assessment of shoulder strength in professional baseball pitchers. J Orthop Sports Phys Ther, 2000, 30(9): 544–551.

21. Edelson G. The development of humeral head retroversion. J Shoulder Elbow Surg, 2000, 9(4): 316–318.

22. Flannigan B, Kursunoglu-Brahme S, Snyder S, et al. MR arthrography of the shoulder: comparison with conventional MR imaging. Am J Roentgenol, 1990, 155(4): 829–832.

23. Fleisig G, Chu Y, Weber A, et al. Variability in baseball pitching biomechanics among various levels of competition. Sports Biomech, 2009, 8(1): 10–21.

24. Fleisig GS, Andrews JR, Dillman CJ, et al. Kinetics of baseball pitching with implication about injury mechanisms. Am J Sports Med, 1995, 23: 233–239.

25. Fleisig GS, Barrentine SW, Zheng N. Kinematic and kinetic comparison of baseball pitching among various levels of development. J Biomech, 1999, 32: 1371–1375.

26. Fleisig GS, Bolt B, Fortenbaugh D, et al. Biomechanical comparison of baseball pitching and long-

toss: implications for training and rehabilitation. J Orthop Sports Phys Ther, 2011, 41(5): 296–303.
27. Fleisig GS, Kingsley DS, Loftice JW, et al. Kinetic comparison among the fastball, curveball, change-up, and slider in collegiate baseball pitchers. Am J Sports Med, 2006, 34(3): 423–430.
28. Fung DT, Wang VM, Andarawis-Puri N, et al. Early response to tendon fatigue damage accumulation in a novel in vivo model. J Biomech, 2010, 43(2): 274–279.
29. Garrison JC, Cole MA, Conway JE, et al. Shoulder range of motion deficits in baseball players with an ulnar collateral ligament tear. Am J Sports Med, 2012, 40(11): 2597–2603.
30. Giphart JE, van der Meijden OA, Millett PJ. The effects of arm elevation on the 3-dimensional acromiohumeral distance: a biplane fluoroscopy study with normative data. J Shoulder Elbow Surg, 2012, 21(11): 1593–1600.
31. Glousman R, Jobe F, Tibone J, et al. Dynamic electromyographic analysis of the throwing shoulder with glenohumeral instability. J Bone Joint Surg Am, 1988, 70(2): 220–226.
32. Hagstrom LS, Marzo JM. Simple versus horizontal suture anchor repair of bankart lesions: which better restores labral anatomy? Arthroscopy, 2013, 29(2): 325–329.
33. Huffman GR, Tibone JE, McGarry MH, et al. Path of glenohumeral articulation throughout the rotational range of motion in a thrower's shoulder model. Am J Sports Med, 2006, 34(10): 1662–1669.
34. Itoi E, Kido T, Sano A, et al. Which is more useful, the "full can test" or the "empty can test" in detecting the torn supraspinatus tendon? Am J Sports Med, 1999, 27(1): 65–68.
35. Jia X, Ji JH, Petersen SA, et al. Clinical evaluation of the shoulder shrug sign. Clin Orthop Relat Res, 2008, 466(11): 2813–2819.
36. Jobe CM. Posterior superior glenoid impingement: expanded spectrum. Arthroscopy, 1995, 11(5): 530–536.
37. Jobe FW, Tibone JE, Perry J, et al. An EMG analysis of the shoulder in throwing and pitching. A preliminary report. Am J Sports Med, 1983, 11(1): 3–5.
38. Joshi M, Thigpen CA, Bunn K, et al. Shoulder external rotation fatigue and scapular muscle activation and kinematics in overhead athletes. J Athl Train, 2011, 46(4): 349–357.
39. Kibler WB. Role of the scapula in the overhead throwing motion. Contemp Orthop, 1991, 22: 525–532.
40. Kibler WB. The role of the scapula in athletic shoulder function. Am J Sports Med, 1998, 26: 325–337.
41. Kibler WB, Sciascia AD, Dome D. Evaluation of apparent and absolute supraspinatus strength in patients with shoulder injury using the scapular retraction test. Am J Sports Med, 2006, 34(10): 1643–1647.
42. Kibler WB, Sciascia AD, Thomas SJ. Glenohumeral internal rotation deficit: pathogenesis and response to acute throwing. Sports Med Arthrosc, 2012, 20(1): 34–38.
43. Kibler WB, Sciascia AD, Uhl TL, et al. Electromyographic analysis of specific exercises for scapular control in early phases of shoulder rehabilitation. Am J Sports Med, 2008, 36(9): 1789–1798.
44. Konda S, Yanai T, Sakurai S. Configuration of the shoulder complex during the arm-cocking phase in baseball pitching. Am J Sports Med, 2015, 43(10): 2445–2451.
45. Laudner KG, Lynall R, Meister K. Shoulder adaptations among pitchers and position players over the course of a competitive baseball season. Clin J

Sport Med, 2013, 23(3): 184–189.

46. Laudner KG, Moline MT, Meister K. The relationship between forward scapular posture and posterior shoulder tightness among baseball players. Am J Sports Med, 2010, 38(10): 2106–2112.

47. Laudner KG, Stanek JM, Meister K. Differences in scapular upward rotation between baseball pitchers and position players. Am J Sports Med, 2007, 35(12): 2091–2095.

48. Laudner KG, Stanek JM, Meister K. The relationship of periscapular strength on scapular upward rotation in professional baseball pitchers. J Sport Rehabil, 2008, 17(2): 95–105.

49. Lee JH, Cynn HS, Yi CH, et al. Predictor variables for forward scapular posture including posterior shoulder tightness. J Bodyw Mov Ther, 2015, 19(2): 253–260.

50. Lee SB, Kim KJ, O'Driscoll SW, et al. Dynamic glenohumeral stability provided by the rotator cuff muscles in the mid-range and end-range of motion. A study in cadavera. J Bone Joint Surg Am, 2000, 82(6): 849–857.

51. Luckin KA, Biedermann MC, Jubrias SA, et al. Muscle fatigue: conduction or mechanical failure? Biochem Med Metab Biol, 1991, 46(3): 299–316.

52. Madsen PH, Bak K, Jensen S, et al. Training induces scapular dyskinesis in pain-free competitive swimmers: a reliability and observational study. Clin J Sport Med, 2011, 21(2): 109–113.

53. Maenhout A, Dhooge F, van Herzeele M, et al. Acromiohumeral distance and 3-dimensional scapular position change after overhead muscle fatigue. J Athl Train, 2015, 50(3): 281–288.

54. Maenhout A, van Cingel R, de Mey K, et al. Sonographic evaluation of the acromiohumeral distance in elite and recreational female overhead athletes. Clin J Sport Med, 2013, 23(3): 178–183.

55. Maenhout A, van Eessel V, van Dyck L, et al. Quantifying acromiohumeral distance in overhead athletes with glenohumeral internal rotation loss and the influence of a stretching program. Am J Sports Med, 2012, 40(9): 2105–2112.

56. Matsuura T, Suzue N, Iwame T, et al. Epidemiology of shoulder and elbow pain in youth baseball players. Phys Sportsmed, 2016, 44(2): 97–100.

57. McFarland EG, Kim TK, Savino RM. Clinical assessment of three common tests for superior labral anterior-posterior lesions. Am J Sports Med, 2002, 30(6): 810–815.

58. Morgan CD, Burkhart SS, Palmeri M, et al. Type II SLAP lesions: three subtypes and their relationships to superior instability and rotator cuff tears. Arthroscopy, 1998, 14(6): 553–565.

59. Muraki T, Yamamoto N, Zhao KD, et al. Effect of posteroinferior capsule tightness on contact pressure and area beneath the coracoacromial arch during pitching motion. Am J Sports Med, 2010, 38(3): 600–607.

60. Muratori LM, Lamberg EM, Quinn L, et al. Applying principles of motor learning and control to upper extremity rehabilitation. J Hand Ther, 2013, 26(2): 94–102.

61. Myers JB, Laudner KG, Pasquale MR, et al. Scapular position and orientation in throwing athletes. Am J Sports Med, 2005, 33(2): 263–271.

62. Newham DJ, McPhail G, Mills KR, et al. Ultrastructural changes after concentric and eccentric contractions of human muscle. J Neurol Sci, 1983, 61(1): 109–122.

63. Oliver G, Weimar W. Scapula kinematics of youth baseball players. J Hum Kinet, 2015, 49: 47–54.

64. Oliver GD, Weimar WH, Plummer HA. Gluteus medius and scapula muscle activations in youth baseball pitchers. J Strength Cond Res, 2015, 29(6): 1494–1499.

65. Pappas AM, Zawacki RM, Sullivan TJ. Biome-

chanics of baseball pitching: a preliminary report. Am J Sports Med, 1985, 13: 216–222.
66. Pink M. Understanding the linkage system of the upper extremity. Sports Med Arthrosc Rev, 2001, 9: 52–60.
67. Pink MM, Perry J. Operative techniques in upper extremity sports injuries. St. Louis: Mosby, 1996.
68. Proske U, Morgan DL. Muscle damage from eccentric exercise: mechanism, mechanical signs, adaptation and clinical applications. J Physiol, 2001, 537(Pt 2): 333–345.
69. Ramappa AJ, Chen PH, Hawkins RJ, et al. Anterior shoulder forces in professional and little league pitchers. J Pediatr Orthop, 2010, 30(1): 1–7.
70. Reagan KM, Meister K, Horodyski MB, et al. Humeral retroversion and its relationship to glenohumeral rotation in the shoulder of college baseball players. Am J Sports Med, 2002, 30(3): 354–360.
71. Reeser JC, Joy EA, Porucznik CA, et al. Risk factors for volleyball-related shoulder pain and dysfunction. PMR, 2010, 2(1): 27–36.
72. Reinold MM, Wilk KE, Macrina LC, et al. Changes in shoulder and elbow passive range of motion after pitching in professional baseball players. Am J Sports Med, 2008, 36(3): 523–527.
73. Reuther KE, Thomas SJ, Tucker JJ, et al. Scapular dyskinesis is detrimental to shoulder tendon properties and joint mechanics in a rat model. J Orthop Res, 2014, 32(11): 1436–1443.
74. Savoie FH 3rd, Field LD, Atchinson S. Anterior superior instability with rotator cuff tearing: SLAC lesion. Orthop Clin North Am, 2001, 32(3): 457–461.
75. Scholz JP, Schoner G. The uncontrolled manifold concept: identifying control variables for a functional task. Exp Brain Res, 1999, 126(3): 289–306.
76. Schwartzberg R, Reuss BL, Burkhart BG, et al. High prevalence of superior labral tears diagnosed by MRI in middle-aged patients with asymptomatic shoulders. Orthop J Sports Med, 2016, 4(1): 2325967115623212.
77. Sein ML, Walton J, Linklater J, et al. Shoulder pain in elite swimmers: primarily due to swim-volume-induced supraspinatus tendinopathy. Br J Sports Med, 2010, 44(2): 105–113.
78. Seitz AL, Reinold M, Schneider RA, et al. No effect of scapular position on 3-dimensional scapular motion in the throwing shoulder of healthy professional pitchers. J Sport Rehabil, 2012, 21(2): 186–193.
79. Solem-Bertoft E, Thuomas KA, Westerberg CE. The influence of scapular retraction and protraction on the width of the subacromial space. An MRI study. Clin Orthop Relat Res, 1993, 296: 99–103.
80. Soslowsky LJ, Thomopoulos S, Tun S, et al. Neer award 1999. Overuse activity injures the supraspinatus tendon in an animal model: a histologic and biomechanical study. J Shoulder Elbow Surg, 2000, 9(2): 79–84.
81. Struminger AH, Rich RL, Tucker WS, et al. Scapular upward-rotation deficits after acute fatigue in tennis players. J Athl Train, 2016, 51(6): 474–479.
82. Struyf F, Nijs J, de Graeve J, et al. Scapular positioning in overhead athletes with and without shoulder pain: a case-control study. Scand J Med Sci Sports, 2011, 21(6): 809–818.
83. Struyf F, Nijs J, Meeus M, et al. Does scapular positioning predict shoulder pain in recreational overhead athletes? Int J Sports Med, 2014, 35(1): 75–82.
84. Suzuki H, Swanik KA, Huxel KC, et al. Alterations in upper extremity motion after scapular-muscle fatigue. J Sport Rehabil, 2006, 15: 71–88.
85. Takenaga T, Sugimoto K, Goto H, et al. Posterior

shoulder capsules are thicker and stiffer in the throwing shoulders of healthy college baseball players: a quantitative assessment using shear-wave ultrasound Elastography. Am J Sports Med, 2015, 43(12): 2935–2942.

86. Tate AR, McClure PW, Kareha S, et al. Effect of the scapula reposition test on shoulder impingement symptoms and elevation strength in overhead athletes. J Orthop Sports Phys Ther, 2008, 38(1): 4–11.

87. Thomas SJ, Swanik CB, Higginson JS, et al. A bilateral comparison of posterior capsule thickness and its correlation with glenohumeral range of motion and scapular upward rotation in collegiate baseball players. J Shoulder Elbow Surg, 2011, 20(5): 708–716.

88. Thomas SJ, Swanik CB, Higginson JS, et al. Neuromuscular and stiffness adaptations in division I collegiate baseball players. J Electromyogr Kinesiol, 2013, 23(1): 102–109.

89. Thomas SJ, Swanik CB, Kaminski TW, et al. Humeral retroversion and its association with posterior capsule thickness in collegiate baseball players. J Shoulder Elbow Surg, 2012, 21(7): 910–916.

90. Thomas SJ, Swanik CB, Kaminski TW, et al. Assessment of subacromial space and its relationship with scapular upward rotation in college baseball players. J Sport Rehabil, 2013, 22(3): 216–223.

91. Thomas SJ, Swanik KA, Swanik C, et al. Glenohumeral rotation and scapular position adaptations after a single high school female sports season. J Athl Train, 2009, 44(3): 230–237.

92. Thomas SJ, Swanik KA, Swanik CB, et al. Internal rotation and scapular posi-tion changes following competitive high school baseball. J Sport Rehabil, 2010, 19(2): 125–135.

93. Thomas SJ, Swanik KA, Swanik CB, et al. Internal rotation and scapular position differences: a comparison of collegiate and high school baseball players. J Athl Train, 2010, 45(1): 44–50.

94. Thomas SJ, Swanik KA, Swanik CB, et al. Glenohumeral rotation and scapular position change following a division I collegiate baseball season. J Sport Rehabil, 2013, 22(2): 115–121.

95. Thomas SJ, Swanik KA, Swanik CB, et al. Internal rotation deficits affect scapular positioning in baseball players. Clin Orthop Relat Res, 2010, 468(6): 1551–1557.

96. Tirman PF, Bost FW, Garvin GJ, et al. Posterosuperior glenoid impingement of the shoulder: findings at MR imaging and MR arthrography with arthroscopic correlation. Radiology, 1994, 193(2): 431–436.

97. Tirman PF, Bost FW, Steinbach LS, et al. MR arthrographic depiction of tears of the rotator cuff: benefit of abduction and external rotation of the arm. Radiology, 1994, 192(3): 851–856.

98. Warner JJ, Micheli LJ, Arslenian LE, et al. Scapulothoracic motion in normal shoulders and shoulders with glenohumeral instability and impingement syndrome: a study using Moiré topographic analysis. Clin Orthop Relat Res, 1992, 285: 191–199.

99. Werner SL, Gill TJ, Murray TA, et al. Relationships between throwing mechanics and shoulder distraction in professional baseball pitchers. Am J Sports Med, 2001, 29(3): 354–358.

100. Wilk KE, Macrina LC, Fleisig GS, et al. Deficits in glenohumeral passive range of motion increase risk of elbow injury in professional baseball pitchers: a prospective study. Am J Sports Med, 2014, 42(9): 2075–2081.

101. Wilk KE, Macrina LC, Fleisig GS, et al. Deficits in glenohumeral passive range of motion increase risk of shoulder injury in professional baseball pitchers: a prospective study. Am J Sports Med,

2015, 43(10): 2379–2385.
102. Williams JG, Laudner KG, McLoda T. The acute effects of two passive stretch maneuvers on pectoralis minor length and scapular kinematics among collegiate swimmers. Int J Sports Phys Ther, 2013, 8(1): 25–33.
103. Woledge RC. Possible effects of fatigue on muscle efficiency. Acta Physiol Scand, 1998, 162(3): 267–273.
104. Wolff J. Das gesetz der transformation der knochen. Berlin: A. Hirshwald, 1892.
105. Yoo JC, Lee YS, Tae SK, et al. Magnetic resonance imaging appearance of a repaired capsulolabral complex after arthroscopic bankart repair. Am J Sports Med, 2008, 36(12): 2310–2316.
106. Yukutake T, Yamada M, Aoyama T. A survey examining the correlations between Japanese little league baseball coaches' knowledge of and compliance with pitch count recommendations and player elbow pain. Sports Health, 2013, 5(3): 239–243.

第7章 肩胛骨运动障碍和盂肱关节不稳定

W. Ben Kibler, Aaron D. Sciascia

解剖和生物力学

从生物力学角度看,盂肱关节是一种由骨、韧带和肌肉组成的闭链结构,手臂和手在完成一些具体任务时需要放置或移动到某个位置,这种闭链结构帮助平衡、稳定和对抗手臂和手在活动过程中可能产生的过多位移[1]。对于几乎所有正常的肩臂功能,盂肱关节的运动学基本都通过这种球窝装配的平衡来实现。

肩胛骨作为盂肱关节中的"盂",是闭链结构中的一个关键元素。肩胛骨在创建和维护球窝运动机制时担任着多重作用。

首先,关节盂必须在三维空间中维持位置的动态稳定,来保持盂肱角度——关节盂凹面和肱骨长轴(从肱骨头到肘部连线)的夹角——在一个"安全范围"有最小的剪切力[2]和最大的球窝凹陷压迫[3,4],并使维持关节稳定所必需的肌肉激活最小化[5]。Jobe估计这个角度为±30°,经生物力学验证研究表明,当盂肱角度测量为±29.3°时,肌肉在保持关节稳定方面最有效[6]。如果盂肱角度保持在这个参数之内,合力矢量就在盂窝中,剪切力是最小的,韧带张力是最小的,肌肉的激活需求也是最小的,这是创建稳定性最有效的关节条件。在这个位置,肩袖中的所有内在肌可以相对直线地向肩关节内拉,最大限度地形成球窝凹陷压迫。

在活动的中段由于缺乏足够的来自骨骼和韧带的静态稳定,动态稳定是非常重要的。动态定位是整个动力链中多个节段综合协调的一部分,其在日常和体育活动中对肩部需求和负荷做出预期反应。

完成这种定位需要肩胛骨的摆位与预期的手臂和肩动作相匹配。因为围绕在肩关节周围的速度、力量和运动常常太频繁和太快,导致身体无法用感觉反馈调节肌肉活动、移动肩胛骨[1,5]。肩胛骨自身的运动只能产生最多40%肩前伸所必需的力量和手臂加速度[5]。大多数的力量来自髋、躯干激活(核心稳定),通过动力链的激活将手臂向前移动,此力量产生互动力矩,让手臂在空中移动[7,8],类似于挥鞭子末期。在正常的肩部运动中,这些预期运动是生物力学闭链的一部分,将肩胛骨和手臂的运动连在一起[1, 5, 8]。

肌肉的激活顺序让身体习得预期的骨摆位，也就是预程序模式，可以定义为依赖力量的激活模式[5, 9]，它集成多条肌肉来移动多个关节[10-12]。这类模式通过前馈感觉信息使骨和关节以最有效的方式摆位。肌肉高度发育，会因受伤或失用而迅速退化。

典型的肌肉激活模式包括稳定对侧髋关节和躯干，作为肩胛骨活动的基础[13]，前后核心稳定用于肩部力量形成[14]，在肩袖激活之前依次激活对侧、同侧腹肌[15]，以及在肩袖激活之前激活肩胛骨稳定肌[16]。

肌肉激活产生动态定位的功能和可观察到的结果被称为肩肱节律（SHR），即手臂和肩胛骨的同步运动。肩肱节律被比喻为"海狮鼻子上的球"，鼻子（关节盂）主动移动来匹配球（肱骨头）的预期运动，使球保持在鼻子的中心。

第二，肩胛骨是稳定的基座，也是所有内在肌和外在肌的起点，这些肌肉在几乎所有的活动范围内让盂肱关节保持动态稳定。协调、平衡的肌肉激活让盂肱关节在各个平面的90%的关节运动中达到最佳稳定性。在向心和离心活动中，最大限度地激活肩袖和三角肌，增加关节凹陷压迫[17-20]。有证据表明，稳定的肩胛骨可以使肌力提高24%[18, 20]。

第三，需要最佳的肩胛骨位置和运动来限制在韧带和关节内的其他被动约束结构上的负荷。肩胛骨前伸增加会造成盂肱下韧带前侧的过度拉伸负荷[21]，增加盂

关节不稳定的风险。同时，前伸时关节盂前倾加大，增加了后上盂唇的压力和剪切力，会造成损伤，并降低盂唇作为垫片及垫圈的功能（它可以使盂肱关节的稳定性最大化）[1, 22]。例如，在网球运动时，改变躯干和肩胛骨的位置会增加关节内压力，这种压力与关节损伤相关联[23]。

综上所述，肩胛骨在盂肱关节稳定性中的作用是直接形成最大的功效以保护相对脆弱的球窝运动，并应对在运动和工作中需要加在肩部的负荷、压力和张力。若肩胛骨发生改变，可能会降低这种功效，导致负荷增加、受伤、功能障碍加重，可能让治疗更加困难。

肩胛骨改变与盂肱关节不稳定相关

肩胛骨静态位置或动态运动的改变统称肩胛骨运动障碍（图7.1），常见于表现为盂肱关节不稳定的患者，占这类患者的67%～80%[2, 24, 25]。肩胛骨运动障碍表现为肩胛骨正常运动学的改变，进而导致肩部正常生物力学和关节稳定性的改变。I型（过度前倾）和II型（过度外旋）运动障碍的位置使盂肱角度超出了"安全范围"，增加了前侧的剪切作用，并增加了盂肱下韧带前侧的拉伸负荷[21, 26]。肩胛骨过度前伸，是I型或II型模式的结果，减少了肩袖激活的最大值，减少了建立动态稳定的"压缩袖"肌肉功能。III型（肩峰上抬缺失）运动障碍位置可造成手臂抬高撞击，形成"不稳定/撞击"连接[27]。然而，通常没有特定的运动障碍模式与特定类型的盂

肱关节不稳定有普遍的关联。在许多病例中，运动障碍被认为是损伤的结果。但在一些情况下，它可能是一个关键原因。在任何情况下，都应该考虑其对最佳肩部稳定性和功能有害。看起来，运动障碍的主要原因包括肌肉柔韧性改变、力量不平衡和/或肌肉激活改变，其可在骨或关节损伤后出现。

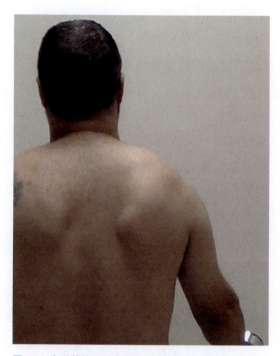

图7.1 在手臂放下时肩胛骨运动障碍的示例

在班卡特损伤伴创伤后前侧或后侧不稳定的患者中，运动障碍是继发于结构损伤的最常见的问题，肩胛骨运动学的完全恢复需要病理结构先恢复。但是，如果运动员为了完成比赛而推迟手术治疗，或者选择非手术治疗，那先恢复肌肉来稳定肩胛骨是整体治疗的一部分[28-31]。

在由于重复微创伤（通常是一个很长的时间过程）导致盂肱关节不稳定的患者

中，下斜方肌和前锯肌的无力和抑制，合并胸小肌和背阔肌的僵硬，是导致肩胛骨运动障碍和肩胛骨前伸的常见原因[24, 32]。

多向不稳定患者已经被证实有肩胛下肌、冈上肌、下斜方肌、前锯肌抑制的表现，合并胸小肌和背阔肌的激活增强[33-35]。这些激活牵拉肩胛骨向前伸，并使关节盂向下倾斜，使大部分由骨骼提供的下方稳定性被消除。激活的背阔肌将肱骨头向下拉，使盂肱关节在中段活动范围形成特征性的不稳定。当患者有不稳定指征时，肩胛骨的运动障碍模式表现为肩胛骨下角突出。

综上所述，肩胛骨运动障碍通常与所有类型的盂肱关节不稳定有关。位置和运动的障碍降低了"海狮"维持"球"在它"鼻子"上的能力，形成并加重了盂肱关节运动学和肌肉激活的改变，损害了肩关节的功能。这些都增加了不稳定，可能降低非手术或手术后的康复效果。应将评价有或没有肩胛骨运动障碍纳入肩关节不稳定综合检查的一部分。

体格检查

盂肱关节不稳定的肩胛骨评估

由于肩胛骨上覆盖着肌肉组织，并缺乏客观、可重复的测量试验，肩胛骨位置和运动的临床评估常常很困难，可以进行一系列的特殊检查（包括位置、运动、力量和动态稳定试验），让检测具有可重复性。

可尝试通过观察两侧肩胛骨的休息位

姿势来评估静态肩胛骨位置。用记号笔标记上、下内侧边界是一个很好的方法。肩胛骨运动障碍模式通常可以通过观察肩胛骨的静态位置论证。已改变的静态位置表现为肩胛骨错位、下内侧缘突出、喙突痛和肩胛骨运动障碍（统称为SICK），其特征被归纳为肩胛骨下沉，实际上这是由肩胛骨前倾引起的。

触诊上斜方肌和下斜方肌的痛点区域，触诊胸小肌和背阔肌的痛点区域，可以识别引起肌肉柔韧性降低、肌肉抑制或过度激活的疼痛区域，这也是临床需要治疗的问题。

临床的肩胛骨运动动态检查，可以通过观察手臂的上抬和下降获得可靠的结果。这些运动需要协调、有序地激活肌肉来保持闭链机制。这一机制失效会引起肩胛骨内旋增加，并伴随内侧缘隆起[26, 36]。临床观察到，有症状的患者肩胛骨内侧缘隆起，与生物力学上的运动障碍有关[37]。该方法可靠（敏感性为0.64~0.84），是测定是否存在运动障碍的依据[38, 39]。患者双手都拿3~5磅（1.36~2.27千克）的重物，将双侧手臂向前屈并上举至最大范围，再放下，重复3~5次[40, 41]。有症状的一侧，若肩胛骨内侧缘突起则记录为"是"，若无突起则记录为"否"。

肩胛骨稳定力量可以通过几种方法进行临床评估。通过夹肩胛骨来评估肩胛骨后缩能力：肩胛骨应后缩并在等长收缩状态保持10秒。在这段时间内，无力的肌肉会出现痉挛。墙式俯卧撑可以估计前锯肌的力量，特别是在"推"（肩胛骨过度前伸）的位置。II型运动障碍会表现出肌肉疲劳。横向滑动测量是一项半动态的复合肩胛骨稳定力量评估[42-45]。此项测试通过观察一些标记点，查看肩胛骨在承受不同的负荷时，为保持肩胛骨位置而激活的肌肉。以3个不同的位置来改变肩胛骨负荷，测量脊柱上一点和双侧肩胛骨内下角，比较两侧差异。位置1是双臂静止在休息位。位置2是双手放在髋部，中立伸展位。位置3是手臂在肩胛骨平面外展，略低于90°，同时内旋到最大。双侧的距离差异大于1.5 cm提示肩胛骨缺乏动态稳定。此项测试也可用于监测康复的进展，随着肩胛骨稳定度的提高，双侧的差异会逐渐减少，降至1.5 cm以下。

肩胛骨辅助试验（SAT）和肩胛骨后缩/复位测试（SRT）是两种复位操作，这些操作可改变损伤的症状，提供关于肩胛骨运动障碍在肩关节损伤后需要恢复的功能障碍中的作用的信息[18, 20, 46, 47]。SAT可帮助评估肩胛骨对撞击和肩袖力量的影响，SRT评估肩胛骨对肩袖力量和盂唇症状的影响。做SAT时，当受试者抬起手臂，测试者施加轻柔的力量辅助肩胛骨上旋和向后倾斜[46, 47]。若撞击症状的疼痛弧减轻，或无痛运动的范围增加，则结果属于阳性。做SRT时，测试者根据标准的徒手肌力测试对冈上肌的力量进行分级[18, 20]，然后测试者将受试者的肩胛骨放在后缩的位置并稳定住。如果冈上肌力量增加，或与盂唇损伤相关的内旋撞击症状减轻，则结果为阳性。在多向不稳定患者中，SRT将消除前伸和下倾的位置，并促进正常的盂肱关节运动学，从而减少不稳定的感觉。虽然这些测试不能诊断肩关节病理学的特定类型，但SAT或SRT阳性表明肩胛骨运动障碍直接导致了症状产生，并表明需要及早进行肩胛骨康复训练，以改善肩胛骨控制。

非手术治疗

盂肱关节不稳定的肩胛骨康复

肩胛骨康复可用于术前、术后和非手术情境中[48, 49]。术前肩胛骨康复旨在重建动力链激活模式，以最大限度地提高激活肩胛骨稳定肌和控制肩胛骨后缩的能力。方法类似于交叉韧带手术的术前准备。术后的肩胛骨康复应在术后的极早期开始。在手臂仍在悬吊状态或其他术后保护状态时，就可以开始躯干和髋部力量增强训练和肩胛骨后缩训练。这些训练为更高级的、特定的肩部运动奠定了一个稳定的基础。随着愈合进程和手臂的外展和旋转活动恢复，通过闭链的轴向负荷和肩胛骨时钟训练增强肩胛骨稳定肌，同时最大限度地减少修复部位的负荷。当适合进行肩袖运动时，肩胛骨稳定和肱骨头下压的综合训练可以重建"压缩袖"的激活功能，使肱骨头从稳定的肩胛骨移开。

肩胛骨康复作为盂肱关节不稳定非手术治疗的一部分，主要与潜在的病理变化有关。创伤后盂肱关节不稳定的患者经常出现韧带和/或骨的损伤，这影响了球窝运动学。因微创伤导致了盂肱关节不稳定的患者，可以通过重建肩肱节律、最大限度地提高凹陷压迫和球窝运动学来恢复功能。多向不稳定是一个非常依赖肌肉的问题，有效的肩胛骨控制和通过康复手段达到的肌肉激活，往往会成功解除症状。

康复指南

肩胛骨专项康复训练

肩胛骨控制康复训练可分为三组：提高肩胛骨肌力的近端动力链训练、减少牵拉肩胛骨力量的柔韧性训练和激活肩胛骨周围肌肉的专项训练。

躯干和髋部的动力链训练从髋部伸展和躯干伸展的最佳位置开始，也在此位置结束。它们包括躯干和髋部的屈伸、旋转和对角运动，进阶训练包括上下台阶和增加负荷。

影响灵活性的特定区域包括喙突前方（胸小肌和肱二头肌短头）、背阔肌和肩部旋转肌群。这些部位的紧张增加了肩胛骨前伸。打开书本训练（图7.2）拉伸喙突周围肌肉；墙角拉伸训练（图7.3）为站立位肩前屈，拉伸背阔肌；卧姿拉伸训练（图7.4）和跨躯干内收训练（图7.5）拉伸肩部旋转肌群。

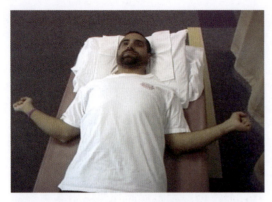

图7.2 打开书本训练拉伸肩关节前部的紧张组织

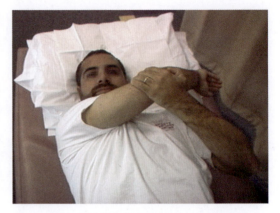

图7.5 跨躯干内收训练拉伸肩关节后部的紧张组织

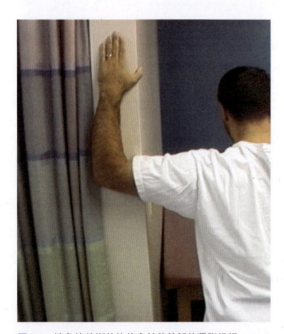

图7.3 墙角拉伸训练拉伸肩关节前部的紧张组织

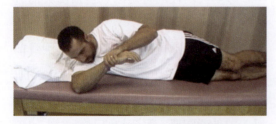

图7.4 卧姿拉伸训练拉伸肩关节后部的紧张组织

肩胛骨周围肌肉强化应强调让肩胛骨处于后缩的位置，因为这是最大限度发挥肩胛骨功能的有效位置。肩胛骨后缩训练可以站立进行，模拟正常的激活顺序，并允许动力链排序。夹肩胛骨、躯干后伸和肩胛骨后缩训练可以在康复早期开始，以达到综合激活的目的。

一些特定的训练已被证明对激活关键的肩胛骨稳定肌（下斜方肌和前锯肌）非常有效，包括低位划船训练（图7.6）和下滑训练（图7.7），它们都是等长收缩训练；还有割草机训练（图7.8）和抢劫姿势训练（图7.9）；另一种有效的训练方法是击剑训练（图7.10）。

还应强调闭链训练，它可以重建闭链机制的正常激活。把手放在固定或可移动的表面上，从远端向近端给手臂和肩胛骨加载负荷，包括有节奏的稳定训练（图7.11）、肩胛骨时钟训练（图7.12）和洗墙训练（图7.13）。

一旦达到了肩胛骨控制，就要增加对肩胛骨及肩袖的训练，如出拳训练（图7.14）

第 7 章 肩胛骨运动障碍和盂肱关节不稳定 · 85

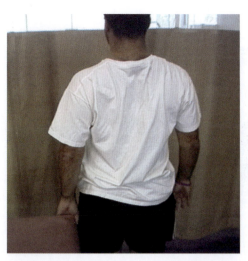

图 7.6 低位划船训练是等长训练，可以增强下斜方肌和前锯肌的力量

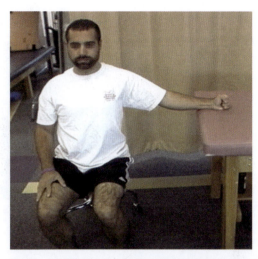

图 7.7 下滑训练也可以增强下斜方肌和前锯肌的力量。训练时让手臂向内收的方向做等长收缩下压

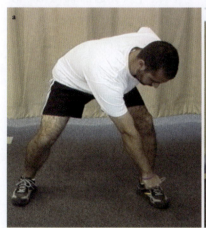 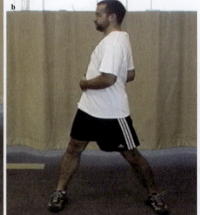 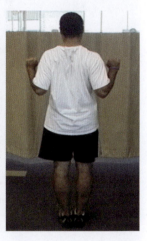

图 7.8 割草机训练用躯干旋转来促进肩胛骨后缩

图 7.9 抢劫姿势训练的训练口令是"肘关节向身后的口袋里放"

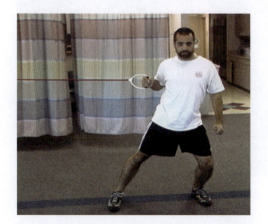 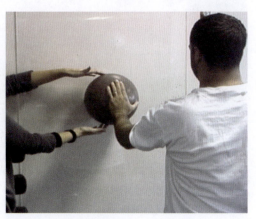

图 7.10 击剑训练是在肩胛骨抗阻后缩时，向侧方迈步

图 7.11 有节奏的稳定训练

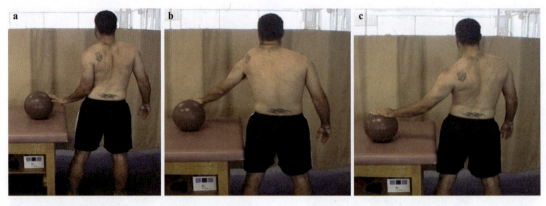

图7.12 肩胛骨时钟训练：后缩（a）、前伸（b）和下压（c）

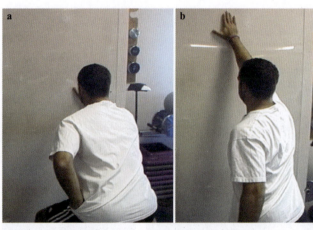

图7.13 洗墙训练是一个利用所有动力链节段的闭链运动

和过肩下砸（图7.15）。这些训练可以促进肩袖激活，使其在稳定的肩胛骨上移动。这些训练可以在外展和屈曲的多个平面进行，可以伴有不同的阻力数量或类型，也可以针对特定的体育运动进行调整。

（连晓文）

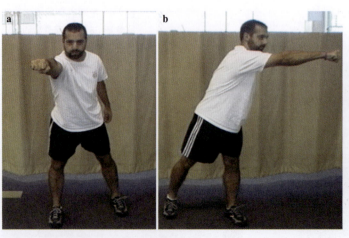

图7.14 出拳训练可以在多个平面进行

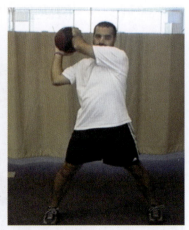

图7.15 过肩下砸

参考文献

1. Veeger HEJ, van der Helm FCT. Shoulder function: the perfect compromise between mobility and stability. J Biomech, 2007, 40(10): 2119–2129.
2. Warner JJ, Micheli LJ, Arslanian LE, et al. Scapulothoracic motion in normal shoulders and shoulders with glenohumeral instability and impingement syndrome. Clin Orthop Relat Res, 1992, 285: 191–199.
3. Lippitt S, Matsen FA 3rd. Mechanisms of glenohumeral joint stability. Clin Orthop Relat Res, 1993, 291: 20–28.
4. Lippitt S, Vanderhooft JE, Harris SL, et al. Glenohumeral stability from concavity-compression: a quantitative analysis. J Shoulder Elbow Surg, 1993, 2(1): 27–35.
5. Happee R, van der Helm FCT. Control of shoulder muscles during goal-directed movements, an inverse dynamic analysis. J Biomech, 1995, 28: 1179–1191.
6. Jobe FW, Tibone JE, Jobe CM, et al. The shoulder. Philadelphia: WB Saunders, 1990.
7. Kibler WB. Biomechanical analysis of the shoulder during tennis activities. Clin Sports Med, 1995, 14: 79–85.
8. Putnam CA. Sequential motions of body segments in striking and throwing skills: description and explanations. J Biomech, 1993, 26: 125–135.
9. Nichols TR. A biomechanical perspective on spinal mechanics of coordinated muscular action. Acta Anat, 1994, 15: 1–13.
10. Nieminen H, Niemi J, Takala EP, et al. Load-sharing patterns in the shoulder during isometric flexion tasks. J Biomech, 1995, 28(5): 555–566.
11. Sporns O, Edelman GM. Solving Bernstein's problem: a proposal for the development of coordinated movement by selection. Child Dev, 1993, 64: 960–981.
12. Zattara M, Bouisset S. Posturo-kinetic organization during the early phase of voluntary upper limb movement. J Neurol Neurosurg Psychiatry, 1988, 51(7): 956–965.
13. Young JL, Herring SA, Press JM, et al. The influence of the spine on the shoulder in the throwing athlete. J Back Musculoskelet Rehabil, 1996, 7: 5–17.
14. Kibler WB, Press J, Sciascia AD. The role of core stability in athletic function. Sports Med, 2006, 36(3): 189–198.
15. Hirashima M, Kadota H, Sakurai S, et al. Sequential muscle activity and its functional role in the upper extremity and trunk during overarm throwing. J Sports Sci, 2002, 20: 301–310.
16. Kibler WB, Chandler TJ, Shapiro R, et al. Muscle activation in coupled scapulohumeral motions in the high performance tennis serve. Br J Sports Med, 2007, 41: 745–749.
17. Kebaetse M, McClure PW, Pratt N. Thoracic position effect on shoulder range of motion, strength, and three-dimensional scapular kinematics. Arch Phys Med Rehabil, 1999, 80: 945–950.
18. Kibler WB, Sciascia AD, Dome D. Evaluation of apparent and absolute supraspinatus strength in patients with shoulder injury using the scapular retraction test. Am J Sports Med, 2006, 34(10): 1643–1647.
19. Smith J, Dietrich CT, Kotajarvi BR, et al. The effect of scapular protraction on isometric shoulder rotation strength in normal subjects. J Shoulder Elbow Surg, 2006, 15: 339–343.
20. Tate AR, McClure P, Kareha S, et al. Effect of the scapula reposition test on shoulder impingement symptoms and elevation strength in overhead athletes. J Orthop Sports Phys Ther, 2008, 38(1): 4–11.

21. Weiser WM, Lee TQ, McQuade KJ. Effects of simulated scapular protraction on anterior glenohumeral stability. Am J Sports Med, 1999, 27: 801–805.
22. Burkhart SS, Morgan CD, Kibler WB. The disabled throwing shoulder: Spectrum of pathology. Arthroscopy, 2003, 19(4): 404–420.
23. Martin C, Kulpa R, Ropars M, et al. Identification of temporal pathomechanical factors during the tennis serve. Med Sci Sports Exerc, 2013, 45(11): 2113–2119.
24. Burkhart SS, Morgan CD, Kibler WB. The disabled throwing shoulder: Spectrum of pathology. Arthroscopy, 2003, 19(6): 641–661.
25. Paletta GA, Warner JJP, Warren RF, et al. Shoulder kinematics with two-plane x-ray evaluation in patients with anterior instability or rotator cuff tears. J Shoulder Elbow Surg, 1997, 6: 516–527.
26. Kibler WB, Uhl TL, Maddux JWQ, et al. Qualitative clinical evaluation of scapular dysfunction: a reliability study. J Shoulder Elbow Surg, 2002, 11: 550–556.
27. Jobe FW, Kvitne RS, Giangarra CE. Shoulder pain in the overhand or throwing athlete the relationship of anterior instability and rotator cuff impingement. Orthop Rev, 1989, 18(9): 963–975.
28. Buss DD, Lynch GP, Meyer CP, et al. Nonoperative Management for In-Season Athletes with Anterior Shoulder Instability. Am J Sports Med, 2004, 32(6): 1430–1433.
29. Owens BD, Dickens JF, Kilcoyne KG, et al. Management of Mid-Season Traumatic Anterior Shoulder Instability in athletes. J Am Acad Orthop Surg, 2012, 20(8): 518–526.
30. Wang RY, Arciero RA. Treating the athlete with anterior shoulder instability. Clin Sports Med, 2008, 27: 631–648.
31. Wilk KE, Macrina LC. Nonoperative and postoperative rehabilitation for glenohumeral instability. Clin Sports Med, 2013, 32: 865–914.
32. Ludewig PM, Reynolds JF. The association of scapular kinematics and glenohumeral joint pathologies. J Orthop Sports Phys Ther, 2009, 39(2): 90–104.
33. Barden JM, Balyk R, Raso VJ. Atypical shoulder muscle activation in multidirectional instability. Clin Neurophysiol, 2005, 116: 1846–1857.
34. Illyes A, Kiss RM. Kinematic and muscle activity characteristics of multidirectional shoulder joint instability during elevation. Knee Surg Sports Traumatol Arthrosc, 2006, 14: 673–685.
35. Morris AD, Kemp GJ, Frostick SP. Shoulder electromyography in multidirectional instability. J Shoulder Elbow Surg, 2004, 13: 24–29.
36. Ludewig PM, Cook TM, Nawoczenski DA. Three-dimensional scapular orientation and muscle activity at selected positions of humeral elevation. J Orthop Sports Phys Ther, 1996, 24(2): 57–65.
37. Uhl TL, Kibler WB, Gecewich B, et al. Evaluation of clinical assessment methods for scapular dyskinesis. Arthroscopy, 2009, 25(11): 1240–1248.
38. Kibler WB, Ludewig PM, McClure PW, et al. Clinical implications of scapular dyskinesis in shoulder injury: the 2013 consensus statement from the "scapular summit". Br J Sports Med, 2013, 47: 877–885.
39. Kibler WB, Ludewig PM, McClure PW, et al. Scapular summit 2009. J Orthop Sports Phys Ther, 2009, 39(11): A1–A13.
40. McClure PW, Tate AR, Kareha S, et al. A clinical method for identifying scapular dyskinesis. J Athl Train, 2009, 44(2): 160–164.
41. Tate AR, McClure PW, Kareha S, et al. A clinical method for identifying scapular dyskinesis. J Athl Train, 2009, 44(2): 165–173.

42. Koslow PA, Prosser LA, Strony GA, et al. Specificity of the lateral scapular slide test in asmptomatic competitive athletes. J Orthop Sports Phys Ther, 2003, 33: 331–336.

43. Odom CJ, Hurd CE, Denegar CR, et al. Intratester and intertester reliability of the lateral scapular slide test and its ability to predict shoulder pathology. J Athl Train, 1995, 30(2): s9.

44. Odom CJ, Taylor AB, Hurd CE, et al. Measurement of scapular assymetry and assessment of shoulder dysfunction using the lateral scapular slide test: a reliability and validity study. Phys Ther, 2001, 81: 799–809.

45. Shadmehr A, Bagheri H, Ansari NN, et al. The reliability measurements of lateral scapular slide test at three different degrees of shoulder abduction. Br J Sports Med, 2010, 44: 289–293.

46. Kibler WB. The role of the scapula in athletic function. Am J Sports Med, 1998, 26: 325–337.

47. Rabin A, Irrgang JJ, Fitzgerald GK, et al. The intertester reliability of the scapular assistance test. J Orthop Sports Phys Ther, 2006, 36(9): 653–660.

48. McMullen J, Uhl TL. A kinetic chain approach for shoulder rehabilitation. J Athl Train, 2000, 35(3): 329–337.

49. Sciascia AD, Cromwell R. Kinetic chain rehabilitation: a theoretical framework. Rehabil Res Pract, 2012, 2012: 853037.

第8章　锁骨骨折

Peter W. Hester, W. Ben Kibler

引言

锁骨骨折占成人骨折的5%，占肩关节骨折的44%[1]。高达81%的骨折位于锁骨的中部1/3，其中一半被认为是"移位"骨折[2]。从既往治疗来看，使用吊带或8字形固定的非手术治疗被认为是首选的治疗标准，并且治疗后的整体功能表现是被普遍接受的[3]。然而，最近的研究表明，非手术治疗可能会产生不太令人满意的结果，包括非手术治疗后骨折畸形愈合和骨不连的发生率高，肌肉力量和耐力不足，以及患者对结果评分的实质性不满[3-6]。手术治疗似乎会产生更好的结果评分[6]，但也有一系列风险，包括公认的手术并发症风险和有时需要进行第二次手术移除内固定。依据这些研究结果，研究人员强调需要鉴别手术适应证（哪类锁骨骨折需要手术修复），以及明确手术结果应该是什么（重建正常肩胛骨位置及其对肩关节运动的功能性影响）（图8.1）。

似乎骨折愈合并不是影响锁骨骨折最佳结果的唯一甚至主要因素。锁骨骨折愈合的最佳结果取决于肩胛骨的最佳功能表现，这需要恢复锁骨功能，因为锁骨能促进肩部运动的正常力学[7-12]。手术指征可能更注重校正由锁骨损伤导致的力学改变，而不仅仅关注锁骨解剖。肩胛骨静态位置和动态运动的评估可以提供与力学改变相关的关键信息，并且表明是否需要对解剖结构进行外科矫正。

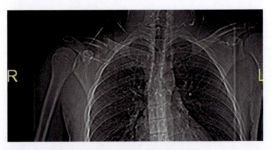

图8.1　右锁骨骨折导致肩胛骨重新摆位

锁骨解剖及力学

锁骨是连接肩胛带与脊柱的支柱[9]。最佳的肩肱节律和上肢功能需要最佳的锁骨解剖结构。锁骨的S形结构允许其大范围地旋转，围绕长轴进行40°~50°的旋转是将肩和手臂放置在功能位置上的关键[13]。在这方面，锁骨的功能类似于手腕的桡骨。任何骨骼正常形状的缺失都可能降低远端关节的功能。

锁骨长度也是一个重要的生物力学因素。正常近端（内侧）到远端（外侧）长度的损失，不管是通过粉碎、成角或结构短缩引起的损失，还是在完整的肩锁关节存在时有损失，都会导致肩内旋和前倾，最常见的特征是肩胛骨前伸[7, 9, 11, 12]。肩胛骨前伸与多种疾病相关，例如撞击综合征、肩袖肌腱病变、肩袖损伤、盂唇损伤和功能性肌肉无力[14-21]。

多重变形力是影响锁骨骨折碎片位置的因素。最受关注的是锁骨的外侧片段，因其附着在肩胛骨上。最初的冲击力可造成骨折碎片移位、锁骨短缩和成角。上肢的重力将拉动锁骨外侧片段向下、向内。将手臂固定在身体前部的吊带中，可以加重这一姿势。

肌肉力量将形成变形力。一般来说，胸锁乳突肌可以在锁骨内侧片段上施加一个向上外旋的力。然而，主要的变形力会通过附着于喙突和肱骨的附件间接地施加在锁骨外侧片段上。胸大肌、胸小肌、背阔肌和前三角肌可对锁骨外侧片段产生一个向下内旋的力。这些力量也可使肩胛骨处于前伸的位置。

总的来说，这些变形力常常使外侧片段叠加在内侧片段上，也可能使外侧片段相对于内侧片段处于在前或后、下或上方向和/或向前旋转的位置（图8.2）。这些位置在三维影像中表现出畸形，而在二维影像中可能表现为无明显异常，但在动态肩关节检查时可清楚地被发现。肩胛骨评估可以证明锁骨畸形，因为肩胛骨位置必须与锁骨外侧片段的位置相符合。肩胛骨出现前伸更加证明了锁骨出现畸形，也可以预测如果不矫正锁骨畸形而使肩胛骨保持该位置是否会发生功能缺损。

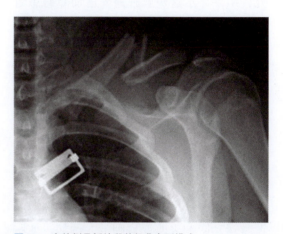

图8.2　内外侧骨折片段的经典变形模式

锁骨骨折和肩胛骨

锁骨骨折短缩、旋转和/或成角之后出现的三维变形导致结构效率丧失，可能导致身体出现运动障碍及活动对身体有更高的要求。有个重点关注解剖学的实验室，其工作人员详细描述了肩胛骨和锁骨骨折畸形愈合的关联[22]。锁骨骨折畸形愈合与力量减退、快速疲劳、疼痛及肢体和肩胛带感觉异常有关（图8.3）。在非手术治疗的中轴锁骨骨折患者中，高达70%的患者发生了明显的临床肩胛骨运动障碍[12]。

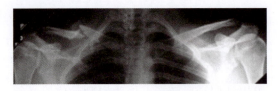

图8.3　在功能受限的情况下，锁骨骨折畸形愈合的临床表现与相关影像学表现

Shields等人[12]最先提出了关于锁骨中段骨折后肩胛胸壁运动障碍发生率的研究，结果显示这些肩胛胸壁运动障碍患者的SICK肩胛骨评分更差。在这项包括24名患者的回顾性研究中，手术组的12名患者中仅有1名患者（8%）出现肩胛胸壁运动障碍，而非手术组的12名患者中有8名患者（67%）出现肩胛胸壁运动障碍。非手术组表现出更多的疼痛、肌力下降，以及因肩胛骨位置变化导致的关节活动度下降。

Ledger等人[22]报道，短缩的锁骨通过调整运动限制来改变肩胛带，例如，使胸锁关节向上的角度增加10°，肩胛骨前伸增加6°。这些将导致肩在伸展、内收及内旋时肌肉力量至少下降10%。

短缩的锁骨不仅减少了附在锁骨上的胸大肌的力矩，更多地表现为在肩关节处于较高外展位时屈曲和外展的肌肉力量下降，而且会对所有肌肉组织产生挑战，因为肩胛骨位置改变可导致软组织的位置发生改变。据Veeger和van der Helm描述，这种位置性力矩会改变肌肉平衡关系[23]。Jupiter等人[24]支持这种不合适的肌腱会失去力学优势的观点。

在模拟锁骨骨折的尸体模型研究中，Hillen等人[8]将簇标记物放置于锁骨、胸骨、肱骨和肩胛骨上。该研究提出关于人群中肩胛骨位置的罕见的解剖学见解。该研究在完整的、被切除的和用钢板固定的锁骨上进行了徒手运动试验。结果表明，长度缩短3.6 cm的锁骨标本在肩关节30°外展位时，肩胛骨前伸增加20°，外旋增加12°，后倾减少7°，以及胸锁关节后缩角度增加——平均每缩短1.2 cm角度就增加1.2°。

在对照组研究中，由于喙锁韧带的稳定作用，肩锁关节未受影响。然而胸锁关节处出现了运动和旋转增加，这意味着有关节疾病发生的风险。

Kibler和Sciascia[9]描述了倾斜角度减少及外旋角度增加是如何改变肩峰位置的。该描述支持继发肩峰下撞击综合征和肩袖功能受限的观念，因为肩峰的前外侧部分被摆放在更前部和外部的位置。

Andermahr等人[7]提出肩胛骨位置的改变意味着关节盂的位置也发生了变化，使得盂肱关节接触力的方向也受到影响，推断盂唇和关节囊会受到不可预期的剪切力影响。Veeger和van der Helm[23]也支持这一观点，因为肩袖的稳定力可能会改变，并且可能会增加盂肱关节的接触力和关节囊与盂唇的剪切力。

延迟手术的时间越长，肩胛骨错位的程度越高，6周内手术恢复情况更好，超过40周则更严重[25, 26]。

做切开复位内固定术（ORIF），平均0.6个月的急性组效果优于平均63个月的延迟组[27]。延迟组的肩关节屈曲耐力下降，急性组的Constant量表评分较好。

X线片解读

X线片用于明确锁骨骨折的诊断并提供关于锁骨粉碎和重叠的信息。然而作为二维工具，它们通常不能准确地显示三维平面的骨畸形或评估肩胛骨位置。仔细观察X线片可能会发现微小的结构改变，这可能表明肩胛骨错位，错位可导致运动障碍和功能受损。在做非手术治疗或手术治疗的决定时，一定要对比类似的图像。

图8.4和8.5显示骨折移位可能在一周内增加，并伴有肩峰投影改变，同时也提示需要进行类似X线片的比较。还要注意肩峰定位的不一致性，这对于理解锁骨外侧片段的旋转程度和角度很有价值（图8.5）。CT等高级影像技术可能有助于确定骨折的严重程度（图8.6）。

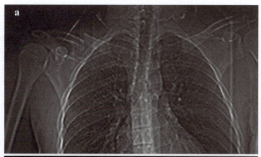

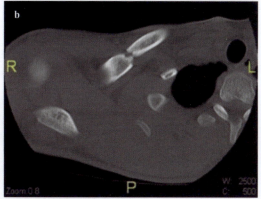

图8.6 患者的骨折CT影像

通过标准化的X线检查，可以观察并实际测量对锁骨畸形进行手术矫正后引起的肩胛骨位置变化。手术前后分别测量肩胛骨内侧到外侧的宽度，显示宽度明显增加，因为肩胛骨前伸减少了（图8.7）。此外，肩胛骨向下移位的程度可以用锁骨内侧片段的下边界与肩胛冈之间的距离来衡量。在手术矫正后，这种"肩胛沟"将会减小，表明肩胛骨位置相对于锁骨恢复正常化（图8.8）。

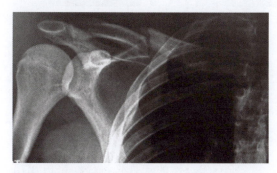

图8.4 患者最初的正位X线片

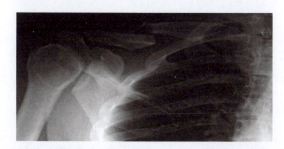

图8.5 患者骨折一周后的X线片。15°的角度变化显示出明显的移位

临床评估

每位锁骨骨折患者都应该评估外侧片段是否旋转不良，以及是否有肩胛骨运动障碍的可能性。在受伤后做早期评估时，患者伤处可能非常疼痛或肿胀，影响评估结果；但是在10~21天之后，就可以准确

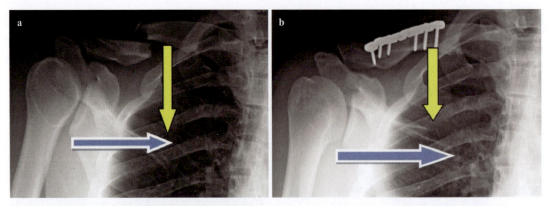

图8.7 与复位后相比，骨折导致的肩胛骨前伸可能在X线片上显示为肩胛骨宽度相对性变窄（蓝色箭头所指），同时锁骨内侧片段下表面到肩胛冈距离相对性增加（黄色箭头所指）。作者称该区域为"肩胛沟"

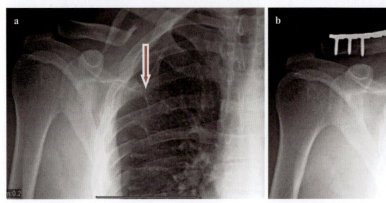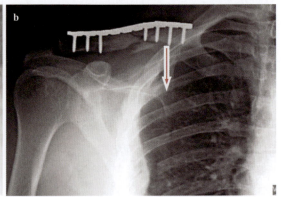

图8.8 "肩胛沟"复位固定

地评估了。肩部姿势的双侧比较可以显示出手臂是否下垂和肩胛骨是否前伸。从后面观察肩部，可找到肩胛骨运动障碍的位置。在3周时，骨折部位形成了足够的骨痂以允许手臂运动。手法稳定有运动障碍并前伸的肩胛骨，使其后缩，这样可以逆转外侧片段的前旋，减轻手臂疼痛，增加手臂活动范围和力量。

在已确定锁骨骨不连和骨折畸形愈合并伴有持续的肩关节症状时，标准肩胛骨评估的原则应作为综合肩关节评估的一部分[28]。重点应放在确定是否存在运动障碍，以及肩胛骨辅助试验和肩胛骨后缩测试对症状有何影响。

治疗指南

所有闭合性的锁骨骨折最初可以用吊带固定来治疗。大约10～21天后进行再评估，包括影像学检查和临床评估。再评估可以准确地评估锁骨骨折位置和肩胛骨位置。此时没有或稍有肩胛骨运动障碍的患者通常在适当的非手术治疗中表现良好。锁骨畸形已形成和/或有肩胛骨运动障碍的患者，应就发现的可能存在的生物力学缺陷向医生进行咨询。

锁骨骨折、骨不连和骨折畸形愈合手术固定的目标

复位及固定旨在恢复肩胛骨位置和肩胛骨旁肌肉和骨骼的定位和平衡，优化肩部活动度、肌力和耐力。急性骨折的早期复位和固定将更好地确保正确愈合，并降低肌肉嵌入骨折断端的风险。这种早期固定还有助于恢复最佳的活动度、肌力和耐力（图8.9）。100%的骨折移位和大于15 mm的骨骼短缩是采取固定治疗的有力适应证。并发肱骨干骨折是进行ORIF的充分适应证。

与髓内皮下单螺钉固定相比，使用钢板和螺钉的ORIF可提供优良的效果并将并发症风险降至更低，不过后期需要移除。手术室中有两种不同的锁骨钢板系统可供使用，有助于医生在了解锁骨的解剖差异后确保最佳的轮廓选择。

术后，患者使用吊带维持3周，同时激活肩胛骨内侧肌肉来保持良好的姿势。3周后允许康复锻炼。

X线检查应在术后1个月、2个月和3个月进行。大多数患者在第3个月和第4个月之间可进行常规活动。

骨折畸形愈合通常是考虑早期进行ORIF的最佳证据。如果患者最初考虑非手术治疗，他们必须了解之后可能会出现的简单功能障碍和日常生活活动能力下降，以及后续手术复杂性增加的情况（图8.10）。

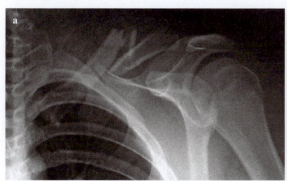
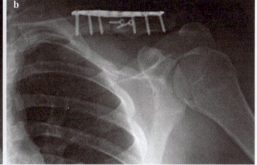

图8.9 这些正位图像可以观察到固定后肩峰位置的变化

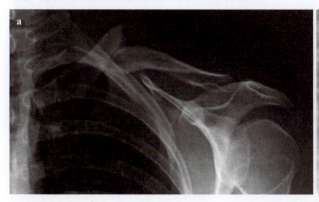
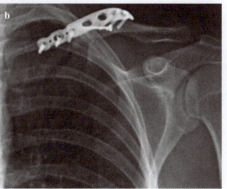

图8.10 职业攀树者锁骨骨折畸形愈合再骨折合并肱骨干骨折，应用ORIF治疗，在术后3个月肩胛骨功能恢复正常，回归正常生活

在前 2～3 周进行 ORIF 是首选，可以最大限度地减少骨痂、粘连和肌肉短缩问题。

总结

锁骨骨折是经常发生于三个平面的三维畸形，其中外侧片段相对于内侧片段更可能出现旋转不良、成角和短缩的情况。附着于外侧片段的肩胛骨可移动到临床上可观察到的运动障碍位置，即肩胛骨前伸。这个运动障碍位置可以提供关于外侧片段错位的关键信息，并提示肩胛骨前伸的不良功能效应。锁骨骨折的 ORIF 手术指征，可以通过询问患者在治疗时是否存在肩胛骨错位来更好地确认。

（苟艳芸）

参考文献

1. Craig EV. The shoulder. Philadelphia: W. B. Saunders, 1990.
2. Rowe CR. An atlas of anatomy and treatment of midclavicular fractures. Clin Orthop, 1968, 58: 29–42.
3. Eichinger JK, Balog TP, Grassbaugh JA. Intramedullary fixation of clavicle fractures: anatomy, indications, advantages, and disadvantages. J Am Acad Orthop Surg, 2016, 24(7): 455–464.
4. Jones GL, Bishop JY, Lewis B, et al. Intraobserver and interobserver agreement in the classification and treatment of midshaft clavicle fractures. Am J Sports Med, 2014, 42(7): 1176–1181.
5. McKee MD, Pedersen EM, Jones C, et al. Deficits following nonoperative treatment of displaced midshaft clavicular fractures. J Bone Joint SurgAm, 2006, 88: 35–40.
6. Zlowodzki M, Zelle B, Cole PA, et al. Treatment of acute midshaft clavicle frac-tures: systematic review of 2144 fractures: on behalf of the evidence-based orthopaedic trauma working group. J Orthop Trauma, 2005, 19(7): 504–507.
7. Andermahr J, Jubel A, Elsner A, et al. Malunion of the clavicle causes significant glenoid malposition: a quantitative anatomic investigation. Surg Radiol Anat, 2006, 28(5): 447–456.
8. Hillen RJ, Burger BJ, Poll RG, et al. The effect of experimental shortening of the clavicle on shoulder kinematics. Clin Biomech, 2012, 27(8): 777–781.
9. Kibler WB, Sciascia AD. Current concepts: scapular dyskinesis. Br J Sports Med, 2010, 44(5): 300–305.
10. Lazarides S, Zafiropoulos G. Conservative treatment of fractures at the middle third of the clavicle: the relevance of shortening and clinical outcome. J Shoulder Elbow Surg, 2006, 15(2): 191–194.
11. Matsumura N, Ikegami H, Nakamichi N, et al. Effect of shortening deformity of the clavicle on scapular kinematics: a cadaveric study. Am J Sports Med, 2010, 38(5): 1000–1006.
12. Shields E, Behrend C, Beiswenger T, et al. Scapular dyskinesis following displaced fractures of the middle clavicle. J Shoulder Elbow Surg, 2015, 24(12): e331– e336.
13. Sahara W, Sugamoto K, Murai M, et al. Three-dimensional clavicular and acromioclavicular rotations during arm abduction using vertically open MRI. J Orthop Res, 2007, 25: 1243–1249.
14. Kibler WB, Kuhn JE, Wilk KE, et al. The disabled throwing shoulder—spectrum of pathology: 10 year update. Arthroscopy, 2013, 29(1): 141–161.

15. Kibler WB, Sciascia AD, Dome D. Evaluation of apparent and absolute supraspinatus strength in patients with shoulder injury using the scapular retraction test. Am J Sports Med, 2006, 34(10): 1643–1647.
16. Lukasiewicz AC, McClure P, Michener LA, et al. Comparison of 3-dimensional scapular position and orientation between subjects with and without shoulder impingement. J Orthop Sports Phys Ther, 1999, 29(10): 574–586.
17. Mihata T, Jun BJ, Bui CN, et al. Effect of scapular orientation on shoulder internal impingement in a cadaveric model of the cocking phase of throwing. J Bone Joint Surg Am, 2012, 94(17): 1576–1583.
18. Reuther KE, Thomas SJ, Tucker JJ, et al. Scapular dyskinesis is detrimental to shoulder tendon properties and joint mechanics in a rat model. J Orthop Res, 2014, 32(11): 1436–1443.
19. Smith J, Kotajarvi BR, Padgett DJ, et al. Effect of scapular protraction and retraction on isometric shoulder elevation strength. Arch Phys Med Rehabil, 2002, 83: 367–370.
20. Tate AR, McClure P, Kareha S, et al. Effect of the scapula reposition test on shoulder impingement symptoms and elevation strength in overhead athletes. J Orthop Sports Phys Ther, 2008, 38(1): 4–11.
21. Weiser WM, Lee TQ, McQuade KJ. Effects of simulated scapular protraction on anterior glenohumeral stability. Am J Sports Med, 1999, 27: 801–805.
22. Ledger M, Leeks N, Ackland T, et al. Short malunions of the clavicle: an anatomic and functional study. J Shoulder Elbow Surg, 2005, 14(4): 349–354.
23. Veeger HEJ, van der Helm FCT. Shoulder function: the perfect compromise between mobility and stability. J Biomech, 2007, 40: 2119–2129.
24. Jupiter JB, Ring D. A comparison of early and late reconstruction of malunited fractures of the distal end of the radius. J Bone Joint Surg Am, 1996, 78(5): 739–748.
25. George DM, McKay BP, Jaarsma RL. The long-term outcome of displaced mid-third clavicle fractures on scapular and shoulder function: variations between immediate surgery, delayed surgery, and nonsurgical management. J Shoulder Elbow Surg, 2015, 24(5): 669–676.
26. Olsen BS, Vaesel MT, Sojeberg JO. Treatment of midshaft clavicular nonunion with plate fixation and autologous bone grafting. J Shoulder Elbow Surg, 1995, 4(5): 337–344.
27. Potter JM, Jones C, Wild LM, et al. Does delay matter? The restoration of objectively measured shoulder strength and patient-oriented outcome after immediate fixation versus delayed reconstruction of displaced mid-shaft fractures of the clavicle. J Shoulder Elbow Surg, 2007, 16(5): 514–518.
28. Kibler WB, Ludewig PM, McClure PW, et al. Clinical implications of scapular dyskinesis in shoulder injury: the 2013 consensus statement from the "scapular summit". Br J Sports Med, 2013, 47: 877–885.

第9章 肩锁关节分离及关节炎

Brent J. Morris, David Dome, Aaron D. Sciascia, W. Ben Kibler

肩锁关节解剖

肩锁关节在肩部功能方面承担了许多关键作用。肩锁关节是提供正常肩部运动的螺旋轴结构的重要组成部分[1, 2]。肩锁关节稳定锁骨支，并可以让锁骨前后移动、上下移动和旋转。

肩锁韧带控制着大部分肩锁关节的前后移动，另一些控制作用来自喙锁韧带。肩锁韧带，尤其是肩锁韧带的后部和上部，提供了水平稳定性，同时在垂直和旋转稳定性方面也发挥作用[3]。

肩锁韧带的上部（56%）和后部（25%）为后向移动提供阻力[4]，肩锁韧带上部如同一条张力带，帮助控制肩峰的侧向倾斜。锥状韧带及其附着在锁骨偏内侧和后侧的部分提供了60%的垂直稳定性[4]，斜方韧带及其附着在锁骨偏外侧和前侧的部分提供了垂直和旋转稳定性。

肩锁关节损伤

肩锁关节损伤一般从二维方式考虑和分类。Rockwood分类[5]已经广泛应用于肩锁关节损伤分类中，它是单纯基于X线片的分类。Rockwood分类通过X线的正位片和腋位片来评估肩锁关节，观察锁骨相对于肩峰向上、向后的移位。可惜的是，Rockwood分类在临床分型和治疗方面的可靠性较差，加上三维CT检查也未提高其在临床分型和治疗方面的可靠性[6]。

肩锁关节损伤应以三维方式考虑肩胛骨在损伤模式中的作用。肩锁关节损伤可以改变正常的肩胛骨运动。锁骨在肩胛骨和手臂的运动中作为可活动的支架，发挥许多关键作用。肩锁关节在控制正常肩肱节律的螺旋轴机制中起统一连接的作用[1, 2, 7, 8]，锁骨和肩胛骨正常运动学的三维属性增进了手臂功能。这些研究表明，当手臂旋转和抬高时，锁骨以胸锁关节为基座，作为一个活动支架沿着锁骨轴线上抬、前伸、后缩和旋转。肩锁关节发挥着稳定但有轻微活动性的连接作用。最后，肩胛骨作为肱骨和手臂的一个活动但稳定的基座，随着手臂运动进行上旋、后倾、外旋动作，并向上、下和向内、外移动[2, 7-9]。韧带断裂失去稳定性，使肩胛骨发生第3种移位——向锁骨的内下方移动。在有症状的肩锁关节分离患者中，他们的很多临床表现与肩胛骨的位置和运动改变有关。锁骨突出主要是由于第3种移位。肩胛骨过度前伸会导致肩关节活动度下降，并表现出外展和屈曲力量下降[10-13]。对有症状的患者，应评估其肩胛骨的静态位置和动态运动，作为指导治疗方案的诊断的一部分[4]。

肩锁关节损伤的临床诊断

临床检查可以识别肩锁关节损伤的三维后遗症情况，并帮助指导治疗方案，而不是单纯依靠X线片和二维分类对肩锁关节损伤进行分型。在肩锁关节损伤患者中，可通过临床检查发现肩胛骨运动障碍，检查具有准确性和可预测性。伴随肩胛骨运动障碍的肩部功能障碍可能包括肩关节活动度下降和力量的减少[1]。我们认为，在手法检查中发现患有肩锁关节上、下和前、后松弛的患者若表现为肩胛骨运动障碍，其一定存在高度损伤。我们认为，有相同疾病的患者若没有肩胛骨运动障碍表现，则其为低度损伤。我们中心的所有肩锁关节损伤患者在手术前都接受了系统的肩胛骨康复治疗。典型的低度损伤可以不通过手术治疗，而高度损伤可能由于生物力学破坏和功能丧失而需要手术治疗。

此外，最近研究人员提出了一项针对III型损伤的新修订方案，将Rockwood III型肩锁关节损伤细分为III A型和III B型，并认识到体格检查的价值和肩胛骨的作用。III A型有稳定的肩锁关节，在越过躯干做上臂水平内收时没有出现锁骨过度抬起，也没有明显的肩胛骨功能障碍。IIIB型的肩锁关节不稳定，具有难治性肩胛骨功能障碍，且在越过躯干做上臂水平内收时出现锁骨过度抬起[14]。

不稳定性肩锁关节损伤的手术治疗：手术方式的分类

非解剖重建技术和解剖重建技术都是被提倡的。非解剖重建技术包括喙肩韧带转移。Cadenat在1917年首次描述了利用肩峰侧后束转移喙肩韧带，将其缝合到锥状韧带和锁骨后上段骨膜的残余部分，来重建喙锁韧带（锥状韧带和菱形韧带）[4, 15]。Weaver-Dunn技术涉及类似的非解剖转移，将喙肩韧带从肩峰侧转移，并且已经出现了许多该技术的改进方案。不幸的是，喙肩韧带的转移不能重建喙锁韧带的解剖结构，而且只能提供完整喙锁复合体25%的强度；也不能修复肩锁复合体[16]。

肩锁关节对盂肱关节和肩胛胸壁功能至关重要。肩锁韧带和喙锁韧带的适当修复对完全稳定肩胛骨及重建平移和旋转功能是必要的。同时固定肩锁韧带和喙锁韧带并不是一个新概念，最早由Baum于1886年报道；然而，目前文献中报道的技术大多不涉及解剖性肩锁韧带和喙锁韧带重建。最近的一项系统性综述表明，在120篇不同的文章中，描述到的162种外科手术方式中只有13种（8%）是解剖重建技术[17]。

已经出现了强调喙锁韧带解剖重建的技术，但所描述的技术通常涉及锁骨远端切除，这样通常不需要对受损的肩锁韧带进行正式的修复或重建。最近的资料表明，肩锁韧带和喙锁韧带的解剖重建都可以帮助恢复平移和旋转[3]，因为喙肩韧带转移伴增强，不能解决肩胛骨在锁骨上前后平移的问题[18]。

三维修复喙锁韧带和肩锁韧带的解剖重建比单独重建喙锁韧带更有优势，因为它能够恢复肩锁关节的所有能力——水平、垂直和旋转的稳定性，它们可以稳定肩胛骨运动和肩肱节律。最近的文献已经注意到喙锁韧带重建后的肩锁关节复位不良和不稳定[19, 20]。静态正位X线片显示锁骨和肩峰"被复位"；然而，腋位或交叉内收位X线片显示复位不良，或检查时可见肩锁关节不稳定。

在肩锁关节重建手术中，经常会有一个问题，即如何处理锁骨远端。一些外科医生选择切除锁骨远端，而另一些外科医生选择保留锁骨远端。肩锁关节损伤中处理锁骨远端的治疗方法随着时间推移而变化。以往的手术技术包括保留锁骨远端和不重建喙锁韧带的刚性而做肩锁关节固定。这些早期的技术会带来持续的疼痛和继发肩锁关节炎[21, 22]。后来，单独切除锁骨远端治疗肩锁关节损伤的方法被提出，但它不能恢复肩锁关节的稳定性，效果较差[4]。锁骨短缩或肩锁关节不稳定可能导致肩胛骨处在病理位置，即前伸和内旋位[3]。我们的技术是：如同其他人提出的保留锁骨远端[4]，以帮助恢复解剖稳定性，并保持最佳的锁骨支架功能和肩胛骨活动度。

我们对不稳定肩锁关节损伤的手术方式

本研究的肩锁重建遵循了Carofino和Mazzocca建立的原则[4, 18, 23]。为了解所述技术的潜在弱点，我们对移植物通道、移植物和韧带附着技术进行了改进。该技术在最近的出版物中得到了完整的描述[24]。

患者被安置成一个略微改进的沙滩椅体位。手术切口沿着锁骨前上缘，从锁骨中部到肩锁关节并穿过肩峰外侧缘。开始时从内侧切开，用电灼法刺激斜方肌筋膜反射。从锁骨远端向肩峰沿着纵轴切开，切口小心地维持在锁骨上，这样能保证原有的常附着在肩峰上的肩锁韧带前部和后部可以被识别和松解，用于修复（图9.1）。这些韧带经常在锁骨下半部分留下瘢痕，它们的松动有助于关节复位。

一种将同种异体移植物"对接"到肩峰的方法已被发现有效且结实。从肩峰缘外侧到关节处的肩峰缘上方钻两个2.4 mm的孔（图9.2a）。轻轻清除肩峰边缘以提供附着处并刺激愈合，将2号聚对二氧杂环己酮（PDS）缝线做成环形缝线传递器（图9.2b），待随后使用。

然后可以切开三角肌来观察喙锁间隔。仔细切开喙突周围以松解瘢痕，为移植物通过创建隧道。器械从内侧向外侧通

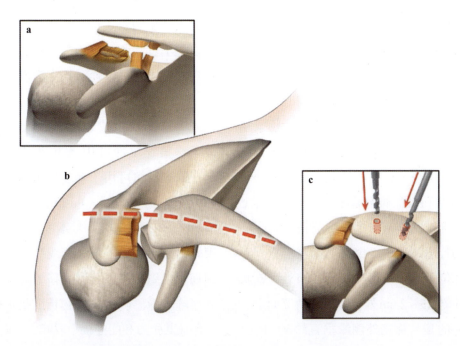

图9.1 （a）高度肩锁韧带和喙锁韧带损伤伴肩锁韧带从锁骨上撕脱和喙锁韧带中段损伤 （b）切口从肩峰外侧到锁骨中轴（虚线） （c）根据锥状韧带和菱形韧带原有的附着点，在锁骨上钻孔

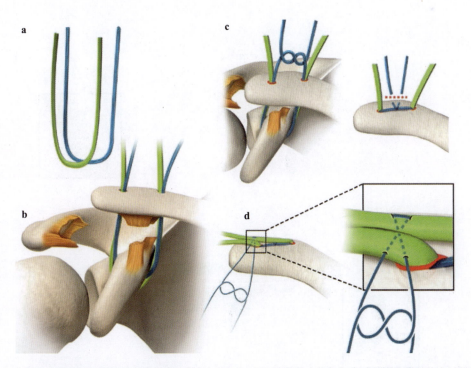

图9.2 （a）重建包括半腱肌的同种异体肌腱（绿色）和5条2号PDS缝线（蓝色） （b）缝线和移植物穿过锁骨上的钻孔 （c）系上PDS缝线，以增加愈合移植物的稳定性（多余的缝线被移除，如红色虚线所示） （d）用所示的缝合方法将移植物尾部固定在一起

过，移植物从外侧向内侧穿梭，将潜在的神经血管结构风险降到最低。

喙锁重建构件包括半腱肌同种异体移植物（6.0 mm×至少260 mm）和5条2号PDS缝线，作为内夹板。每个移植物末端都有一个25 mm的棒球式端头。这一结构通过喙突下方，并经过解剖定位的锁骨4.5 mm钻孔处。锥状钻孔位于锁骨后上缘，对准锥状结节。锥状结节是一个容易触及的标志，位于喙突内侧缘正上方。菱形钻孔位于锥状钻孔前方约1 cm处、锥状钻孔外侧1.5~2 cm处，视患者情况而定，其针对的是与喙突外侧缘垂直约30°的斜方韧带嵴（图9.3）。然后移植物的两端相互对接通过，将肩峰拉向锁骨，对关节进行手法复位。缝线系在锁骨上，为喙锁重建提供初始的稳定性。拉紧移植物，然后将多重不可吸收的缝线缝在锁骨上。喙锁重建的稳定性可以通过检查有没有表现出上、下松弛感来评估。

肩锁韧带重建包括上、前、后三部分。移植物尾部可用于重建肩锁韧带上部，原有组织可用于修复韧带前、后部。将两个生物相容锚（PushLock, Arthrex, Naples, FL）用双层1号不可吸收缝线置入锁骨的前上、后上部，缝线穿过活动的肩锁韧带组织，但不扎紧。移植物尾部被带到肩峰边缘。确保移植物长度是正确的，以保证其张力和能连接上肩峰，并放置1号不可吸收缝线通过（图9.4）。缝线穿过先前的肩峰钻孔，系在肩峰外侧，连接移植物尾部，重建肩锁韧带上部。然后将前后

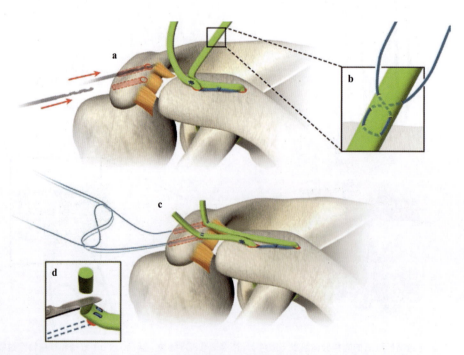

图9.3 （a）钻孔穿过外侧肩峰，将移植物尾部固定到骨中。缝线被放置在每个移植物尾部，见（b），协助让移植物正确地固定到先前准备好的肩峰边缘（c）上。多余的移植物尾部组织被切除，见（d）。

的原生组织绑紧,完成修复(图9.5)。评估整个结构的稳定性——没有表现出上、下松弛和前、后松弛。缝合三角肌,逐层闭合伤口,并使用吊带和绷带。

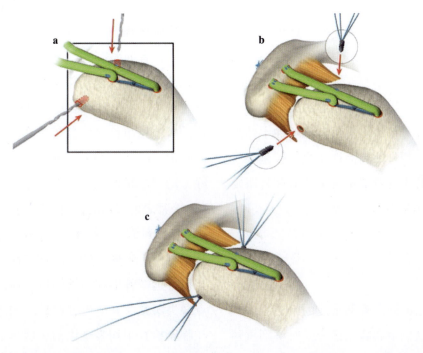

图9.4 (a)在锁骨前上方和后上方钻孔 (b)将用于修复原有的肩锁韧带的锚放进孔内 (c)缝线穿过但不打结

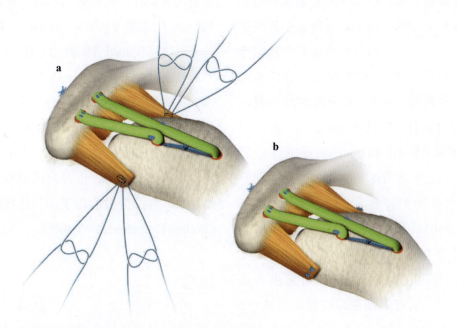

图9.5 (a)修复原有韧带的前部和后部 (b)将其固定在锁骨上

肩锁重建术后康复

术后，所有患者均用吊带和绷带4周。3周内不允许内旋、外展，6周内不允许主动前屈。在前3周，患者可以进行主动的肩胛骨后缩和下压。所有患者在术后第3周进行正式的物理治疗，并执行标准化的闭链训练方案，旨在最小化盂肱关节的剪切力，并通过肩部和肩胛骨训练增加本体感觉反馈。肩胛骨的灵活性和稳定性是通过在这本书的康复章节中讨论的肩胛骨康复方案来加强的。

结局

关于喙锁韧带解剖重建的报道很多，但关于肩锁韧带和喙锁韧带同时解剖重建的报道却很少。Carofino和Mazzocca描述了用半腱肌移植、环绕喙突来完成肩锁韧带和喙锁韧带的解剖重建，将其用挤压螺钉固定在锁骨上，用移植物的剩余端重建肩锁韧带后上部[4]。该文章提及了17名患者，至少随访6个月，平均随访21个月。美国肩肘外科医生评分（ASES）、简单肩关节测试（SST）和Constant量表评分显示，术前、术后肩部功能评分有显著性差异。17名患者中有3名（17.6%）报告失败。

我们的研究人群包括23名患者。15名患者（年龄 = 42 ± 18岁；男性10名，女性5名）需要手术治疗，其中1名患者是双侧重建，所有人都是高度损伤。另有5名低度损伤患者和3名高度损伤患者不需要手术。这强化了肩胛骨运动障碍作为肩锁功能受损的指标有助于确定手术适应证的观点。手术患者平均随访3 ± 1.5年（范围1.5 ~ 5年）。所有15名患者的16个肩部在初次临床检查时均有前、后松弛，其中64%的患者同时有上、下松弛。无上、下松弛的患者肩峰完全移位到锁骨下，伴随固定缺失。4名患者之前做过肩锁关节重建手术包括单纯喙锁韧带重建（2）、钩板内固定（1）和喙锁韧带重建伴锁骨远端切除（1）。在其余12个肩中，8个是受伤后前3个月之内重建的，而4个是损伤后治疗了4个月到6年。术后，有1名患者失去了解剖复位，表现为前、后稳定性丧失，这是锁骨远端骨溶解和跌倒后肩锁韧带附着点缺失所致。其他患者在最近的随访中，在临床检查中均表现出前、后与上、下的动态稳定性和对称的肩胛骨活动。确定静态稳定性的X线检查表明，喙锁距离平均为1 cm（范围为0.59 ~ 1.31 cm），跌倒后失去肩锁复位的患者距离为1.31 cm。患者上肢功能（DASH）评分从术前51分（范围11 ~ 98分）到最终13分（范围0 ~ 43分），显示出显著改善（$P < 0.001$），平均DASH评分变化为38 ± 27分。手术无并发症发生，没有感染，也没有因缝线、移植物复位或移除失败而再手术。这些结果与Carofino和Mazzocca的相似[4]。

结论

进行肩锁韧带和喙锁韧带解剖重建的

肩锁关节解剖重建术可恢复肩锁关节的解剖和肩胛骨力学，效果良好。我们尝试将临床经验与对肩锁关节功能的三维理解相结合，以更好地分级和治疗肩锁关节损伤。肩胛骨运动障碍的存在与否，不是手术适应证或禁忌证的绝对标准，但是从我们的数据表明，肩胛骨运动障碍可以作为肩肱节律和肩功能障碍的标志，它的确可以作为一个具有一致性的、有价值的信息，用于确定手术的适应证。

（连晓文）

参考文献

1. Gumina S, Carbone S, Postacchini F. Scapular dyskinesis and SICK scapula syndrome in patients with chronic type III acromioclavicular dislocation. Arthroscopy, 2009, 25(1): 40–45.
2. Oki S, Matsumura N, Iwamoto W, et al. Acromioclavicular joint ligamentous system contributing to clavicular strut function: a cadaveric study. J Shoulder Elbow Surg, 2013, 22(10): 1433–1439.
3. Beitzel K, Obopilwe E, Apostolakos J, et al. Rotational and translational stability of different methods for direct acromioclavicular ligament repair in anatomic ac-romioclavicular joint reconstruction. Am J Sports Med, 2014, 42(9): 2141–2148.
4. Carofino BC, Mazzocca AD. The anatomic coracoclavicular ligament reconstruction: surgical technique and indications. J Shoulder Elbow Surg, 2010, 19: 37–46.
5. Rockwood CA, Wirth MA. Fractures in adults. Philadelphia: Lippincott-Raven, 1996.
6. Cho CH, Hwang I, Seo JS, et al. Reliability of the classification and treatment of dislocations of the acromioclavicular joint. J Shoulder Elbow Surg, 2014, 23: 665–670.
7. Sahara W, Sugamoto K, Murai M, et al. Three-dimensional clavicular and acromioclavicular rotations during arm abduction using vertically open MRI. J Orthop Res, 2007, 25: 1243–1249.
8. Teece RM, Lunden JB, Lloyd AS, et al. Three-dimensional acromioclavicular joint motions during elevation of the arm. J Orthop Sports Phys Ther, 2008, 38: 181–190.
9. Ludewig PM, Phadke V, Braman JP, et al. Motion of the shoulder complex during multiplanar humeral elevation. J Bone Joint Surg Am, 2009, 91(2): 378–389.
10. Kebaetse M, McClure PW, Pratt N. Thoracic position effect on shoulder range of motion, strength, and three-dimensional scapular kinematics. Arch Phys Med Rehabil, 1999, 80: 945–950.
11. Kibler WB, Sciascia AD, Dome D. Evaluation of apparent and absolute supraspinatus strength in patients with shoulder injury using the scapular retraction test. Am J Sports Med, 2006, 34(10): 1643–1647.
12. McKee MD, Pedersen EM, Jones C, et al. Deficits following nonoperative treatment of displaced midshaft clavicular fractures. J Bone Joint Surg Am, 2006, 88: 35–40.
13. Smith J, Kotajarvi BR, Padgett DJ, et al. Effect of scapular protraction and retraction on isometric shoulder elevation strength. Arch Phys Med Rehabil, 2002, 83: 367–370.
14. Bak K, Mazzocca A, Beitzel K, et al. Shoulder concepts 2013. Heidelberg: Springer, 2013.
15. Cerciello S, Edwards TB, Morris BJ, et al. The treatment of type III acromiocla-vicular dislocations with a modified Cadenat procedure: surgical technique and mid-term results. Arch Orthop Trauma Surg, 2014, 134: 1501–1506.

16. Lee SJ, Nicholas SJ, Akizuki KH, et al. Reconstruction of the coracoclavicular ligaments with tendon grafts: a comparative biomechanical study. Am J Sports Med, 2003, 31: 648–655.
17. Beitzel K, Cote MP, Apostolakos J, et al. Current concepts in the treatment of acromioclavicular joint dislocations. Arthroscopy, 2013, 29(2): 387–397.
18. Mazzocca AD, Santangelo SA, Johnson ST, et al. A biomechanical evaluation of an anatomical coracoclavicular ligament reconstruction. Am J Sports Med, 2006, 34(2): 236–246.
19. Baker JE, Nicandri GT, Young DC, et al. A cadaveric study examining acromio-clavicular joint congruity after different methods of coracoclavicular loop repair. J Shoulder Elbow Surg, 2003, 12: 595–598.
20. Jerosch J, Filler T, Peuker E, et al. Which stabilization technique corrects anatomy best in patients with AC separation? An experimental study. Knee Surg Sports Traumatol Arthrosc, 1999, 7: 365–372.
21. Sage FP, Salavtore JE. Injuries of the acromioclavicular joint: a study of results in 96 patients. South Med J, 1963, 56: 486–495.
22. Urist MR. Complete dislocation of the acromioclavicular joint. J Bone Joint Surg Am, 1963, 45: 1750–1753.
23. Mazzocca AD, Arciero RA, Bicos J. Evaluation and treatment of acromioclavicular joint injuries. Am J Sports Med, 2007, 35(2): 316–329.
24. Kibler WB, Sciascia AD, Morris BJ, et al. Treatment of symptomatic acromioclavicular joint instability by a docking technique: clinical indications, surgical technique, and outcomes. Arthroscopy, 2017, 33: 696–708.

第 10 章　肩骨关节炎

Brent J. Morris, T. Bradley Edwards, Thomas W. Wright

引言

肩胛骨运动异常或肩胛骨运动障碍是指肩胛骨在正常休息位或运动时出现异常[1]。我们对肩胛骨运动障碍的研究取得重大进展，得益于现有的观测方法已经得到了科学数据的支持。肩胛骨运动障碍的定义已被全世界理解并接受，且影响广泛。我们对肩胛骨的理解已经非常深入，远远超越最初对翼状肩胛和神经系统疾病的理解。我们开始探索包括肩骨关节炎在内的其他肩胛骨疾病，并试图发现更多的因果关系。

肩胛骨有效地建立了肩袖功能和肩部运动平台。肩胛骨运动障碍是肩胛骨运动节律异常，可能会影响肩关节功能。据报道，多达67%～100%的肩关节损伤患者出现肩胛骨运动障碍[2-4]。肩胛骨运动障碍与多种肩关节疾病相关，包括撞击综合征、肩关节不稳、前关节囊松弛、盂唇损伤、肩袖力弱、锁骨骨折和肩锁关节损伤等[5-10]。

尽管越来越多的证据表明肩胛骨运动障碍与多种肩关节疾病有关，但是关于肩胛骨运动障碍与肩骨关节炎的相关研究非常有限。这一章我们将回顾肩胛骨运动障碍与肩骨关节炎的关系，并讨论潜在的意义。

肩胛骨运动障碍与原发性盂肱关节骨关节炎：发病、预防、早期后方半脱位和后关节盂侵蚀的治疗

肩胛骨运动障碍与原发性盂肱关节骨关节炎患病率的关系并未被证实。盂肱关节骨关节炎与关节内移位和关节活动受限有关，但是这类患者的肩胛肱骨运动、肩胛胸壁运动会如何受到影响并不清楚。目前尚不清楚肩胛骨运动障碍是否可以在肩关节置换术后得以解决。

我们经验性地认为，原发性盂肱关节骨关节炎患者存在肩胛骨运动障碍。前瞻性研究是有必要的，我们希望通过理解肩胛骨规律与盂肱关节骨关节炎，发现潜在的治疗方法，以提高患者的治疗效果。

在盂肱关节骨关节炎患者中，发生离心性后方关节盂侵蚀的患者的治疗难度最

大。后方半脱位和关节盂侵蚀现象很久以前就被关注[11]。Walch等人[12]提出了依据CT结果对原发性盂肱关节骨关节炎进行分类的方法，包括B2型关节盂或关节盂后倾伴有后方侵蚀、双凹征（图10.1）。

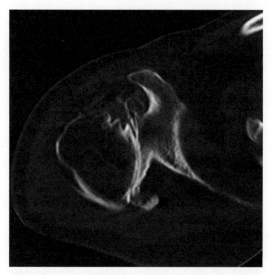

图10.1 关节CT显示离心性关节盂后方侵蚀合并双凹征，与Walch B2分型一致

肩胛骨运动障碍与肩胛骨的异常前伸有关[10]。肩胛骨前伸导致肩胛骨后倾减少[10]。盂肱关节骨关节炎患者异常前伸的肩胛骨会加剧后方半脱位，并导致可怕的B2型关节盂。目前的难题在于确认肩胛骨前伸是否是病变的罪魁祸首，或是骨关节炎导致的肩关节疼痛引起了肩胛骨前伸。因此需要进一步的研究来明确疾病的发生、发展过程。

早期骨关节炎年轻患者的静态后方半脱位是外科处理的难点[13]。原发性肩关节炎伴后方半脱位被认为是盂肱关节骨关节炎的第一阶段，早于关节盂后方侵蚀[13]。肱骨头后方半脱位是离心性关节盂后方侵

蚀的原因[14]。医生们尝试过不同的外科手术方式，包括后方骨移植、后方关节囊紧缩、后方关节囊缝合等，随访结果显示所有患者的骨关节炎和持续性或复发性后方脱位仍有发生[13]。

越来越多的文献评价了B2型关节盂。然而，目前文献没有关注到肩胛骨在关节盂磨损中的动态作用。静态三维研究对于理解关节盂侵蚀非常重要，然而更好地理解肩胛骨的动态作用是研究深入的关键。肩胛骨显然不是一个静态结构，它有较大的活动范围。McClure等人[15]测量了人体在运动中的肩胛骨三维运动数据，可以帮助我们理解正常肩胛骨的运动。三维运动传感器被固定在健康志愿者的肩胛骨上。在健康人群中，盂肱关节与肩胛胸壁的平均运动比例为1.7∶1[15]。在肩胛骨平面的上举过程中，肩胛骨平均发生了50°的上旋、30°的后倾和24°的外旋[15]。因此，虽然关节盂的细微改变很重要，但是我们也应该考虑到在肩关节活动范围内肩胛骨运动的巨大变化。

一篇近期发表的队列研究发现，通过三维CT重建，与正常关节盂相比，B2型关节盂在发病前即有明显的后倾[16]。该研究的结论是，发病前较大的关节盂后倾与后方不稳定有关，并且可能是离心性关节盂磨损的原因。这篇研究并没有考虑肩胛骨的动态作用与关节盂磨损的关系。

一项独立的3D对比研究评估了肩骨关节炎与非关节炎的肩肱关系[17]。研究目的是为了更好地理解骨关节炎患者肩关节的

离心负荷，结论是后方离心负荷与临床不良结局相关，可能与全肩关节置换术后关节盂不能发挥原有功能有关[17-21]。有研究者认为，肩骨关节炎没有增加原发的关节盂后倾向病理变化的发展[17]。这个研究小组没有观察肩胛骨的动态运动，但是他们认识到：要了解肩关节的生物力学关系，必须要进行肩肱评估[17]。在手术干预之前进行肩胛骨的稳定训练，可能有助于改善肩胛骨运动障碍和该类患者前伸的肩胛骨位置。

早期后方半脱位、后方关节盂侵蚀和原发性盂肱关节骨关节炎患者手术治疗的意义

轻度后方半脱位、后唇撕裂和早期盂肱关节骨关节炎的患者群体仍然面临挑战（图10.2和10.3）。他们尚未完全准备好进行全肩关节置换术，最佳治疗方案仍充满不确定性。Walch等人[13]无法确定一种成功的针对肩关节静态后方脱位的复杂病例的治疗方法。

基于对肩胛骨的理解，我们改进了轻度后方脱位和早期骨关节炎患者的治疗方案，但此方案目前还缺乏证实结果的随访数据。我们相信，这一类患者可能最终都会发展成可怕的B2型。术前，我们评估肩胛骨并确定是否存在肩胛骨运动障碍，同时进行矫正性查体，包括肩胛骨辅助试验和肩胛骨后缩测试。我们发现，患者在检查过程中都会出现后方关节线疼痛伴动态盂唇剪切试验阳性。我们利用肩关节X线片评估骨关节炎和后方半脱位，用MRI进一步评估盂肱关节骨关节炎、盂唇病变和后方脱位的程度，用CT额外评估关节盂的形态。肩胛骨运动障碍患者要接受为期6周的肩胛骨稳定性训练。我们有一个综合性

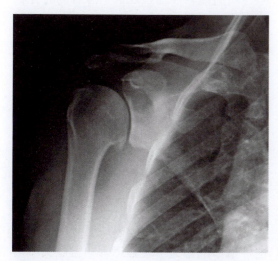

图10.2 X线片显示早期骨关节炎，关节间隙变窄，肱骨头前下方骨赘

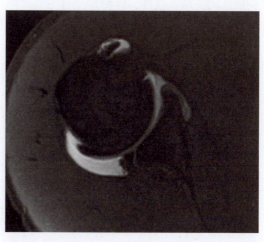

图10.3 MRI轴向位显示轻度后方脱位伴有后方盂唇巨大撕裂

训练方案将在康复章节详述。

外科干预措施有关节镜下修复上盂唇和后方盂唇（经典的四铆钉修复）、盂肱关节清理术（包括有指征的摘除肱骨骨赘和肱二头肌腱固定术）。如果患者肩关节外旋受限，就要进行关节镜下前关节囊松解。术后肩胛骨康复是关键，维持肩关节的活动范围对预防盂肱关节僵硬很重要。

肩胛骨运动障碍与肩袖病变：肩肱节律、盂肱关节与肩胛胸壁运动的关系

肩胛骨运动障碍与肩袖病变发生率的关系尚未明确。最新的研究评估了反向肩关节置换手术（RSA）后患者的肩肱与肩胛胸壁运动，但是还缺乏术前信息。与原发性盂肱关节骨关节炎相似，目前尚不清楚RSA能否解决肩胛骨运动障碍。照已有情况来看，在RSA后肩关节的运动限制会导致盂肱关节运动减少，并提出更多的肩胛胸壁运动要求。此外，即使是全肩关节置换术，也不太可能恢复正常的盂肱关节运动。

RSA后的生物力学明显不同于全肩关节置换术。de Wilde等人[22]是第一批评估RSA后患者肩胛骨的研究者。他们评估了4名因肱骨近端肿瘤行RSA的患者的肩胛胸壁运动节律，发现术后肩胛骨外旋和前伸的角度增加。

Kwon等人[23]对17名RSA后6个月以上的患者进行肩关节运动分析，并与12名健康人进行对照。利用3D电磁运动捕捉系统测量肩胛胸壁和盂肱关节的运动[23]。大部分运动发生在盂肱关节，但RSA组患者的肩胛胸壁运动大幅度增加[23]。研究者们得出结论，肩关节运动学显著改变，并且在RSA后利用增加的肩胛胸壁运动来实现肩部抬高[23]。

Walker等人[24]应用3D荧光成像评估了28名RSA后一年以上的患者，RSA组的肩肱节律（1.3∶1）明显低于正常（3∶1），表明RSA组的肩胛胸壁运动增加，盂肱关节运动减少。之前同一队列研究发现，与对照组相比，上斜方肌与三角肌的肌电活动明显增加[24, 25]。研究者假设如果改良康复方案，注重肩胛骨的稳定性，会优化RSA后的康复效果[24]。

RSA的意义

基于先前研究RSA后的肩胛骨作用的引用，肩袖损伤患者的盂肱关节功能受限，我们经验性地发现这些患者同时存在肩胛骨运动障碍。RSA后肩胛胸壁运动增加可以改善功能。肩胛骨功能优化可以避免盂肱关节和假体承受的剪切力增大。随着球窝关节固定技术的发展，灾难性的关节盂破坏已经非常少见了。但是在美国还缺乏肩胛骨功能可能有助于保持球窝寿命的长期研究。在肩袖损伤的患者中，我们曾经遇到过罕见的肩胛胸壁融合患者。之前讨论的肩胛骨原则适用于该患者。在这种情形下，为了缓解患者的盂肱关节疼痛，我们考虑进行RSA，但是，继发于肩

胛胸壁运动的丧失和球窝的失效，预计会增加盂肱关节的剪切力。

总结

肩胛骨运动障碍和肩骨关节炎关系的证据有限，我们已经注意到原发性盂肱关节骨关节炎患者和肩袖损伤关节病患者的肩胛骨运动障碍。肩胛骨原则在肩骨关节炎中的应用可为肩骨关节炎患者术前和术后肩胛骨运动障碍的识别和治疗提供依据。我们假设具有挑战性的B2型关节盂可能会因肩胛骨异常前伸而加剧。对于肩胛骨后方半脱位伴有后方盂唇撕裂的患者，建议进行肩胛骨康复治疗，盂唇修复术后进行肩胛骨康复对这类患者有好处。静态3D研究对于我们了解肩骨关节炎和关节盂侵蚀很重要。然而，更好地理解肩胛骨动态作用是关键的，未来要持续推进研究。肩胛骨显然不是一个静态结构，它有较大的活动范围。未来肩胛骨动态模型可能是可行的，使我们可以依据患者的特殊情况和肩胛骨的运动来制订手术方案。各研究的相同发现可以指导术前、术后康复，为患者进行获益最大的、使假体使用时间最久的肩胛骨治疗方案。

（马钊）

参考文献

1. Kibler WB, McMullen J. Scapular dyskinesis and its relation to shoulder pain. J Am Acad Orthop Surg, 2003, 11: 142–151.
2. Warner JJ, Micheli LJ, Arslanian LE, et al. Scapulothoracic motion in normal shoulders and shoulders with glenohumeral instability and impingement syndrome. Clin Orthop Relat Res, 1992, 285: 191–199.
3. Gumina S, Carbone S, Postacchini F. Scapular dyskinesis and SICK scapula syndrome in patients with chronic type III acromioclavicular dislocation. Arthroscopy, 2009, 25(1): 40–45.
4. Paletta GA, Warner JJP, Warren RF, et al. Shoulder kinematics with two-plane x-ray evaluation in patients with anterior instability or rotator cuff tears. J Shoulder Elbow Surg, 1997, 6: 516–527.
5. Mihata T, McGarry MH, Kinoshita M, et al. Excessive glenohumeral horizontal abduction as occurs during the late cocking phase of the throwing motion can be critical for internal impingement. Am J Sports Med, 2010, 38(2): 369–382.
6. Weiser WM, Lee TQ, McQuade KJ. Effects of simulated scapular protraction on anterior glenohumeral stability. Am J Sports Med, 1999, 27: 801–805.
7. Burkhart SS, Morgan CD, Kibler WB. The disabled throwing shoulder: Spectrum of pathology. Arthroscopy, 2003, 19(4): 404–420.
8. Kibler WB, Kuhn JE, Wilk KE, et al. The disabled throwing shoulder-spectrum of pathology: 10 year update. Arthroscopy, 2013, 29(1): 141–161.
9. Lintner D, Noonan TJ, Kibler WB. Injury patterns and biomechanics of the athlete's shoulder. Clin Sports Med, 2008, 27(4): 527–552.
10. Kibler WB, Sciascia AD, Wilkes T. Scapular dyskinesis and its relation to shoulder injury. J Am Acad Orthop Surg, 2012, 20(6): 364–372.
11. Neer CS, Watson KC, Stanton JF. Recent experience in total shoulder replacement. J Bone Joint Surg Am, 1982, 64(3): 319–337.

12. Walch G, Badet R, Boulahia A, et al. Morphologic study of the glenoid in primary glenohumeral osteoarthritis. J Arthroplast, 1999, 14(6): 756–760.
13. Walch G, Ascani C, Boulahia A, et al. Static posterior subluxation of the humeral head: an unrecognized entity responsible for glenohumeral osteoarthritis in the young adult. J Shoulder Elbow Surg, 2002, 11: 309–314.
14. Kidder JF, Rouleau DM, Pons-Villanueva J, et al. Humeral head posterior subluxation on CT scan: validation and comparison of 2 methods of measurement. Tech Should Elbow Surg, 2010, 11: 72–76.
15. McClure PW, Michener LA, Sennett BJ, et al. Direct 3-dimensional measurement of scapular kinematics during dynamic movements in vivo. J Shoulder Elbow Surg, 2001, 10: 269–277.
16. Knowles NK, Ferreira LM, Athwal GS. Premorbid retroversion is significantly greater in type B2 glenoids. J Shoulder Elbow Surg, 2016, 25: 1064–1068.
17. Jacxsens M, van Tongel A, Henninger HB, et al. A three-dimensional comparative study on the scapulohumeral relationship in normal and osteoarthritic shoulders. J Shoulder Elbow Surg, 2016, 25(10): 1607–1615.
18. Boileau P, Avidor C, Krishnan SG, et al. Cemented polyethylene versus uncemented metal-backed glenoid components in total shoulder arthroplasty: a prospective, double-blind, randomized study. J Shoulder Elbow Surg, 2002, 11: 351–359.
19. Ho JC, Sabesan VJ, Iannotti JP. Glenoid component retroversion is associated with osteolysis. J Bone Joint Surg, 2013, 95(12): e82.
20. Iannotti JP, Norris TR. Influence of preoperative factors on outcome of shoulder arthroplasty for glenohumeral osteoarthritis. J Bone Joint Surg, 2003, 85(2): 251–258.
21. Walch G, Moraga C, Young A, et al. Results of anatomic nonconstrained prosthesis in primary osteoarthritis with biconcave glenoid. J Shoulder Elbow Surg, 2012, 21: 1526–1533.
22. de Wilde LF, Plasschaert FS, Audenaert EA, et al. Functional recovery after a reverse prosthesis for reconstruction of the proximal humerus in tumor surgery. Clin Orthop Relat Res, 2005, 430: 156–162.
23. Kwon YW, Pinto VJ, Yoon J, et al. Kinematic analysis of dynamic shoulder motion in patients with reverse total shoulder arthroplasty. J Shoulder Elbow Surg, 2012, 21: 1184–1190.
24. Walker D, Matsuki K, Struk AM, et al. Scapulohumeral rhythm in shoulders with reverse shoulder arthroplasty. J Shoulder Elbow Surg, 2015, 24: 1129–1134.
25. Walker D, Wright TW, Banks SA, et al. Electromyographic analysis of reverse total shoulder arthroplasties. J Shoulder Elbow Surg, 2014, 23: 166–172.

第11章 肩胛骨肌肉撕脱

W. Ben Kibler, Aaron D. Sciascia

病理解剖及临床表现

肩胛骨肌肉的直接损伤并不广为人知，也没有很好的分类。只有一例个案报告记录了菱形肌的创伤性撕脱，症状与翼状肩胛有关，通过手术固定得以解决[1]。因此，手臂因受到创伤而导致肩胛骨或其周围出现症状的患者，在没有得到准确诊断的情况下，症状可能会持续数月或数年。这可能会对功能方面产生有害影响。病理解剖表现为下斜方肌和菱形肌从脊柱和肩胛骨内侧缘发生了生理性脱离。随着针对该类患者的临床经验的积累，可以看出该类患者的临床病史和体格检查非常相似。该类病症的显著特征包括：

1. 位于肩胛骨内侧缘的稳定结构有过创伤或破坏，并且最初两周内有早期症状；
2. 沿着肩胛骨内侧缘相应区域的高强度疼痛；
3. 疼痛部位通常有可触及的明显缺陷；
4. 在需要对抗手臂位置（前屈、过头运动、推拉）的肩胛骨控制体位中表现无力和手臂功能障碍；
5. 在临床检查中，通过手法稳定肩胛骨，症状有明显但短暂的缓解；
6. 一组非常一致的手术发现，所有这些特征存在于大部分患者中，形成了该类病症的临床诊断标准。

多种病因被报道为初次发现。绝大多数病例发病出现在急性创伤性张力负荷后，几乎一半涉及座椅安全带约束的交通事故，但也有许多其他原因，如直接的打击创伤，投掷、接物或举起重物时手臂完全伸展，拉重物，扣篮后挂在篮筐上，还有电击（触电或心脏电除颤）。肩胛骨内侧缘的疼痛随着病情的发展而加剧，在休息时平均6分（疼痛评分，满分10分），在活动时平均8分（疼痛评分，满分10分）。由于疼痛时间长、强度高，疼痛可能演变为一种由中枢介导的慢性疼痛反应[2]，对功能和治疗反应有广泛的影响。因为增加了损伤组织的张力，所以手臂离开躯干的应用如手臂前屈或过头受到很大的限制。因为缺乏下斜方肌活动，所以上斜方肌活动增加和痉挛造成了偏头痛样头痛。颈部和肩关节的合并症状可能是由于运动学障碍而出现的，这通常会成为治疗重点，包括手术治疗颈部椎间盘疾病、肩关节撞击综合征或肩关节内部紊乱，可是很少有良好的结果。

体格检查也显示出一系列与之相吻合的发现，包括肩胛骨内侧缘的局部压痛，这通常是一种明显的、可触及的软组织损伤，可能是由于肌肉撕脱或萎缩、肩胛骨静态位置改变及动态运动学障碍（包括弹响肩）造成肩关节撞击综合征和前屈无力，肩锁关节和/或胸锁关节压痛。通过一些肩胛骨纠正动作练习后，临床症状可以减少或减轻。

当因创伤性损伤导致肩胛骨内侧缘疼痛时，临床人员必须努力排除肩胛骨肌群撕脱的可能性。如果临床表现为肩胛骨疼痛伴肩袖无力，通过稳定肩胛骨和限制手臂前屈和过头旋转可以得到改善，这些均与下斜方肌和菱形肌的失活相吻合[3-5]。这些肌肉是手臂抬高≥90°时稳定肩胛骨后缩的关键肌肉[5-7]，这些肌肉失活见于临床上的肩袖无力[8, 9]和撞击综合征[3, 10]。虽然可能存在盂肱关节损伤，但必须注意不要立即假定为盂肱关节损伤；当患者感到肩胛骨内侧缘疼痛时，内部排列不良是主要的病理。最近一份报告报道了在一组被确定为有一个或多个肩胛骨肌肉撕脱的患者中，所有因撞击症状而接受肩峰下减压术的患者均未获得肩部或肩胛骨疼痛的缓解，这表明主要问题出在肩胛骨上[11]。

影像学

目前，该诊断仍属临床诊断。影像学检查对显示手术中发现的撕裂、松动或瘢痕增生没有帮助。在关于这种情况的第一份报告中，尽管所有78名患者都进行了多次影像学检查，但只有两份CT结果和一份MRI结果显示出损伤。方法问题可能可以解释这一失误：切割的角度没有很好地显示损伤区域，切割的厚度不够精确，或者评估这些病变的最佳MRI可视化方法尚不可知。所有的MRI扫描都是在慢性期进行的，因此几乎看不到急性损伤的征象。组织的松散附着可能会导致读片时对撕裂辨别不清。最近随访的两名患者在受伤后两周内进行了MRI扫描，显示菱形肌附着区出现急性破坏和积液。手术时没有液体或炎症，而这些是损伤区域的典型影像学标记；分离的下斜方肌松弛地挂在肩胛冈上，而不是从肩胛冈上脱离，因此，在扫描过程中没有发现分离。菱形肌是最常通过致密的瘢痕组织与肩胛骨边缘相连的肌肉。诊断性超声由于具有较好的检测增厚组织的能力，可能是一种较好的成像方法。在发现更有效的成像方法之前，应使用特定的纳入标准、病史和体格检查结果来确定临床诊断。因为这些标准已成功地识别出那些在手术中会表现出病理变化，并且对手术治疗有反应的患者。

总之，尽管影像学不能成功地定义病理解剖，但是损伤机制、临床病史和临床检查与纳入、排除标准高度吻合，它们构成临床诊断的基础，从而确定病变，形成治疗方法，并与预期结局相关联。

肩胛肌再附着术

肩胛骨肌肉撕脱的初步解决方法包括识别和治疗伴随或代偿肌肉损伤和随之产生运动障碍的肌肉不平衡和肌肉无力，并在颈部和肩部找出其他可能存在的病理解剖。然而，大多数符合临床诊断纳入标准的患者需要用手术来解决肌肉撕脱的问题。为了让撕脱的肩胛骨稳定肌重新附着，制订以下步骤[11, 12]。患者俯卧位，接受全身麻醉，患侧手臂垂向一侧，在胸前放置毛巾卷以便识别肩胛骨内侧缘。随后标记肩胛骨内侧缘和肩胛冈表面。切口沿着肩胛骨内侧缘从上到下，从肩胛冈到最大压痛区或损伤区域的顶端。它通常位于肩胛冈向下 6 ~ 8 cm 处，但可以延伸到整个内侧边缘。如果患者陈诉疼痛下及肩胛骨下角，那么切口应向下延伸到肩胛骨下角这个区域。切开软组织，露出下斜方肌和菱形肌附着处。下斜方肌跨过肩胛冈，而菱形肌作为定位的向导（图 11.1）。这种损伤可以被理解为下斜方肌和/或菱形肌撕脱，肌肉通过瘢痕组织松散附着，或通过致密的瘢痕组织连接。一旦确定了受影响的肌肉，瘢痕或结缔组织就应该被清除，使肌

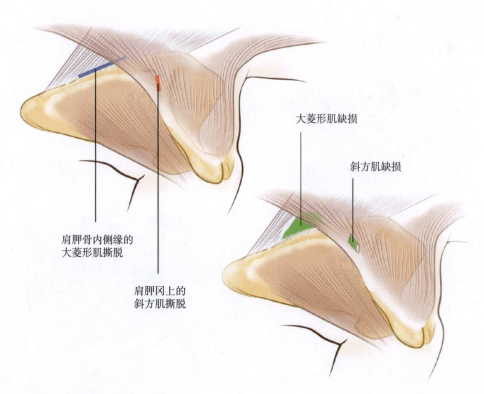

图 11.1 大菱形肌和下斜方肌撕脱伤示意图

肉移开重新附着（图11.2a）。使冈下肌附着在距肩胛骨内侧缘和肩胛冈约1 cm处，以便在距内侧缘2 cm和肩胛冈1 cm处钻孔。孔的位置是从背侧到腹侧（图11.2b）。孔与孔间隔6~8 mm，每组孔沿着肩胛骨内侧缘与肩胛冈间隔10~15 mm。孔的总数取决于修复的长度，通常肩胛冈上只有一组孔。这一组孔从上到下位于距肩胛骨内侧缘20~25 mm处。如果出现大面积的下斜方肌损伤情况，那么应放置两组钻孔。随后下斜方肌和菱形肌被移动到肩胛骨和肩胛冈的背侧。褥式缝合：从背侧到腹侧通过肌肉和对孔中的一个，然后从腹侧到背侧反向通过另一个孔，肌肉先穿过菱形肌（图11.3a）。褥式缝合允许菱形肌重新附着在肩胛骨背侧表面，距离肩胛骨内侧缘约1 cm。然后下斜方肌被重新连接到肩胛冈上（图11.3b）。缝线在肩胛骨处于外旋位时向下系牢，接着使用修复缝线沿肩胛骨内侧缘重新连接冈下肌，然后闭合筋膜和皮下组织。图11.4提供了术前损伤与术后修复的对比图。

术后，手臂被保护在中立旋转位4周，但鼓励患者立即做柔和的肩胛骨后缩运动。在这段恢复期，由于对侧肩胛骨肌肉被"串扰（crosstalk）"，无论是手术还是非手术的手臂，常见的任务如使用移动设备、驾驶或其他重复性的手臂动作都会造

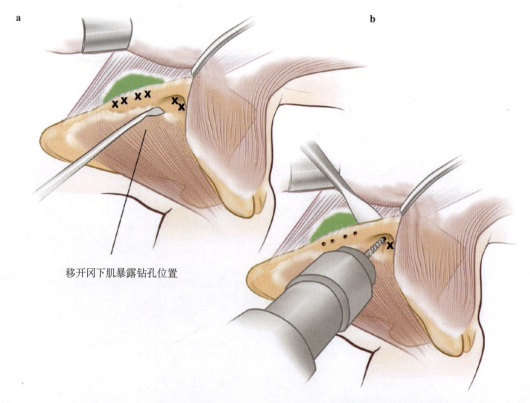

图11.2 （a）钻孔前将冈下肌从肩胛骨内侧缘移开 （b）在肩胛骨内侧缘和肩胛冈上钻孔（成对）

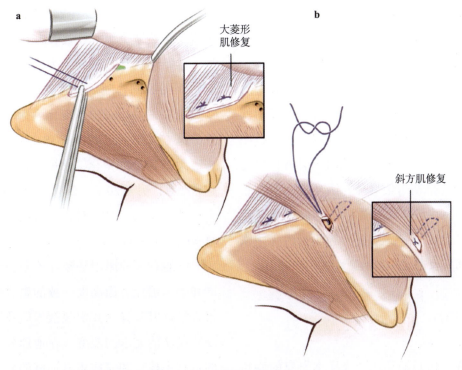

图11.3 (a) 大菱形肌修复示意图 (b) 下斜方肌修复示意图

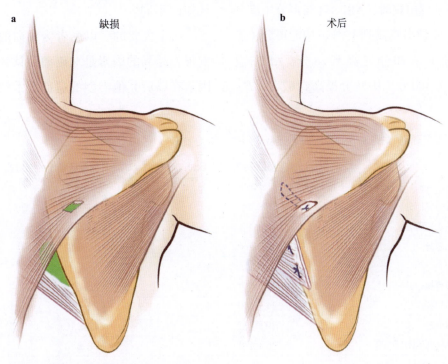

图11.4 术前损伤与术后修复对比图

成疼痛和肌肉痉挛。此外,手术后的固定一定伴随典型的退化、萎缩,这导致手臂容易疲劳,从而增加疼痛和痉挛。因此,患者被告知在手术后3~4周取下吊带之前不要执行这些任务。在第4周,开始使用外展不超过90°的手部稳定动作进行闭链的肌肉激活。到6~8周时,患者伤口已经愈合,早期力量增强,活动范围允许超过90°,并且开始接受标准的肩胛骨强化训练。最大力量如果在6~9个月内无法恢复,可能反映了肌肉的慢性失用和萎缩。

术后结局

在一份长期随访的大样本研究的原始报告中,研究者描述了手术的治疗结局,整个组都恢复良好,疼痛和功能得到了显著改善[11]。出院时,ASES疼痛得分(满分50分)从18分提高到35分,功能得分(满分50分)从20分提高到28分,ASES总分(满分100分)从38分提高到62分($P < 0.001$)。这些结果至少在2年的随访中仍然维持。虽然整个组都恢复良好,但患者自报告的结局仍存在差异。为了更仔细地观察结局的不同,随后的评估以ASES总分(>10分)的最小可检测变化为标准进行了亚分组[13]。78名患者中有58名(74%)报告了大于10分的变化,并被认为有显著的临床改善。另外20名(26%)在ASES上没有达到至少10分的改变,并且被认为没有显著改善(表11.1)。

可能有多种原因导致在诊断、纳入标准和手术治疗方面高度一致的患者们的自报告结局有差异,其中包括术后及恢复活动阶段功能需求的改变,在地理分布不同的组别中执行和完成康复训练的差异性,慢性损伤对肌肉力量和激活的影响,以及患者对临床问题及其功能恢复的期望和认知的不同。

一个主要的、以患者为导向的、能影响报告结局的因素是对疼痛的认知。这个因素在以后其他类型的肩部手术中已得到

表11.1 对肩胛肌再附着术有反应者与无反应者的ASES比较

	有反应者($n = 58$)	无反应者($n = 20$)
	手术前	
ASES疼痛得分	16 ± 11	27 ± 12*
ASES功能得分	18 ± 11	24 ± 9
ASES总分	34 ± 16	50 ± 12*
	手术后	
ASES疼痛得分	38 ± 10*	26 ± 12
ASES功能得分	31 ± 11*	21 ± 10
ASES总分	69 ± 18*	42 ± 16
自手术前到手术后的变化	35 ± 18*	-8 ± 14

*得分增加显著($P < 0.001$)

注意[14-18]。一项初步研究使用疼痛灾难化程度量表（PCS）评估了31名术后患者的疼痛认知[19]。这个由13个项目组成的自报告量表评估了患者对疼痛影响日常生活的态度，其最大分值为65分（得分越低，疼痛灾难化的特征越少）。21名患者被归为非灾难化患者（<30分）。10名患者被归类为灾难化患者（≥30分），这意味着他们会持续地意识到疼痛，他们认为这个疼痛会对他们的身体功能产生负面影响。这种患者感知在很多方面影响了报告的结局。

灾难化患者中只有3名患者对手术结果表示满意，而7名患者对结果表示不满意或不确定。疼痛灾难化对ASES总分也有影响。非灾难化患者的平均ASES总分比灾难化患者高29分（表11.2）。对手术不满意且疼痛灾难化的患者，其ASES疼痛得分较非灾难化患者低12～17分，而灾难化患者与非灾难化患者在ASES功能得分上的差异仅为4～6分。

这些发现表明，疼痛感知可能是收集患者自报告结局数据时的一个重要因素。

在对报告结局不太满意的患者中，疼痛感知有所不同。这种患者的特异性特征可能在受伤之前就已经存在，可能受到许多其他因素的影响（压力、焦虑、以前的经历，等等），或者是由于痛觉感受器、脊髓和大脑的神经可塑性变化，从而导致慢性疼痛[15]。这可能是非常重要的原因，因为诊断往往是延迟的，所以患者经历了长时间的损伤和疼痛。

这些发现有以下临床意义。第一，认识到患者对疼痛的总体反应及对疼痛灾难化的特定效应可能对治疗产生很大影响，医生应在诊断过程中评估患者的自报告结局，并在适当时将其作为综合治疗计划的一部分。第二，从临床经验来看，通过再附着过程使肌肉张力得到再平衡是肩胛骨内侧缘疼痛缓解的主要因素，在术后早期可感受到这种缓解。因此，应尽早发现这类损伤，以尽量减少撕脱对疼痛和肌肉抑制产生的有害影响。大多数患者对手术结果表示满意，是因为疼痛感降低，日常活动能力恢复。

表11.2 在肩胛肌再附着术后非灾难化患者和灾难化患者之间的ASES比较

	非灾难化（n = 21）	灾难化（n = 10）	P值
ASES疼痛得分	43 ± 8	27 ± 12	<0.001
ASES功能得分	40 ± 9	27 ± 12	0.005
ASES总分	83 ± 15	54 ± 18	<0.001
未满足ASES的MDC>10	1[a]	6	0.047

[a]患者初始ASES总分=90，最近随访ASES总分=88
MDC：最小可检测变化

总结

肩胛骨肌肉撕脱是一种临床可识别的综合征，其病史和检查结果相对一致，可用于诊断和治疗。它的具体发病率尚不清楚，但随着我们对它的认识的深入改进，这种诊断可能会相对普遍。在几乎所有的病例中，手术治疗可以显著减轻疼痛，但若功能有变化，也可能无法恢复正常。影响功能活动能力的因素可能包括慢性疼痛后遗症、长期肌肉萎缩、肌肉激活模式的改变及其他的手术后遗症。患者的报告，特别是对疼痛的感知，可能对结局的评估有很大影响。认识到该情况可以使早期的识别、评估和治疗成为可能，从而缩短功能障碍时间，减少功能失代偿，并可能获得更好的功能结局。

（张鑫）

参考文献

1. Hayes JM, Zehr DJ. Traumatic muscle avulsion causing winging of the scapula. J Bone Joint Surg Am, 1981, 63: 495–497.
2. Latremoliere A, Woolf CJ. Central sensitization: a generator of pain hypersensitivity by central neural plasticity. J Pain, 2009, 10: 895–926.
3. Cools AM, Witvrouw EE, Declercq GA, et al. Scapular muscle recruitment pattern: Trapezius muscle latency with and without impingement symptoms. Am J Sports Med, 2003, 31: 542–549.
4. Ludewig PM, Cook TM. Alterations in shoulder kinematics and associated muscle activity in people with symptoms of shoulder impingement. Phys Ther, 2000, 80(3): 276–291.
5. Ludewig PM, Reynolds JF. The association of scapular kinematics and glenohumeral joint pathologies. J Orthop Sports Phys Ther, 2009, 39(2): 90–104.
6. Bagg SD, Forrest WJ. A biomechanical analysis of scapular rotation during arm abduction in the scapular plane. Am J Phys Med Rehabil, 1988, 67: 238–245.
7. Ludewig PM, Cook TM, Nawoczenski DA. 3-Dimensional scapular orientation and muscle activity at selected positions of humeral elevation. J Orthop Sports Phys Ther, 1996, 24: 57–65.
8. Lukasiewicz AC, McClure P, Michener LA, et al. Comparison of 3-dimensional scapular position and orientation between subjects with and without shoulder impingement. J Orthop Sports Phys Ther, 1999, 29(10): 574–586.
9. Smith J, Dietrich CT, Kotajarvi BR, et al. The effect of scapular protraction on isometric shoulder rotation strength in normal subjects. J Shoulder Elbow Surg, 2006, 15: 339–343.
10. Kebaetse M, McClure PW, Pratt N. Thoracic position effect on shoulder range of motion, strength, and three-dimensional scapular kinematics. Arch Phys Med Rehabil, 1999, 80: 945–950.
11. Kibler WB, Sciascia AD, Uhl TL. Medial scapular muscle detachment: clinical presentation and surgical treatment. J Shoulder Elbow Surg, 2014, 23(1): 58–67.
12. Kibler WB. Sports medicine surgery. Philadelphia: Elsevier Saunders, 2010.
13. Michener LA, McClure PW, Sennett BJ. American shoulder and elbow surgeons standardized assessment form, patient self-report section: Reliability, validity, and responsiveness. J Shoulder Elbow Surg, 2002, 11: 587–594.
14. Coronado RA, Simon CB, Valencia C, et al. Ex-

perimental pain responses support peripheral and central sensitization in patients with unilateral shoulder pain. Clin J Pain, 2014, 30(2): 143–151.
15. Dean BJF, Gwilym SE, Carr AJ. Why does my shoulder hurt? A review of the neuroanatomical and biochemical basis of shoulder pain. Br J Sports Med, 2013, 47: 1095–1104.
16. Gwilym SE, Oag HCL, Tracey I, et al. Evidence that central sensitisation is present in patients with shoulder impingement syndrome and influences the outcome after surgery. J Bone Joint SurgBr, 2011, 93(4): 498–502.
17. Valencia C, Fillingim RB, Bishop M, et al. Investigation of central pain processing in postoperative shoulder pain and disability. Clin J Pain, 2014, 30(9): 775–786.
18. Valencia C, Kindler LL, Fillingim RB, et al. Investigation of central pain processing in shoulder pain: converging results from 2 musculoskeletal pain models. J Pain, 2012, 13(1): 81–89.
19. Sullivan MJL, Bishop S, Pivik J. The pain catastrophizing scale: development and validation. Psychol Assess, 1995, 7: 524–532.

第12章 神经损伤和翼状肩胛

John E. Kuhn

引言

肩胛骨是上肢功能和力量的基础。就像工地里的起重机一样，肩胛骨必须固定在"地基"上，这样手臂才能抬起和移动重物。如果起重机驾驶室的底座不牢固，起重机就会倾斜。如果肩胛骨没有固定在胸壁上，它也会倾斜。在起于或止于肩胛骨的17块肌肉中，那些像起重机的机架一样，将肩胛骨固定在躯干上的肌肉包括胸小肌、肩胛舌骨肌、肩胛提肌、前锯肌、斜方肌和大、小菱形肌（表12.1）。

表12.1 肩胛骨肌群

肩胸肌群
肩胛提肌
肩胛舌骨肌
胸小肌
大菱形肌
小菱形肌
前锯肌
斜方肌
肩肱肌群
肩袖
冈下肌
肩胛下肌
冈上肌

（续表）

小圆肌
其他
肱二头肌长头
肱二头肌短头
喙肱肌
三角肌
大圆肌
肱三头肌长头

与肩胛骨相连的17块肌肉中，肩胸肌群（7块）为稳定肩胛骨提供了基础，它们使上肢能够活动。如果这些肌肉不能正常工作，将发生翼状肩胛。

翼状肩胛形成的原因有很多[1]，包括静态来源（最常见的是肩胛骨软骨瘤）（图12.1）、动态来源（肩胛骨运动障碍）、创伤性肌肉撕脱[2]，以及最常见的神经损伤。这一章将着重讲述翼状肩胛的神经学原因。

胸长神经损伤和前锯肌麻痹

胸长神经支配前锯肌。这条神经通常起于C_5、C_6和C_7的前支。需要注意的是，C_5和C_6的神经根穿过中斜角肌，并可能在这里卡压；然后神经向下延伸至臂丛和腋窝血管后面，沿着胸壁一侧支配前锯肌（图12.2）。胸长神经因长度和体表位置特殊，易发生神经失用性牵拉损伤。

病史

胸长神经的损伤通常发生于牵伸过程[1]，特别是在运动时。神经可能因压迫而损伤，很少有穿透性损伤。患者可能直到几天或几周后才会注意到症状。通常主诉为上肢力量丧失，长期如此可能导致其他肩胛骨肌肉疼痛，特别是胸小肌和肩胛提肌。因为这些肌肉为了代偿前锯肌无力而过于活跃。

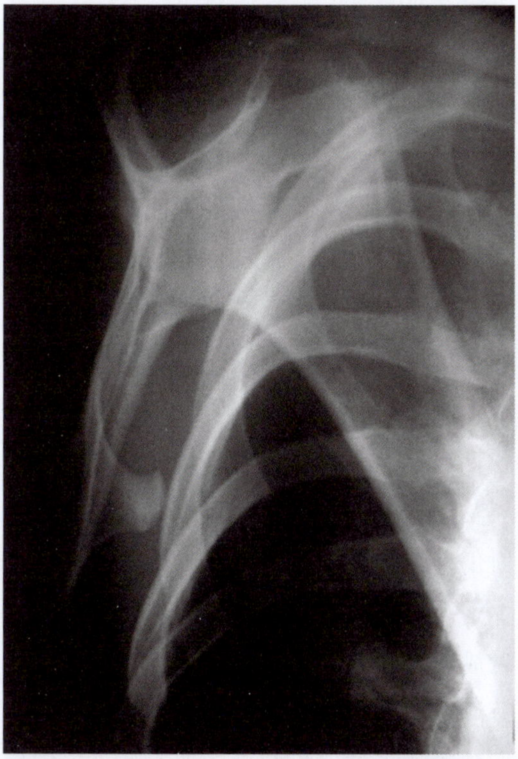

体格检查

前锯肌无力时，肩胛提肌、菱形肌和斜方肌将主要负责牵拉肩胛骨向内和向上（图12.3）。肩胛提肌（肩胛骨的内上角）和胸小肌（喙突的内侧面）的起点处可能存在压痛。伸肘抗阻肩屈曲可能会加重翼状肩胛。

影像学

对于神经损伤，X线和MRI并不是特别有帮助。这些检查对静态来源（肩胛骨软骨瘤、肋骨或肩胛骨骨折畸形愈合）或结构性来源（肌肉撕脱伤）更有用。

图12.1 肩胛骨软骨瘤。这是最常见的肩胛骨肿瘤，可能是翼状肩胛的一个静态来源

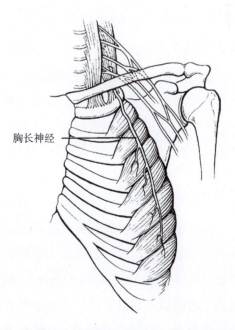

图12.2 胸长神经的解剖位置（来源：Warner JJP, Iannotti JP, Gerber C. Eds. Complex and revision problems in shoulder surgery. Philadelphia: Lippincott-Raven Publishers, 1997.）

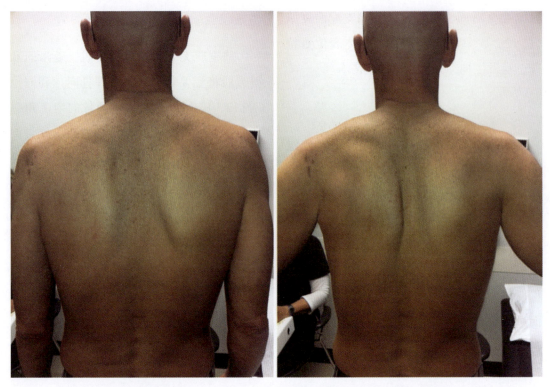

图12.3 左侧前锯肌麻痹导致翼状肩胛。(a)休息位:注意斜方肌和菱形肌主要负责牵拉肩胛骨向上和向内 (b)外展位:手臂上抬或外展加重翼状肩胛

肌电图分析

肌电图可以检测胸长神经的损伤[3]。神经损伤的表现包括潜伏期增加,前锯肌出现纤颤和锐波。随意收缩时,运动单元动作电位减少。

鉴别诊断

由前锯肌麻痹引起的翼状肩胛的鉴别诊断包括翼状肩胛的静态来源(肩胛骨软骨瘤、肩胛骨或肋骨骨折畸形愈合)、肌肉损伤(前锯肌或其他肌肉)或其他神经损伤(副神经、肩胛背神经和/或臂丛神经或颈神经根)。

治疗

由于胸长神经损伤多为神经失用性损伤,可自行恢复,建议保守治疗。然而,这条神经太长了,恢复时间可能长达2年。恢复情况可以通过连续肌电图分析进行跟踪,每3个月内就进行1次。约80%的患者长期情况良好,翼状肩胛恢复,屈曲和外展功能正常;然而,许多患者在长期随访时仍有疼痛[4]。

手术松解锁骨上区域的胸长神经是一种成功的治疗方法[5],也有松解神经远端部分的报道[6]。重要的是要认识到,如果在早期就进行了神经松解术,那么并不确定这些患者是否有自发恢复。神经松解术的结果显示，神经恢复相对较快。

对于那些在 18~24 个月后前锯肌麻痹仍没有恢复的患者，或者在连续肌电图分析中显示 12 个月后也没有发现恢复的患者，可以进行肌肉转移手术。Marmor 和 Bechtol[7] 描述了应用阔筋膜延伸转移胸大肌至肩胛骨下角的手术（图 12.4）。已经有一些对肌腱间接移植可能失败的担忧，导致一些人建议将肌腱直接移植到肩胛骨上（直接转移）[8, 9]。此外，由于肌肉方向靠近前锯肌，许多研究者建议仅使用胸大肌的胸骨头，减少瘢痕，改善腋窝的美观度[8, 10]。Elhassan 和 Wagner[11] 描述了这种移植的不同之处，一部分肱骨保留在胸大肌胸骨头肌腱上，这使得肩胛骨可以骨性愈合。

结局

将胸大肌的胸骨头转移到肩胛骨是有帮助的，大约 90% 的患者可以得到良好到极好的结果[8, 10, 12, 13]。手术失败和翼状肩胛复发是已知的并发症，使用直接转移的话可能较少发生[12]。

副神经损伤和斜方肌麻痹

副神经穿过颈内静脉支配胸锁乳突肌，然后进入颈后三角，供应斜方肌（图 12.5）。它的位置相当浅，在胸锁乳突肌的后部，

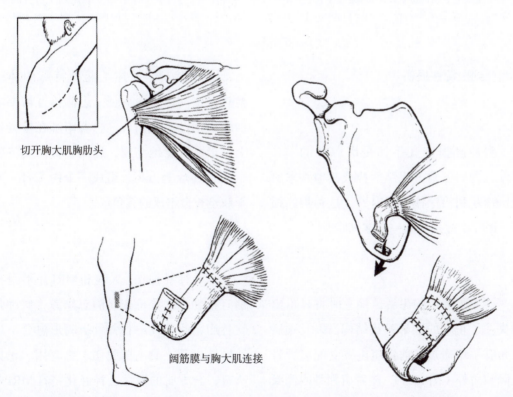

图 12.4　胸大肌移植。如图所示，正如 Marmor 和 Bechtol 所描述的，使用阔筋膜延伸，间接转移胸大肌[7]。直接转移是将肌腱直接连接肩胛骨（来源：Warner JJP, Iannotti JP, Gerber C. Eds. Complex and revision problems in shoulder surgery. Philadelphia: Lippincott-Raven Publishers, 1997.）

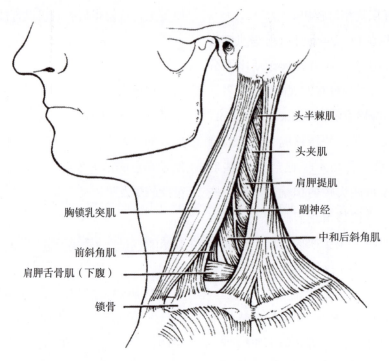

图 12.5 副神经的解剖位置。这条神经位于颈后三角的浅表,手术中易发生医源性损伤(来源:Warner JJP, Iannotti JP, Gerber C. Eds. Complex and revision problems in shoulder surgery. Philadelphia: Lippincott-Raven Publishers, 1997.)

容易受到医源性损伤。

病史

副神经损伤几乎都是医源性的[14],通常是颈后三角淋巴结活检或其他手术所致。诊断和治疗往往延迟[14],这种神经损伤是医疗事故索赔的一个常见原因[15]。

体格检查

斜方肌麻痹的患者,检查时将显示出其失去了正常的颈部蹼状结构,以及颈后三角有手术瘢痕。前锯肌主要支配肩胛骨下降和向外(图12.6)。随着肩胛骨内侧缘升高,将导致翼状肩胛。手臂抗阻屈曲时症状加重。

Levy等人[16]描述了两种特殊的体格检查:主动抬臂滞后征,患侧抬臂需要增加腰椎前凸;三角征,患者俯卧在检查台上,最大限度地前屈,患侧手臂需要将躯干从检查台上抬高,组成一个由手臂、躯干和检查台组成的三角形。

影像学

对于神经损伤,X线和MRI并不是特别有帮助。这些检查对静态来源(肩胛骨软骨瘤、肋骨或肩胛骨骨折畸形愈合)或结构性来源(肌肉撕脱伤)更有用。正如所料,斜方肌的慢性去神经化将在MRI上显示异常,包括斜方肌萎缩和在STIR序列图像中的高强度信号。术后患者可在神经

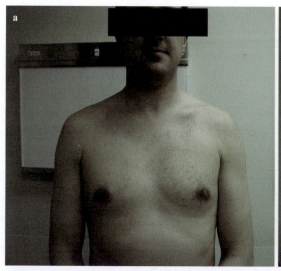 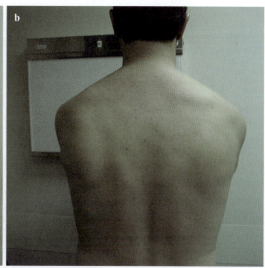

图12.6 由于左侧斜方肌麻痹导致翼状肩胛。(a) 休息位：注意患者左侧颈部蹼状结构减少 (b) 前锯肌主导控制肩胛骨向外和下降

周围发现瘢痕[17]。

肌电图分析

患侧肌电图将显示低振幅的SAN复合肌肉动作电位（CMAP），刺激强度需要比健侧更高才能获得。上斜方肌肌电图显示出密集的纤颤电位，在大约一半的损伤中存在自主运动单元电位（MUPs）[18]。

鉴别诊断

虽然形成翼状肩胛的原因有很多[1]，但是在颈后三角进行淋巴结活检或手术的患者，其翼状肩胛与其他原因形成的不同。

治疗

神经撕裂的外科修复已经取得了一些成功，最好在1年内（早期）进行[19-23]。有文献[24]描述胸外侧神经向副神经转移。不幸的是，副神经损伤通常诊断较晚，神经手术可能不成功。

有一些副神经损伤和斜方肌麻痹的患者可以保守治疗；然而，将手臂举过肩困难或主利手受影响的患者，保守治疗可能效果不佳[25]。这类患者可以采用Eden和Lange所述的肩胛提肌和菱形肌转移[26, 27]（图12.7）。在这个手术中，肩胛提肌从肩胛骨内上角的止点处分离出来，并向外侧转移到肩胛冈上；而大菱形肌和小菱形肌则从肩胛骨的内侧缘分离出来，并转移到冈下窝的外侧。Elhassan和Wagner[13]描述了这种技术的一种改良方法，将菱形肌分离并转移到肩胛冈的不同部位。

结局

在大约75%的患者中，这些手术可以得到良好到极好的结果[22, 23, 28, 29]。较差的结果可能出现在50岁以上的患者和伴有其他肩关节疾病的患者中[22, 29]。

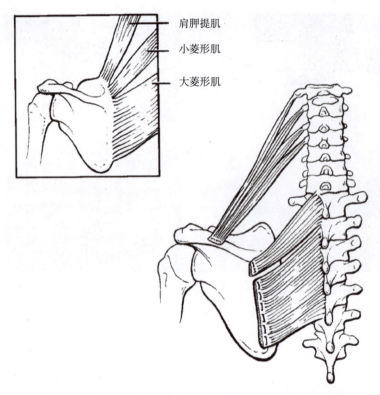

图12.7　斜方肌麻痹转移手术。肩胛提肌转移到肩胛冈外侧，菱形肌转移到冈下窝外侧（来源：Kuhn JE. Disorders of the shoulder: diagnosis and management. Philadelphia: Lippincott Williams & Wilkins, 1999.）

肩胛背神经损伤和菱形肌麻痹

肩胛背神经起源于C_5和C_4腹支，然后穿过中斜角肌，深入肩胛提肌，沿着肩胛骨内侧缘向下支配菱形肌。

肩胛背神经损伤很少见，仅在少数病例报道中有描述[30-32]，但可作为肩关节手术中的斜角肌间阻滞并发症出现[33]。

肩胛背神经损伤的患者，其肩胛骨内侧缘可能有疼痛感。研究慢性疼痛的专家已经发现肩胛背神经卡压综合征，其特征是肩胛骨内侧疼痛，可放射到上肢，并伴有不同程度的功能障碍[34]。

翼状肩胛发生在肩胛骨内侧缘和肩胛骨下角处，患者把手放在髋部并抵抗阻力推肘将加重翼状肩胛[35]。鉴别诊断包括C_5神经根损伤，它也会导致菱形肌无力。

由于这种情况非常罕见，在文献中很少考虑外科治疗。通常推荐保守治疗，但是对于完全的神经损伤，可以尝试神经修复。作者曾做过一例将大圆肌从肱骨转移到胸椎棘突的手术，效果良好。

总结

翼状肩胛的形成原因有很多；然而，神经损伤造成肌肉麻痹是最常见的。因胸长神经损伤造成前锯肌麻痹是最常见的，其次是因副神经损伤造成斜方肌麻痹，最不常见的是因肩胛背神经损伤造成菱形肌麻痹。及早发现这些损伤并迅速开始治疗是很重要的。虽然大多数前锯肌麻痹的患者会自行恢复，但副神经损伤通常是医源性的，可能需要早期手术干预。治疗这些损伤的方法多种多样，其中大多数在使用时能显著减轻疼痛和改善功能。

（刘燕平）

参考文献

1. Kuhn JE, Plancher KD, Hawkins RJ. Scapular winging. J Am Acad Orthop Surg, 1995, 3(6): 319–325.
2. Kibler WB, Sciascia AD, Uhl TL. Medial scapular muscle detachment: clinical presentation and surgical treatment. J Shoulder Elbow Surg, 2014, 23(1): 58–67.
3. Kaplan PE. Electrodiagnostic confirmation of long thoracic nerve palsy. J Neruol Neruosurg Psychiatry, 1980, 43: 50–52.
4. Pikkarainen V, Kettunen J, Vastamäki M. The natural course of serratus palsy at 2 to 31 years. Clin Orthop Relat Res, 2013, 471(5): 1555–1563.
5. Nath RK, Lyons AB, Bietz G. Microneurolysis and decompression of long thoracic nerve injury are effective in reversing scapular winging: long-term results in 50 cases. BMC Musculoskelet Disord, 2007, 8: 25–31.
6. Le Nail LR, Bacle G, Marteau E, et al. Isolated paralysis of the serratus anterior muscle: surgical release of the distal segment of the long thoracic nerve in 52 patients. Orthop Traumatol Surg Res, 2014, 100(4 Suppl): S243– S248.
7. Marmor L, Bechtol CO. Paralysis of the serratus anterior due to electric shock relieved by transplantation of the pectoralis major muscle: a case report. J Bone Joint Surg Am, 1963, 45: 156–160.
8. Streit JJ, Lenarz CJ, Shishani Y, et al. Pectoralis major tendon transfer for the treatment of scapular winging due to long thoracic nerve palsy. J Shoulder Elbow Surg, 2012, 21(5): 685–690.
9. Tauber M, Moursy M, Koller H, et al. Direct pectoralis major muscle transfer for dynamic stabilization of scapular winging. J Shoulder Elbow Surg, 2008, 17(1 Suppl): 29S–34S.
10. Connor PM, Yamaguchi K, Manifold SG, et al. Split pectoralis major transfer for serratus anterior palsy. Clin Orthop Relat Res, 1997, 341: 134–142.
11. Elhassan BT, Wagner ER. Outcome of triple-tendon transfer, an Eden-Lange variant, to reconstruct trapezius paralysis. J Shoulder Elbow Surg, 2015, 24(8): 1307–1313.
12. Chalmers PN, Saltzman BM, Feldheim TF, et al. A comprehensive analysis of pectoralis major transfer for long thoracic nerve palsy. J Shoulder Elbow Surg, 2015, 24(7): 1028–1035.
13. Elhassan BT, Wagner ER. Outcome of transfer of the sternal head of the pectoralis major with its bone insertion to the scapula to manage scapular winging. J Shoulder Elbow Surg, 2015, 24(5): 733–740.
14. Camp SJ, Birch R. Injuries to the spinal accessory nerve: a lesson to surgeons. J Bone Joint Surg Br, 2011, 93(1): 62–67.
15. Morris LG, Ziff DJ, DeLacure MD. Malpractice litigation after surgical injury of the spinal accessory nerve: an evidence-based analysis. Arch Otolaryngol Head Neck Surg. 2008, 134(1): 102–107.
16. Levy O, Relwani JG, Mullett H, et al. The active elevation lag sign and the triangle sign: new clinical signs of trapezius palsy. J Shoulder Elbow Surg, 2009, 18(4): 573–576.

17. Li AE, Greditzer HG 4th, Melisaratos DP, et al. MRI findings of spinal accessory neuropathy. Clin Radiol, 2016, 71(4): 316–320.
18. Laughlin RS, Spinner RJ, Daube JR. Electrophysiological testing of spinal accessory nerve in suspected cases of nerve transection. Muscle Nerve, 2011, 44(5): 715–719.
19. Göransson H, Leppänen OV, Vastamäki M. Patient outcome after surgical management of the spinal accessory nerve injury: a long-term follow-up study. SAGE Open Med, 2016, 4: 2050312116645731.
20. Kim DH, Cho YJ, Tiel RL, et al. Surgical outcomes of 111 spinal accessory nerve injuries. Neurosurgery, 2003, 53(5): 1106–1112, discussion 1102–1103.
21. Park SH, Esquenazi Y, Kline DG, et al. Surgical outcomes of 156 spinal accessory nerve injuries caused by lymph node biopsy procedures. J Neurosurg Spine, 2015, 23(4): 518–525.
22. Teboul F, Bizot P, Kakkar R, et al. Surgical management of trapezius palsy. J Bone Joint Surg Am, 2004, 86(9): 1884–1890.
23. Teboul F, Bizot P, Kakkar R, et al. Surgical management of trapezius palsy. J Bone Joint Surg Am, 2005, 87: 285–291.
24. Maldonado AA, Spinner RJ. Lateral pectoral nerve transfer for spinal accessory nerve injury. J Neurosurg Spine, 2016, 29: 1–4.
25. Friedenberg SM, Zimprich T, Harper CM. The natural history of long thoracic and spinal accessory neuropathies. Muscle Nerve, 2002, 25: 535–539.
26. Eden R. Zur Behandlung der Trapeziuslähmung mittelst Muskelplastik. Dtsch Z Chir, 1924, 184: 387–397.
27. Lange M. The operative treatment of irreparable trapezius paralysis. Istanbul Tip Fak Mecmuasi, 1959, 22: 137–141.
28. Bigliani LU, Compito CA, Duralde XA, et al. Transfer of the levator scapulae, rhomboid major, and rhomboid minor for paralysis of the trapezius. J Bone Joint Surg Am, 1996, 78: 1534–1540.
29. Romero J, Gerber C. Levator scapulae and rhomboid transfer for paralysis of trapezius. The Eden-Lange procedure. J Bone Joint Surg Br, 2003, 85(8): 1141–1145.
30. Argyriou AA, Karanasios P, Makridou A, et al. Dorsal scapular neuropathy causing rhomboids palsy and scapular winging. J Back Musculoskelet Rehabil, 2015, 28(4), 883–885.
31. Burdett-Smith P. Experience of scapula winging in an accident and emergency department. Br J Clin Pract, 1990, 44: 643–644.
32. Akgun K, Aktas I, Terzi Y. Winged scapula caused by a dorsal scapular nerve lesion: a case report. Arch Phys Med Rehabil, 2008, 89(10): 2017–2020.
33. Saporito A. Dorsal scapular nerve injury: a complication of ultrasound-guided interscalene block. Br J Anaesth, 2013, 111(5): 840–841.
34. Sultan HE, Younis El-Tantawi GA. Role of dorsal scapular nerve entrapment in unilateral interscapular pain. Arch Phys Med Rehabil, 2013, 94: 1118–1125.
35. Moore KL, Dalley AF. Clinically orientated anatomy. 4th ed. Philadelphia: Lippincott Williams & Wilkins, 1999.

第13章 神经问题的康复方案

Martin J. Kelley, Michael T. Piercey

由于前锯肌或斜方肌功能的丧失，胸长神经麻痹（LTNP）和副神经麻痹（SANP）的康复对医生来说是大挑战。钝挫伤、穿透性创伤、挤压、拉伸、牵引、病毒感染或医源性创伤等任一原因引起的神经损伤均可导致胸长神经或副神经单独或合并发生麻痹[1-16]。肩胛背神经损伤可能累及菱形肌，但由于这种情况较罕见，本文不直接讨论。LTNP或SANP患者的主诉常为颈、胸、肩或肩胛区疼痛，上肢感觉减退、无力或不稳定，肩关节主动活动范围减少，最明显的是LTNP患者的肩关节屈曲和SANP患者的肩关节外展[1, 2, 5-12, 15-18]。然而，在大多数情况下，患者将经历1~3周的肩胛区疼痛，然后疼痛消失但出现受累区域无力。这些损伤通常导致受累肢体的某些功能受限制，特别是提物或抗阻；然而，大多数人都能轻松自如地完成大多数活动。症状的严重程度可能会有所不同，神经失用或轴突断伤患者往往会在24个月内通过神经再生解决[9, 11, 12, 14-18]。为了正确地指导LTNP或SANP患者，医生必须对肩胛骨解剖、力学、正常肌肉活动有较深的了解，并能正确地完成全面的肩胛骨评估。

胸长神经起源于C_5、C_6、C_7神经根，穿过中斜角肌，经过臂丛后面进入腋下，在第2肋周围形成角度，并下降到胸壁的前外侧表面，只支配前锯肌[4, 8, 9, 12-14, 16, 19, 20]。前锯肌是一块大的扇形肌肉，呈多指状排列，分为3个部分，起于第1~9肋外侧，止于肩胛骨内侧缘[6, 9, 12, 16, 18-21]。总的来说，前锯肌负责肩胛骨前伸和上旋，使肩胛骨在肩部运动时保持适当的关节盂位置，同时保持与胸壁的接触[4, 6, 9, 12, 14, 16, 18, 22-27]。Ekstrom等人[21]的研究表明，前锯肌下部与肩胛骨上旋的关系更为密切，而上部则在前伸时更活跃。鉴于胸长神经的敏感路径和前锯肌的多个指状突起，要考虑到一部分前锯肌可能受到LTNP的影响，而其余部分仍然可以完好无损。这可能发生在神经再生过程中，当上纤维活跃而下纤维不活跃时，导致前伸多于上旋。

副神经从颈后三角向下，支配胸锁乳

突肌，并继续沿肩胛骨内侧缘浅表至肩胛提肌、沿深部至斜方肌内侧，仅支配斜方肌[1, 2, 7-9, 12, 15, 28]。斜方肌起源于 C_7 至 T_{12} 的棘突，扇形，分为3部分。上部起于锁骨外侧 1/3，中部起于肩峰内侧、肩胛冈上方，下部起于肩胛冈下方[7, 9, 12, 15]。斜方肌对过头运动中肩胛骨的稳定，以及肩胛骨上提、后缩和旋转至关重要，尤其是肩胛骨外展[1, 7, 10, 12, 15, 22, 24-26, 28-30]。

在正常情况下，根据 Inman[24] 的研究，肌肉力偶是正确的肩肱力学所必需的。来自上斜方肌、肩胛提肌和前锯肌的力，通过肩胛骨上旋来抵消肩胛带的重量[21, 22, 24, 25, 30-32]。旋转力由中斜方肌、下斜方肌和菱形肌提供，向内侧牵拉肩峰，前锯肌向前外侧牵拉肩胛骨下角[22-25, 30, 32]。当肩胛骨旋转肌的运动控制受损时，如 LTNP 时的前锯肌或 SANP 时的斜方肌，力偶不平衡导致异常运动学，如肩胛骨运动障碍，并导致正常功能组织的张力过度负荷[23, 25, 31-33]。

评估

通常，由于前锯肌或斜方肌张力和活动的中断，LTNP 或 SANP 可导致静态肩胛骨错位[8, 15, 16]。首先，在坐位或站立位时，应评估姿势，因为胸椎和颈椎的定向将直接关系到肩胛骨休息位和肩胛骨运动[25]。特别是必须认识到是否存在脊柱侧弯，以避免混淆静态和动态异常。一个常见的右胸椎侧凸的人会有胸椎右旋，导致肋角（肋骨隆起）明显，因此内侧缘突出、肩胛骨略高，改变了肩胛骨的休息位。因为肩胛骨在另一边处于一个不同形状的"平台"上，所以它将不对称地移动，但这不能与真正的运动障碍混淆。

LTNP 患者的内侧缘明显突起，肩胛骨通常较低。SANP 患者的斜方肌明显萎缩，从外表看，上斜方肌萎缩最明显。SANP 患者的肩胛骨（及整个肩胛带）会下沉、外展和向下旋转[1, 5, 8-10, 12, 15, 16, 25, 28]。

肩胛骨肌肉评估流程可用于确定是否存在神经麻痹、运动控制、运动障碍或其他病理现象（图 13.1）。这些特定的测试也可以帮助追踪随着时间推移神经再支配的情况。测试者必须首先确定受试者是否有明显的运动障碍。肩胛骨运动障碍测试[34, 35]可以确定"是"，观察到异常的模式或运动障碍；或者"否"，观察到正常的肩胛骨运动。矢状面运动障碍可能提示 LTNP。内侧翼通常发生在 90°附近，尤其是下降时。通常下斜方肌变得非常活跃，在有效的活动范围内可见，它试图通过后缩肩胛骨来进行代偿。运动障碍或不能在冠状面无痛上抬超过 90°都可能是 SANP 的表现，但不论是何种表现，都要进一步考虑 LTNP 或 SANP 的存在（图 13.2）。

第 13 章 神经问题的康复方案 · 133

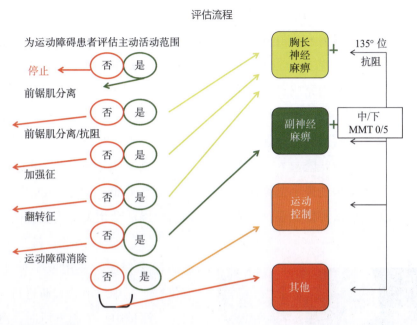

图 13.1 肩胛骨肌肉评估流程

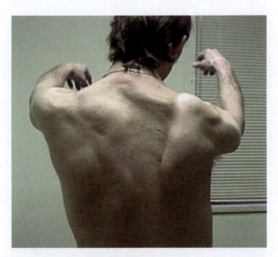

图 13.2 同时有 LTNP 和 SANP 的患者

为了评估是否存在 LTNP，应该进行无阻力和有阻力的前锯肌分离试验、加强征和徒手肌力测试。前锯肌分离试验是在受试者手臂位于肱骨外旋的一侧时完成的，受试者主动前伸和上抬肩胛骨[19, 25, 32, 36]。

如果患者不能将肩胛骨移至未受累侧相同位置或肩胛骨下角、内侧缘突出，则认为是阳性结果。为了进一步观察前锯肌，测试者可以在肩前部增加向后的阻力，以评估肩胛骨内侧缘是否容易后移及程度（图13.3）。如果受试者在矢状面前屈至 90°时出现翼状肩胛，则认为是加强征。此时，代偿性斜方肌活动因拮抗抑制而被迫停止，肩胛骨位置完全取决于前锯肌活动（图13.4）。当受试者完成墙卧撑时，若肩关节屈曲到 90°，也可能出现加强征[8, 9, 16, 19, 25]。受试者仰卧完成前锯肌徒手肌力测试，受试测肩部和肘部屈曲 90°，手臂前伸[37, 38]。测试者的力沿着肱骨轴通过尺骨鹰嘴突施加。在进行这项试验时，必须注意胸小肌，评估其潜在的代偿性使用。专门针对前锯肌下部进行肌力评估的话，可以在肩关节上抬到125°时在肱骨和肩胛骨外侧缘施加内收的力，或者在肩关节前屈125°时施加伸展的力[21, 36]。当完成这些肌力测试的任一个时，使用手持测力计可以帮助量化结果[38]。必须观察肩胛骨或触诊肩胛骨，以确定是否发生翼状隆起。上述每一项试验的阳性结果都可能提示前锯肌存在功能障碍，如果翼状肩胛伴加强征，则存在LTNP。

SANP是否存在是由翻转征和中、下斜方肌徒手肌力测试来提示的。翻转征测试：受试者站立，手臂在一侧，肘关节屈曲至90°，测试者在观察肩胛骨的同时，徒手抵抗肩关节外旋[1, 7, 9]（图13.5）。如果在施加阻力时肩胛骨内侧缘"翻"出胸壁，则结果为阳性[1, 7]。可见斜方肌萎缩及肩胛带降低，提示SANP；然而，这必须与肌肉活动相关，才能全面检查斜方肌功能[1, 5, 7, 8, 12, 15]。为此，按照Kendall[37]所述的标准程序，使用或不使用手持式测力仪[38]，对中、下斜方肌进行徒手肌力测试。当测试中、下斜方肌时，测试者必须触诊确认肌肉是否激活。SANP患者的中、下斜方肌都是完全弛缓的，且看不到菱形肌的激活，因为在不适当的测试位置菱形肌不能激活。测试者必须将受试者的肩胛骨后缩并向后移动，然后提示受试者保持手臂完全外旋。有些病患的副神经近端部分受影响，除了斜方肌，还可能累及胸锁乳突肌[7]，应完成胸锁乳突肌的徒手肌力测试[7, 37]。

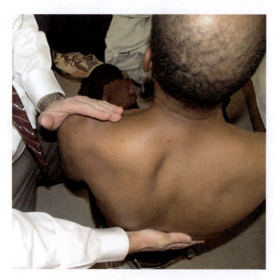

图13.3 抗阻分离前锯肌

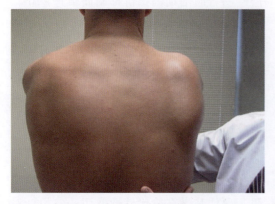

图13.4 加强征：左侧阴性，右侧阳性

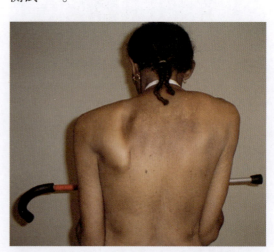

图13.5 翻转征

当通过评估肌肉和神经完整性来确定损伤时，测试者试图通过放置手、提醒或教学来纠正运动障碍。通常情况下，盂肱关节不稳定的患者会通过激活胸小肌或选择性地使前锯肌失活引起肩上抬，伴肩胛骨下降或前倾。测试者应提醒患者将肩胛骨或肩胛带轻微抬高和前伸。这将激活前锯肌，抑制胸小肌，消除运动障碍。

康复原则

一旦医生认识到LTNP和/或SANP的存在，应根据上述试验结果建立客观基准值。干预应立即开始，方法根据损伤程度、神经再生阶段和相关功能限制而有所不同。医生应对患者进行这方面的知识宣教，即LTNP和/或SANP患者的神经再生过程不能加快，患者需要有极大的耐心。如果强迫受影响的肌肉募集，就会对正在愈合的神经施加不必要的应力，产生不适当的代偿策略，相关的组织被激惹，患者可能变得沮丧。医生必须认识到关键原则，即创造一种环境，鼓励使用现有的肌肉系统来改善症状和增加功能，而不是对所有的相关结构施加过度应力。

相关症状或功能受限管理

前锯肌和斜方肌是静态肩胛骨稳定肌，应教导LTNP和/或SANP患者与此损伤相关的肩胛骨、肩胛带和脊柱姿势，考虑颈椎、胸椎和腰椎的方向，并强调适当使用腰托。具体来说，由于前锯肌和斜方肌活动减少，应避免过度的肩胛骨前伸、前倾和内旋[39, 40]。姿势不佳常常导致胸小肌或肩胛提肌、上斜方肌过度活动[8, 9, 26, 41]。应调整体位以最大限度地减少肩胛骨错位和肩下垂对肌肉的影响[2, 23, 25, 31, 32]。当身体直立时，将患肢放在枕头上或外套口袋里，减轻患肢的重量[6]。重要的是教患者如何复制最佳位置，以保持每次的操作一致。在慢性、严重的病例中，可以制作一种矫形器，既支持所涉及的肢体，又允许自由活动[9, 16, 18]（图13.6）。

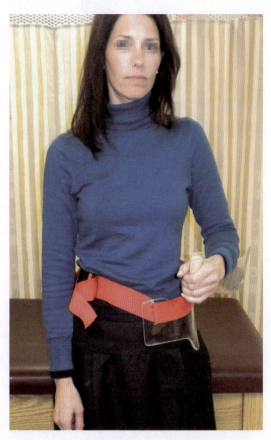

图13.6 上肢支撑矫形器

除了姿势调整，还可以通过热疗法、软组织技术和/或拉伸来解决肌肉组织的过度活动[31]，如颈椎后缩、脊柱松动、胸部伸展和仰卧位胸小肌牵伸等技术可能是有益的；然而，必须避免头和患侧肩分离，尽量减少它对神经再生产生负面影响的可能性。活动修正有助于进一步的症状管理[6, 9, 12, 14, 18]。一些动作，如伸够或提物动作可能会给受影响的、正在愈合的神经和相关的受累肌肉带来过度的应力，易形成不恰当的代偿策略，使未受累的结构处于发生撞击或肌腱变性症状的危险之中[14, 31]。医生应确保全肩存在被动活动范围[3, 5, 8, 9, 12, 14, 16]。如果没有，应手法松动盂肱关节和肩胛胸壁。但应小心操作，例如，对盂肱关节的下滑手法可能牵拉神经。为了提高被动活动范围，可能需要向患者提供家庭训练方案，包括椅子牵伸，仰卧位使用体操棒进行被动前屈和被动外旋等[9]。

代偿策略

针对完全瘫痪或单一肩胛肌显著无力的康复方案，一个重要方面是改善代偿性和原发性肩胛肌活动。换句话说，就是提高患者募集未受影响的（代偿性）肩胛肌的能力，然后针对受影响的原发性肌肉进行活动。因此，我们可以考虑设计两个阶段的康复训练，一个阶段与未受影响的（代偿性）肌肉激活相关，另一个阶段与受影响的（原发性）肌肉激活相关（表13.1和

13.2）。这些训练可能是相同的或类似的，并且可能有重叠，重点在于训练对象是代偿性肌肉还是原发性肌肉。

表 13.1　胸长神经麻痹阶段性康复训练

阶段 1
肩胛骨后缩
肩胛骨后缩伴屈肘和伸肘
侧卧位前屈
俯卧位，90°位进行水平外展训练
应用弹力带进行肩胛骨后缩伴外旋训练
应用弹力带进行肩胛骨后缩伴划船训练
应用弹力带进行肩胛骨后缩伴反手训练
肩胛骨后缩和上抬（朝肩胛骨平面）
应用弹力带进行肩胛骨后缩伴正手训练
阶段 2
前锯肌分离
仰卧位 +*
侧卧位 +，支撑臂掌心朝上抬起
站立位 +，伴球上掌心朝上
俯卧位，球上闭链 +
前锯肌分离，+ 伴抬臂，掌心朝上和屈肘
前锯肌分离，+ 伴抬臂，掌心朝上和伸肘
墙上前锯肌训练
使用弹力带进行前锯肌训练
四点跪位俯卧撑 +
PNF：D1 屈曲模式

*"+"指肩胛骨前伸，下同。

表 13.2　副神经麻痹阶段性康复训练

阶段 1
菱形肌分离
前锯肌分离
肩胛骨上抬
菱形肌分离、后缩伴屈肘和伸肘
应用弹力带进行菱形肌分离、后缩伴划船训练
应用弹力带进行菱形肌分离、后缩伴外旋训练

（续表）

站立位+，伴球上掌心朝上
前锯肌分离，+伴抬臂，掌心朝上和屈肘
前锯肌分离，+伴抬臂，掌心朝上和伸肘
使用弹力带进行前锯肌训练
阶段2
肩胛骨后缩
仰卧位，中斜方肌等长收缩
仰卧位，下斜方肌等长收缩
应用弹力带进行肩胛骨后缩伴外旋训练
应用弹力带进行肩胛骨后缩伴划船训练
俯卧位，过头抬起
应用弹力带进行肩胛骨后缩伴反手训练

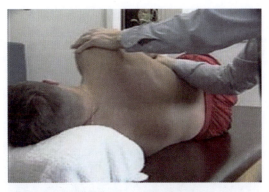

图13.7　徒手抗阻促进中斜方肌和菱形肌的活动

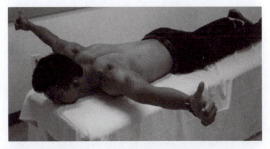

图13.8　俯卧位，90°位进行水平外展训练

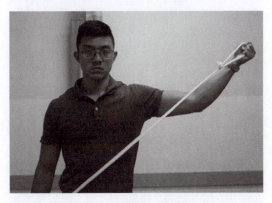

图13.9　肩胛骨后缩，反手使用弹力带

LTNP患者应该训练菱形肌和斜方肌，在没有前锯肌的情况下最大限度地稳定肩胛骨[6, 9, 12, 16]。教患者简单的肩胛骨后缩动作是必要的，患者在简单的功能活动中可以获得近端稳定，如拿起3.7 L牛奶。进阶到远端负荷如划船训练时，可广泛激活斜方肌[31, 42]。菱形肌在肩外展90°和轻微伸展时，伴肱骨内旋和施加作用力于内收和屈曲时，最容易被激活[43]。这些肌肉可以通过徒手抗阻技术进一步定位[32]（图13.7）。一些研究者发现，在完成侧卧外旋、侧卧前屈、俯卧水平外展伴外旋、俯卧伸展练习和俯卧过头抬起动作时，使用最少的上斜方肌或前锯肌可以很好地激活中、下斜方肌[27, 29-31, 41, 42, 44-47]（图13.8）。一旦患者很容易控制菱形肌和斜方肌，保持正确的肩胛骨中立位置至少5秒，菱形肌和斜方肌的使用就可以逐渐整合到更大、更具挑战性的运动模式中[48]（图13.9）。

SANP患者需要训练菱形肌和前锯肌来代偿斜方肌[5, 10]，包括前锯肌分离，仰卧肩胛骨前伸，前锯肌分离伴肩胛骨前伸加抬臂、掌心向上、伸肘，四点跪位俯卧撑伴肩胛骨前伸[42, 44, 47, 49]（图13.10）。可以使用徒手抗阻技术，特别注意菱形肌激活。一且患者能够表现出对前锯肌和菱形肌的正确控制，那么患者就可以在使用菱形肌和前锯肌保持肩胛骨稳定的基础上，执行更大、更复杂的运动模式（图13.11）。

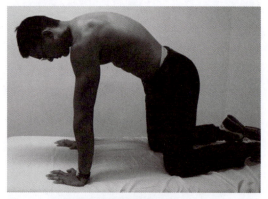

图13.10　四点跪位俯卧撑伴肩胛骨前伸

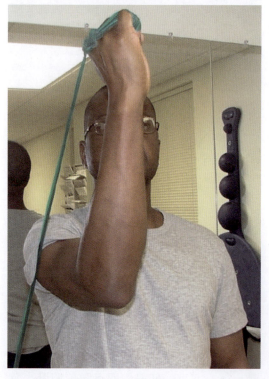

图13.11　使用弹力带进行前锯肌训练

如果疼痛得到适当的控制，关节达到全范围被动活动度，且患者能够正确地实施代偿性运动策略，医生就必须等待神经再生发生，并观察受影响肌肉的活动恢复。每间隔3～6周，随着患者体征或症状改善，重新评估上述测试以监测进展[8]。神经再生的体征应在LTNP和/或SANP发病后12周内明显。如果前锯肌和/或斜方肌在12周后仍然完全缺失，可以考虑手术治疗，特别是怀疑是神经断伤，但通常选择保守治疗6～12个月的情况[8, 9, 15, 16]。需要重申的是，大多数LTNP和SANP患者在24个月内就能治愈，无须手术干预[9, 12, 14-18]。为了使患者的治疗获得成功，医生必须给患者提供全面的教育，患者必须完全理解，必须执行医生布置的家庭训练方案，必须保持耐心，因为神经再生依赖时间。

受累肌肉再训练

一旦出现神经再生的体征，就可以逐渐开始训练前锯肌和/或斜方肌。应选择能成功收缩受累肌肉的运动，以培养适当的运动习惯[32]。直到能连贯完成正确的动作后，这些训练才可以进阶。为了促进运动控制，每天每隔一小时完成一次医生布置的特定家庭训练方案[32]。解决LTNP的前锯肌激活开始于前锯肌分离，要求患者站立位，手臂放在一侧，肱骨保持外旋位，同时肩胛骨前伸并轻微上抬[36]（图13.12）。随着前锯肌获得更大的运动控制，肩胛骨前屈伴前伸训练可以先健侧卧位后仰卧位，先屈肘后伸肘，以增加杠杆臂。在桌上向前滚动球伴肩胛骨前伸训练，可进阶至一个倾斜的表面，最后进阶到墙上。在矢状面，手臂放在墙上向上滑动伴外旋，将显著激活前锯肌（图13.13）。过头前屈伴前伸进阶至垂直位抵抗重力然后抗阻，再进阶至仰卧位肩胛骨前屈伴前伸、D1屈曲模式、肩胛骨平面屈曲至125°和俯卧撑伴前伸[21, 42, 44, 49]（图13.14）。随着SANP患者表现出神经再生，可以开始训练斜方肌。划船可以训练斜方肌整体[42]，然后进阶至仰卧位中、下斜方肌等长训练、侧卧位肩胛骨外旋和前屈，重点是促进斜方肌活动（图13.15）。最后，俯卧位肩水平外展伴外旋、俯卧位伸展和俯卧位抗重力过头抬起[29-31, 36, 42, 44]（图13.16）。

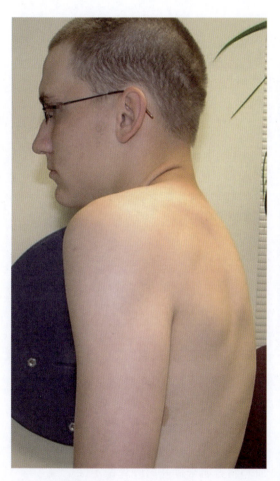

图13.12　前锯肌分离

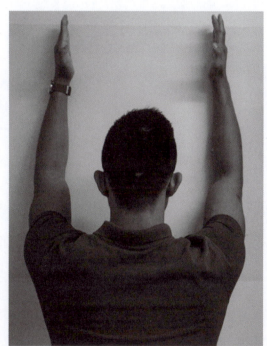

图13.13　墙上前锯肌训练

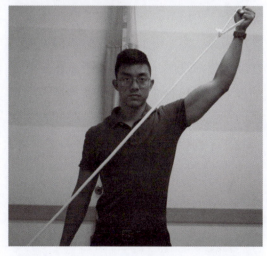

图13.14　D1屈曲模式

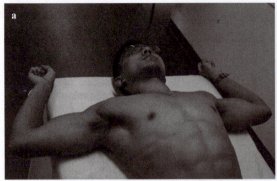
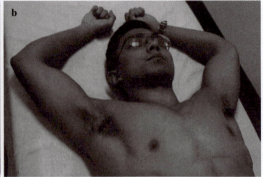

图13.15 中斜方肌（a）和下斜方肌（b）等长训练

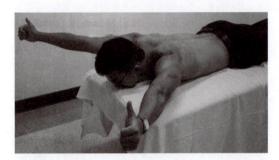

图13.16 俯卧位，过头抬起

结论

LTNP 和 / 或 SANP 患者的康复需要系统性和规律化。虽然医生不能加速神经再生的过程，但是医生可以创造一种环境，鼓励使用现有的肌肉组织来改善症状和增加功能，并且不会对所有相关结构造成过度的应力。为了确定所涉及的结构和监测神经再生的进展，有必要进行具体、全面的评估和定期的再评估。随着神经再生和肌肉再激活的体征变得明显，受影响的肌肉应进行循序渐进的训练。

附件

见表13.3、13.4、13.5和13.6。

表13.3 胸长神经麻痹患者的代偿策略

阶段1
俯卧位，划船
俯卧位，肩水平外展伴外旋
俯卧位，肩水平外展伴内旋
俯卧位，过头抬起，伴下斜方肌训练
站立位，耸肩
肩展30°后伸
坐位，划船
肩内收伴伸展
侧卧位，肩外旋
阶段2
俯卧位，伸展
俯卧位，肩外展90°伴外旋
侧卧位，肩屈曲
坐位，肩胛骨平面屈曲至80°
坐位划船
坐位，肩外展90°
割草机训练

在前锯肌缺失的情况下，应训练菱形肌和斜方肌来提高肩胛骨稳定性。

表13.4 胸长神经麻痹患者受累肌肉再训练

阶段3
坐位，肩屈曲至125°
坐位，肩胛骨平面屈曲至125°
坐位，对角线模式（肩屈曲、水平内收、外旋）
坐位，高划船

（续表）

墙上俯卧撑
仰卧位，肩屈曲 90° +
肩胛骨上抬伴抗阻外旋
阶段 4
肩部推举
墙上俯卧撑 +
桌上俯卧撑 +
肘部俯卧撑 +
膝部俯卧撑 +
地上俯卧撑 +

激活前锯肌来解决 LTNP。

表 13.5　副神经麻痹患者的代偿策略

阶段 1
墙上俯卧撑 +
桌上俯卧撑 +
肘部俯卧撑 +
膝部俯卧撑 +
地上俯卧撑 +
仰卧位，肩屈曲 90° +
阶段 2
坐位，肩屈曲至 125°
坐位，肩胛骨平面屈曲至 125°
肩部推举
肩外展 30° 伴伸展
肩内收伴伸展
坐位，肩外展

训练菱形肌和前锯肌来代偿斜方肌。

表 13.6　副神经麻痹患者受累肌肉再训练

阶段 3
坐位，对角线模式（肩屈曲、水平内收、外旋）
割草机训练
坐姿划船
高划船
低划船
侧卧位，肩屈曲
侧卧位，肩外旋

（续表）

肩胛骨上抬伴抗阻外旋
阶段 4
站立位，耸肩
俯卧位，肩外展至 90° 伴外旋
俯卧位，伸展
俯卧位，肩水平外展伴内旋
俯卧位，肩水平外展伴外旋
俯卧位，过头抬起，在下斜方肌力线方向
侧卧位，肩外旋

SANP 患者表现出神经再生，可以开始训练斜方肌。

（刘燕平）

参考文献

1. Chan PK, Hems TE. Clinical signs of accessory nerve palsy. J Trauma, 2006, 60(5): 1142–1144.

2. Donner TR, Kline DG. Extracranial spinal accessory nerve injury. Neurosurgery, 1993, 32(6): 907–910, discussion 11.

3. Duncan MA, Lotze MT, Gerber LH, et al. Incidence, recovery, and management of serratus anterior muscle palsy after axillary node dissection. Phys Ther, 1983, 63(8): 1243–1247.

4. Ebraheim NA, Lu J, Porshinsky B, et al. Vulnerability of long thoracic nerve: an anatomic study. J Shoulder Elbow Surg, 1998, 7(5): 458–461.

5. Ewing MR, Martin H. Disability following radical neck dissection, an assessment based on the postoperative evaluation of 100 patients. Cancer, 1952, 5(5): 873–883.

6. Gregg JR, Labosky D, Harty M, et al. Serratus anterior paralysis in the young athlete. J Bone Joint Surg Am, 1979, 61(6A): 825–832.

7. Kelley MJ, Kane TE, Leggin BG. Spinal accessory nerve palsy: associated signs and symptoms. J Or-

thop Sports Phys Ther, 2008, 38(2): 78–86.

8. Kuhn JE, Plancher KD, Hawkins RJ. Scapular winging. J Am Acad Orthop Surg, 1995, 3(6): 319–325.

9. Martin RM, Fish DE. Scapular winging: anatomical review, diagnosis, and treatments. Curr Rev Muscoskelet Med, 2008, 1(1): 1–11.

10. McGarvey AC, Osmotherly PG, Hoffman GR, et al. Scapular muscle exercises following neck dissection surgery for head and neck cancer: a comparative electromyographic study. Phys Ther, 2013, 93(6): 786–797.

11. Pikkarainen V, Kettunen J, Vastamäki M. The natural course of serratus palsy at 2 to 31 years. Clin Orthop Relat Res, 2013, 471(5): 1555–1563.

12. Safran MR. Nerve injury about the shoulder in athletes. Am J Sports Med, 2004, 32(4): 1063–1076.

13. Vastamäki M, Kauppila LI. Etiologic factors in isolated paralysis of the serratus anterior muscle: a report of 197 cases. J Shoulder Elbow Surg, 1993, 2(5): 240–243.

14. Watson CJ, Schenkman M. Physical therapy management of isolated serratus anterior muscle paralysis. Phys Ther, 1995, 75(3): 194–202.

15. Wiater JM, Bigliani LU. Spinal accessory nerve injury. Clin Orthop Relat Res, 1999, 368: 5–16.

16. Wiater JM, Flatow EL. Long thoracic nerve injury. Clin Orthop Relat Res, 1999, 368: 17–27.

17. Friedenberg SM, Zimprich T, Harper CM. The natural history of long thoracic and spinal accessory neuropathies. Muscle Nerve, 2002, 25(4): 535–539.

18. Warner JJ, Navarro RA. Serratus anterior dysfunction: recognition and treatment. Clin Orthop Relat Res, 1998, 349: 139–148.

19. Bertelli JA, Ghizoni MF. Long thoracic nerve: anatomy and functional assessment. J Bone Joint Surg Am, 2005, 87(5): 993–998.

20. Cuadros CL, Driscoll CL, Rothkopf DM. The anatomy of the lower serratus anterior muscle: a fresh cadaver study. Plast Reconstr Surg, 1995, 95(1): 93–97, discussion 8–9.

21. Ekstrom RA, Bifulco KM, Lopau CJ, et al. Comparing the function of the up-per and lower parts of the serratus anterior muscle using surface electromyography. J Orthop Sports Phys Ther, 2004, 34(5): 235–243.

22. Bagg SD, Forrest WJ. Electromyographic study of the scapular rotators during arm abduction in the scapular plane. Am J Phys Med, 1986, 65(3): 111–124.

23. Cools AM, Witvrouw EE, Declercq GA, et al. Evaluation of isokinetic force production and associated muscle activity in the scapular rotators during a protraction-retraction movement in overhead athletes with impingement symptoms. Br J Sports Med, 2004, 38(1): 64–68.

24. Inman VT, Saunders JB, Abbott LC. Observations of the function of the shoulder joint. Clin Orthop Relat Res, 1996, 330: 3–12.

25. Kibler WB. The role of the scapula in athletic shoulder function. Am J Sports Med, 1998, 26(2): 325–337.

26. Ludewig PM, Cook TM, Nawoczenski DA. Three-dimensional scapular orientation and muscle activity at selected positions of humeral elevation. J Orthop Sports Phys Ther, 1996, 24(2): 57–65.

27. Maenhout A, van Praet K, Pizzi L, et al. Electromyographic analysis of knee push up plus variations: what is the influence of the kinetic chain on scapular muscle activity? Br J Sports Med, 2010, 44(14): 1010–1015.

28. Jobe CM, Kropp WE, Wood VE. Spinal accessory nerve in a trapezius-splitting surgical approach. J Shoulder Elbow Surg, 1996, 5(3): 206–208.

29. de Mey K, Cagnie B, Danneels LA, et al. Trapezius muscle timing during selected shoulder rehabilitation exercises. J Orthop Sports Phys Ther, 2009, 39(10): 743–752.

30. Moseley JB, Jobe FW, Pink M, et al. EMG analysis of the scapular muscles during a shoulder rehabilitation program. Am J Sports Med, 1992, 20(2): 128–134.

31. Cools AM, Dewitte V, Lanszweert F, et al. Rehabilitation of scapular muscle balance: which exercises to prescribe? Am J Sports Med, 2007, 35(10): 1744–1751.

32. Magarey ME, Jones MA. Dynamic evaluation and early management of altered motor control around the shoulder complex. Man Ther, 2003, 8(4): 195–206.

33. Cools AM, Witvrouw EE, Declercq GA, et al. Scapular muscle recruitment patterns: trapezius muscle latency with and without impingement symptoms. Am J Sports Med, 2003, 31(4): 542–549.

34. McClure P, Tate AR, Kareha S, et al. A clinical method for identifying scapular dyskinesis. J Athl Train, 2009, 44(2): 160–164.

35. Uhl TL, Kibler WB, Gecewich B, et al. Evaluation of clinical assessment methods for scapular dyskinesis. Arthroscopy, 2009, 25(11): 1240–1248.

36. Ekstrom RA, Soderberg GL, Donatelli RA. Normalization procedures using maximum voluntary isometric contractions for the serratus anterior and trapezius muscles during surface EMG analysis. J Electromyogr Kinesiol, 2005, 15(4): 418–428.

37. Kendall FP, McCreary EK, Provance P. Muscles, testing and function: with posture and pain. 4th ed. Baltimore: Williams & Wilkins, 1993.

38. Michener LA, Boardman ND, Pidcoe PE, et al. Scapular muscle tests in subjects with shoulder pain and functional loss: reliability and construct validity. Phys Ther, 2005, 85(11): 1128–1138.

39. Thigpen CA, Padua DA, Michener LA, et al. Head and shoulder posture affect scapular mechanics and muscle activity in overhead tasks. J Electromyogr Kinesiol, 2010, 20(4): 701–709.

40. Wegner S, Jull G, O'Leary S, et al. The effect of a scapular postural correction strategy on trapezius activity in patients with neck pain. Man Ther, 2010, 15(6): 562–566.

41. Castelein B, Cagnie B, Parlevliet T, et al. Scapulothoracic muscle activity during elevation exercises measured with surface and fine wire EMG: a comparative study between patients with subacromial impingement syndrome and healthy controls. Man Ther, 2016, 23: 33–39.

42. Ekstrom RA, Donatelli RA, Soderberg GL. Surface electromyographic analysis of exercises for the trapezius and serratus anterior muscles. J Orthop Sports Phys Ther, 2003, 33(5): 247–258.

43. Smith J, Padgett DJ, Kaufman KR, et al. Rhomboid muscle electromyography activity during 3 different manual muscle tests. Arch Phys Med Rehabil, 2004, 85(6): 987–992.

44. Castelein B, Cagnie B, Parlevliet T, et al. Optimal normalization tests for mus-cle activation of the levator scapulae, pectoralis minor, and rhomboid major: an electromyography study using maximum voluntary isometric contractions. Arch Phys Med Rehabil, 2015, 96(10): 1820–1827.

45. Castelein B, Cagnie B, Parlevliet T, et al. Superficial and deep scapulothoracic muscle elecromyographic activity during elevation exercises in the scapular plane. J Orthop Sports Phys Ther, 2016, 46(3): 184–193.

46. Kibler WB, Sciascia AD, Uhl TL, et al. Electromyographic analysis of specific exercises for scapular control in early phases of shoulder rehabilitation. Am J Sports Med, 2008, 36(9): 1789–1798.

47. Townsend H, Jobe FW, Pink M, et al. Electromyographic analysis of the glenohumeral muscles during a baseball rehabilitation program. Am J Sports Med, 1991, 19(3): 264–272.
48. de Mey K, Danneels LA, Cagnie B, et al. Conscious correction of scapular orientation in overhead athletes performing selected shoulder rehabilitation exercises: the effect on trapezius muscle activation measured by surface electromyography. J Orthop Sports Phys Ther, 2013, 43(1): 3–10.
49. Ludewig PM, Hoff MS, Osowski EE, et al. Relative balance of serratus anterior and upper trapezius muscle activity during push-up exercises. Am J Sports Med, 2004, 32(2): 484–493.

第14章　肩胛骨弹响综合征

George F. Lebus, Zaamin B. Hussain, Jonas Pogorzelski, Peter J. Millett

病理生理

肩胛骨弹响综合征（SSS）以前被描述为在肩胛带运动的过程中，凹形肩胛骨在凸形胸廓上的病理运动，由肩胛胸壁异常生物力学产生的声音和可触知的捻发音可能通过胸腔放大[1]。这种不正常的接触可能是由于常见的解剖结构异常，也可能是由于正常肩胛胸壁的过度使用。目前认为SSS的三种主要病因类型为慢性滑囊炎、肌肉功能障碍和解剖结构异常[2]。

慢性过度使用，特别是从事过头运动的运动员，在没有诱发解剖结构异常的情况下会产生滑囊和周围肌肉组织的炎症，这会导致反应性滑囊炎和随后的瘢痕形成。肩胛胸壁有6个已知的滑囊，2个通常被认为是生理性的，4个小的（或外膜的）滑囊不一定存在，可能与病理运动有关[3]。两个主要的滑囊是前锯肌和胸壁之间的下锯滑囊及前锯肌和肩胛下肌之间的上锯滑囊（图14.1）。这两个滑囊是公认的，已经在关节镜检查和尸体研究中反复发现。另外4个外膜滑囊是在肩胛骨上角的下锯滑囊、上锯滑囊和在肩胛骨下角的滑囊，以及在肩胛骨内侧和上覆斜方肌之间的一个更浅的滑囊。SSS中最常累及的滑囊是在肩胛骨上角的滑囊[4]。在SSS这样的慢性炎症环境中，刺激会导致滑囊炎和瘢痕形成的恶性循环，从而产生撞击、疼痛和进一步的炎症。继发瘢痕的滑囊纤维化会导致疼痛，甚至在没有明显的骨质或软组织解剖异常的情况下，可导致机械性的、可闻及的弹响症状[2]。

肌肉功能失调也可导致SSS[5]，并可表现为生物力学异常、解剖结构变异或两者兼而有之。肩胛骨周围肌肉的协调性可能被肌肉无力、肩关节疾病、创伤或医源性神经损伤破坏，导致肩胛骨周围力偶的破坏和肩胛骨运动异常，从而导致肩胛骨和胸腔异常接触[3, 6]。在这种情况下，手臂前屈可能导致肩胛骨后倾，从而压缩肩胛骨下角和肋弓之间的空间[7]。与此相反，由于胸小肌病理性紧张造成的肩胛骨异常前倾可能会压迫肩胛骨上部和胸壁之间的空间[8]。肌肉萎缩、纤维化或插止点异常可能产生异常的肩胛骨生物力学，导致SSS。

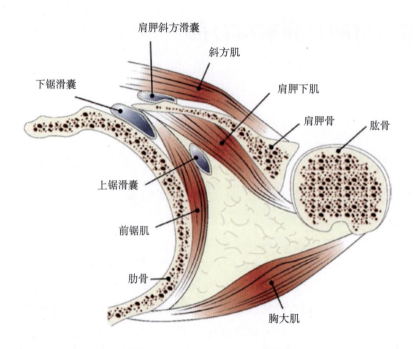

图 14.1 图示为肩胛骨在轴向平面的解剖[30]。两个主要的滑囊——上锯滑囊和下锯滑囊，是多数肩胛胸壁滑囊炎的主要病理来源，可以被甄别

最后，软组织的解剖变化，包括肩胛骨内侧缘的肩胛下肌较薄，可能导致肩胛骨对胸廓的摩擦[9, 10]。尸体研究中描述了肩胛下肌起点和前锯肌止点之间存在位于肩胛骨肋面内上方的裸露区域，并且可能在某些情况下发挥作用[6, 11]。导致SSS的骨骼异常包括解剖结构变异、创伤后状况和肿块病变。对89例肩胛骨弹响综合征进行研究的研究者认定，43%的病例存在骨骼异常[12]。解剖结构变异是最常见的骨结构异常亚组，涉及肩胛骨、胸廓或脊柱。最近的影像学分析表明，肩胛骨形态是弯曲型时，肩胛骨内侧缘向前成角和肩肋距离减少可能与SSS有关[13]。Luschka结节是肩胛骨上角或纤维软骨的突出部分，也被证明与SSS有关[14]。此外，在某些情况下，切除第一根肋骨治疗胸廓出口综合征会导致SSS[15]。关于脊柱异常，过度的胸椎后凸或脊柱侧弯可能是导致肩胛胸壁异常的原因[4]。尽管存在这些相关性，但许多解剖结构变异的患者无症状，因此必须考虑其临床表现[16]。创伤后状况包括肩胛骨或其下肋骨骨折畸形愈合，以及重复性肩胛骨周围肌肉损伤引起的反应性骨刺，这些都会破坏正常的关节[9, 17-19]。此外，肿瘤如骨软骨瘤、弹力纤维瘤和极少的软骨肉瘤也可能是病因，必须排除[20]。肩胛骨上最常见的良性肿瘤是骨软骨瘤[21]，它在文献中已被充分证实是SSS的病因，其中一份报告[12]表明肿块病变占SSS发病的16%。背部弹力纤维瘤可能会特别影响肩胛骨内下角的腹面，引起占位效应和异常生物力学[22]。

临床表现

SSS患者可能出现一系列症状，从轻度不适到有严重疼痛的肩部假性麻痹，伴有可闻及的捻发音。产生这种巨大差异主要是因为病因多样。

病史

肩胛骨滑囊炎或SSS患者通常会主诉疼痛、可触及的骨摩擦感或在运动时可听见弹响，尤其是上肢做抬举过头动作时。这些症状可能因人而异。应询问患者相关疼痛或不适的准确位置、性质和强度，以及其相关症状和加重、缓解因素。Cobey等人[18]的研究显示，SSS患者存在类似症状家族史，提示肩胛骨弹响可能存在遗传倾向。此外，还应注意患者期望的活动类型和以前的水平，以便进行适当的目标设定，有目的地进行康复训练。

体格检查

体格检查应从视诊患者姿势开始，因为已知明显的脊柱后凸会降低肩胛骨的协调性，并可能引起肩胛骨弹响，伴有或不伴有疼痛性滑囊炎[4]。所有患者都应进行颈椎评估，以排除因$C_5 \sim C_8$神经压迫引起的牵涉痛综合征[23, 24]。然后，对双侧肩胛骨进行动态评估，关注手臂经过一系列主动和被动运动时肩胛骨出现的任何不对称、运动障碍、翼状肩胛或可听见的捻发音等。值得注意的是，过头类项目运动员通常会出现优势侧肩胛骨下降、前伸和下旋，但这可能与他们的主诉无关[25]。

此外，肩胛骨运动障碍是肩胛胸壁滑囊炎患者的常见表现，可能是肩胛骨周围肌肉运动不平衡的结果，如前锯肌、斜方肌、肩胛提肌或胸小肌无力或紧张。翼状肩胛可由前锯肌无力引起，最常见的原因是胸长神经麻痹；也可由斜方肌无力或萎缩引起，原因是副神经麻痹。内上方的斜方肌和肩胛提肌紧张可能表现为颈部僵硬，可通过肌肉长度检查进行诊断。前面的胸小肌紧张可引起肩胛骨下降和前伸，可以通过观察患者处于仰卧位置时肩部距离检查台的高度差异来诊断，受影响的肩胛带比健侧的肩胛带高出床面更多[26, 27]。在同一位置评估胸小肌紧张度的另一种方法是将手放在肩前部，施加适度的从前向后的力，推压肩部至检查台时感觉到明显阻力的话提示胸小肌腱短缩。过头类项目运动员出现SICK时，医生应警惕其他相关诊断，包括GIRD、后上关节撞击或SLAP损伤，有可能是通过肩胛骨错位或运动异常的病理生理学改变导致了肩胛骨弹响[1]。

在肩胛骨周围区域触诊可发现与外膜下锯或上锯滑囊炎一致的局部压痛区域。肩胛骨的内上角和内下角是疼痛性滑囊的最常见位置[28]。将手臂置于"鸡翅"姿势，肱骨内旋，手背置于腰骶关节上方，使肩胛骨向外倾斜，可以实现深层触诊[28, 29]。一些患者在做激惹动作的时候，可产生肩胛骨捻发音。在这类情况下，在患者进行激惹动作时触诊肩胛骨有助于确定病变部位[30]。此外，在检查活动范围的过程中，在肩胛骨体上施加从后向前的力也可能导致肩胛骨体和后胸廓之间的捻发音更明显，并加重患者的症状[31]。

肩胛骨周围肌肉力量测试也应在单个肌肉上进行，以确定任何可能导致生物力学失衡、肩胛骨运动障碍或翼状肩胛，以及随之而来的弹响的原因。测试者应施加不同程度的阻力，并将所有阻力测试与对侧对比。斜方肌是通过让患者抗阻耸肩来评估的，然而检查肩胛提肌和菱形肌最好的方法是将患者的手放在同侧髂嵴上，随后使患者的手肘抗阻后推。检查前锯肌则是让患者进行墙壁俯卧撑，测试者视诊和触诊肩胛骨内侧缘。前锯肌无力将加剧肩胛骨内侧缘突起。患者手臂放在体侧抗阻后推，测试者触诊肩胛骨内下角，以此评估背阔肌。

影像学

X线检查

当怀疑肩胛骨弹响综合征时，首先应该进行X线检查，包括正位、Y位和腋位，以便临床医生排除骨骼异常。即使有足够的X线片，仍可能遗漏骨性解剖异常[32]。

CT

当X线检查或临床检查怀疑骨骼病变时，应做CT，以进一步明确病变[32]。年轻患者应避免常规CT，除非有影像学证据提示肩胛胸壁存在骨性或软骨性病变。

MRI

MRI对于识别可能导致肩胸捻发音或滑囊炎的软组织结构最为有用，例如纤维瘢痕组织（图14.2）、炎性组织或肌腱疾病。此外，组织成分分析可用于区分恶性和良性软组织病变[33]。

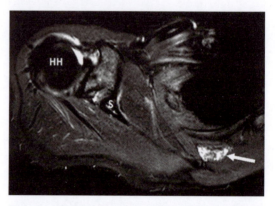

图14.2　SSS患者术前MRI（T_2加权）显示在肩胛骨内上角和胸廓之间产生炎症的纤维瘢痕组织（白色箭头）。HH代表肱骨头，S代表肩胛骨

肌电图

肌电图可用于评估原因不明的翼状肩胛或肩胛骨周围肌肉无力患者的肌肉神经支配是否正常。内侧肩胛翼可能由胸长神经损伤后前锯肌萎缩或无力所致，外侧肩胛翼可能由斜方肌萎缩、无力或副神经功能障碍所致。大多数胸长神经麻痹是创伤导致的，大多数副神经麻痹是颈部或面部手术的医源性损伤导致的[34]。关节镜通道位置异常可能是引起副神经功能障碍的一个极其罕见的原因，但应在适当的情况下考虑[2]。

诊断性注射

一般来说，局部注射麻醉剂和类固醇可以起到诊断和治疗作用。注射后疼痛的暂时缓解证实了滑囊炎的诊断，同时也精确定位了病变的滑囊。尽管患者能立即见到疗效，但这种效果很难长时间维持，虽然有报道称局部注射有长期疗效[35]。局部注射时，患者的体位是俯卧，肩关节伸展、内旋、内收成"鸡翅"姿势。消毒后，将无菌洞巾覆盖在肩胛骨内侧的皮肤上、压痛最明显处，针平行于肩胛骨前缘插入。医生必须明白，注射方向不正确会刺入胸腔。据文献报道，超声定位辅助肩胛骨注射可获得良好的结果[36]。

非手术治疗

除了存在恶性肿块病变的情况，无论SSS的病因为何，都需要先进行非手术治疗。如果SSS是在没有解剖结构异常的情况下由长期过度使用引起的，手术前应尝试6个月至1年的非手术治疗，预计成功率较高[37, 38]。如果SSS是由解剖结构损伤引起的，也仍然需要先进行保守治疗[4]，尽管手术切除或矫正异常解剖结构的治愈率更高[14, 39]。非手术治疗方案包括运动纠正、非甾体类抗炎药物、物理治疗和滑囊注射（类固醇和局部麻醉剂）。如果主要病因是过度使用和生物力学不平衡，患者必须首先纠正运动，以此来打破滑囊炎和瘢痕形成的恶性循环。物理治疗应侧重于肩胛骨周围肌肉强化和改善肩带生物力学。存在不良姿势的患者应进行减少后凸、促进直立姿势和强化上胸肌肉组织的训练。由于肩胛骨负责肩胛带的静态稳定，耐力训练对肩胛骨的稳定性至关重要。这种训练包括多重复的低强度训练。强化肩胛下肌和前锯肌减少了肩胛骨前倾，缓解了滑囊的压迫。肩胛骨内收和姿势性耸肩练习是加强肩胛骨稳定肌的关键，训练对象包括前锯肌、菱形肌和肩胛提肌。具体练习包括Scaption训练（肩胛骨平面的哑铃负重外展训练，可强化肩袖和三角肌）、俯卧撑和俯卧撑+、划船和机械划船，以及球上等长肩胛骨稳定练习。肩胛骨外展和上抬会增加深层肌肉组织的压力和张力，因此应避免[40]。

手术治疗

适应证

非手术治疗后效果不佳的患者可考虑手术治疗。外科手术可为注射后症状暂时缓解的患者或有导致症状的解剖结构异常的患者提供更可靠的疗效[38, 41]。在大多数情况下，可行关节镜手术，然而，对于较大的肿块病变，切开手术可以提供更好的视野并直接切除，防止肿瘤细胞不必要的扩散。关节镜手术提供了更快的术后恢复和康复过程[30, 42]。具体的手术方法因患者的主诉和解剖结构异常而异，但通常手术都需要切除病变滑囊，伴或不伴肩胛骨内上角的部分切除。一些报道证明仅切除滑囊就有良好的疗效[43]；然而，部分肩胛骨切除加上滑囊切除更为常见，尤其是在有机械性捻发音的情况下[29, 44]。

关节镜手术

手术前，应确认患者最疼痛的部位，最大限度地提高手术成功率。在对患者进行麻醉诱导之前，可以用记号笔标记这些疼痛部位。患者采取俯卧位，健侧手臂放在身体侧面（图14.3a）。后背铺巾，并将手术侧用无菌弹力绷带包裹。手术侧的手放于背部，有效地将肩关节置于"鸡翅"姿势，使其伸展并接近最大内旋。这个体位通过增加肩胛骨和胸壁之间的潜在空间来帮助建立通道。可以通过在外侧肩上施加一个向内的力来做进一步的分离，使鞘管在肩胛骨体上安置。骨性标志包括肩胛骨内侧缘和肩胛冈。通道（图14.3b）位于肩胛骨内侧缘内侧3 cm处，并保持在肩胛冈下方，以降低肩胛背神经和动脉主要分支受伤的风险。这种内侧入口的进入方式允许关节镜平行于胸壁进入滑囊，从而降低胸腔破裂的风险。

在肩胛骨下角内侧3 cm处做一个初始观察通道，引入一个30°关节镜（图14.3b）。灌洗液体压力通常保持在50 mmHg或以下。第二个通道（图14.3b）通过三角形定位，位于肩胛骨内侧3 cm处、肩胛冈内侧汇合处的下方。一旦视野足够，就进行诊断性内镜检查。从下方检查肋间肌和肋骨，从外侧检查肩胛下肌，从内侧检查菱形肌和肩胛提肌。穿刺针沿着肩胛骨内上缘放置协助定位。使用刨刀或射频消融器清除滑囊和纤维组织，暴露肩胛骨上缘骨质，不切除肩胛下肌的肌性部分。接下来，用钝性穿刺头穿过上后锯肌（图14.4a），进入上锯滑囊。

用射频探头或关节镜刀移除肌肉来暴露肩胛骨内上角（图14.4b、c）。如果暴露肩胛骨内上角后肩胛骨的捻发音或弹响

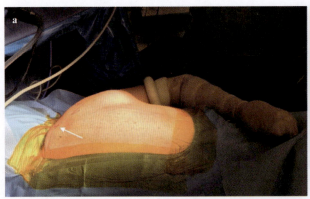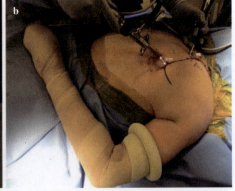

图14.3 （a）右侧肩胛骨和手臂的术中图片，摆成"鸡翅"位。术前，最大压痛点做位置标记（白色箭头）（b）术中右侧肩胛骨的图片，包括肩胛骨内侧缘的骨性标志被标记。入路放置在肩胛骨内侧3 cm处，以最大限度地降低神经血管结构损伤的风险

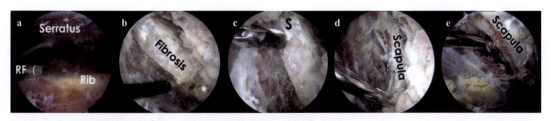

图 14.4 （a）射频（RF）装置移除在肩胸间隙产生炎症的滑囊组织。头端是后上锯肌（Serratus），尾端为肋弓（Rib）（b）纤维瘢痕组织（Fibrosis）被射频装置切除（c）关节镜刀用来切除更多的软组织以松解肩胛骨（S）边缘（d）完成后，肩胛骨（Scapula）内上角可见，部分被切除（e）肩胛骨（Scapula）内上角切除后的最终图片

仍存在，放置穿刺针以标记计划切除的范围。用一个高速钻进行关节镜下的肩胛骨成形术（图 14.4d），移除大约 2 cm（上下径）×3 cm（内外径）的三角形骨段。切除范围是通过关节镜下切除的肩胛骨边缘凸度来确定的。按常规，在患者仍处于麻醉状态时，对肩胛骨进行动态检查，以确保有足够的切除范围，而不会遗留机械性捻发音。如果切除部位太靠外侧，肩胛上神经可能会被损伤，因此，使用关节镜切除肩胛骨不应该超过穿刺针标记的范围。从两个通道视野确认切除充分且平滑（图 14.4e）。因为肩胛骨很薄，所以通常使用锉刀来打磨切除的边缘。在整个活动范围内对手臂进行动态测试，以确保不会出现机械性捻发音[31]。

上方辅助通道可以用来协助切除肩胛骨内上方。这个通道应位于肩胛骨内上角和外侧肩峰之间距离的内 1/3 和外 2/3 的交界处，以保护肩胛上神经和动脉。套管针从内侧和尾侧方向进入，外科医生应该将其密切靠近肩胛骨前部，以避免刺破胸腔[44]。最后，常规关闭入路，术后使用悬吊（表 14.1）。

表 14.1 关节镜下肩胸滑囊切除术拾珍和隐患

	拾珍	隐患
通道	放在肩胛骨内侧缘的内侧 3 cm 处	通道位置太靠外有损伤肩胛背神经和动脉的风险
	在肩胛冈下方	位置太向上有损伤副神经的风险
切除滑囊	以基本平行胸壁的角度切除	过于垂直的角度可能会刺穿胸腔
切除骨头	用穿刺针标记准备切除部分的最外端，在切除前清除骨骼以便达到足够的视野	切除位置太靠外会使肩胛上神经处于危险之中。切除太多可能导致肌肉被破坏和功能障碍
出血	在完成前降低泵压力以获得较好的止血效果	不足的止血方法可能导致术后疼痛性血肿

开放手术

手术前，应定位并标记患者疼痛的精确位置，以便进行手术计划，因为手术可能因患者疼痛的位置而有所不同。肩胛胸壁滑囊炎的最常见部位是肩胛骨内上角[28]。因此，对于大多数患者而言，开放手术通常需要在肩胛骨内上缘进行垂直切口（图

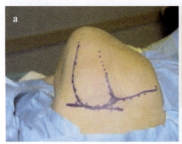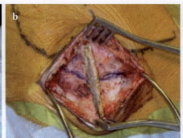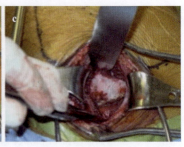

图14.5 （a）术中图片显示了皮肤上标记的上内侧缘、肩胛冈和内侧缘骨性标志，也标记了用于肩胛胸壁滑囊炎开放手术的上内侧缘垂直切口位置 （b）皮肤切口回缩，向下剥离至斜方肌筋膜和肌肉，与其纤维平行横向分开 （c）斜方肌纤维向头端回缩，抬高骨膜下的菱形肌、肩胛提肌、冈上肌和冈下肌，暴露出骨切除的部位

14.5a）。患者置于俯卧位，横向分离肌肉与纤维，向下剥离至斜方肌筋膜和肌肉（图14.5b）。斜方肌纤维向头端回缩，显示出深层的止于肩胛骨内侧缘的菱形肌和肩胛提肌。仔细地沿着肩胛骨内上角，在骨膜下提起这些肌肉及冈上肌、冈下肌，从而暴露骨切除的位置（图14.5c）。摆锯切除肩胛骨内上角，随后进行滑囊切除术（图14.6a、b）。骨切除（图14.6c）总长度通常为 2 cm（上下径）×3 cm（内外径）。在骨切除后，术中进行动态评估，以确认肩胛骨和胸壁之间没有撞击。一旦切除充分，通过肩胛骨内侧缘的骨隧道修复菱形肌和肩胛提肌（图14.7a）。然后以标准的分层方式[4, 30]缝合切口（图14.7b、c），术后患者使用吊带。

在肩胛骨下角的滑囊炎是第二常见肩胛胸壁滑囊炎，切口斜于肩胛骨下侧。切口建立后，向下剥离至筋膜，顺着纤维方向切开下斜方肌和背阔肌，从而暴露并切除滑囊。仔细地除去肩胛骨下缘的任何骨突，然后以标准方式关闭切口[4]。

术后康复

术后康复的过程取决于手术是关节镜手术还是开放手术。对于需要进行骨切除和肌肉修复的开放手术患者，肩部通常固定4周，以便肌肉愈合。之后不久可以开始肩胛骨的被动运动，强调肩胸松动，8周时开始主动运动，12周时开始肌力训练[30]。接受开放手术且不需要通过骨隧道修复肌肉的患者，康复过程可以更快，被动运动在术后立即开始，主动运动在3～4周后，在患者能耐受的情况下可以开始肌力训练[42]。接受关节镜手术的患者在术后具有最少的限制并且恢复最快。他们使用吊带24～48小时，然后在医生允许的情况下开始上肢的被动和主动运动。早期肩胛胸壁松动非常重要。物理治疗主要关注胸部姿势、肩胛骨协调性和力量。关节镜手术1周后可以进行完全主动运动，预期术后2～4周可完全康复；然而，即使患者似乎已经完全恢复，重返运动和过头活动也应该延迟到术后2～3个月进行，以加强切口愈合[30, 42]。

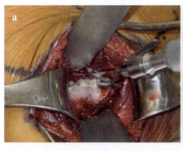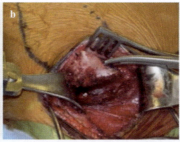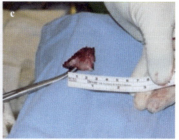

图14.6 （a）用锯来割除内上角 （b）取出被切除的骨性部分 （c）被取出的骨性部分一般是2 cm（上下径）×3 cm（内外径）

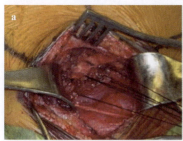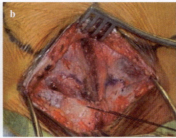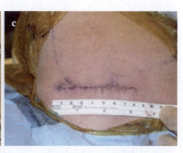

图14.7 （a）切除之后，通过肩胛骨内侧缘的骨隧道仔细修补菱形肌和肩胛提肌 （b）切口以标准分层的方式关闭 （c）切口长度显示为8 cm

手术结局

关节镜手术

几项研究报告了关节镜手术与开放手术或半开放手术对比的相似临床结果。1999年，Harper等人[45]是最早使用关节镜做肩胛骨部分切除术的研究者，他们报告了7名患者在平均7个月的随访中疼痛和功能有显著改善。Lehtinen等人[43]评估了16名经关节镜手术或开放手术的滑囊炎患者，在平均3年的随访中，81%的患者满意，简单肩关节测试为9.8，两种手术方法的患者满意度无统计学差异[43]。后来，Pearse等人[39]报告了13名因滑囊炎或撞击综合征而在关节镜下手术的患者的结果，其中3名进行了额外的肩胛骨内上段切除术。平均随访18.5个月，13名患者中有9名（69.2%）显示疼痛和功能改善，术后平均Constant量表评分为87分（范围58~95分）。Millett等人[31]至少随访2年的研究显示，在关节镜手术（包括或不包括肩胛骨成形术）后，23名患者的疼痛和功能均有所改善。然而，尽管有改善，但这些患者的满意度中位数只有6/10。两名患者未进行肩胛骨成形术，尽管这两名患者症状有所改善，但他们不如那些接受了骨切除的患者满意。研究者推测关节镜下骨切除可以允许更完整的滑囊切除。Blond和Rechter[46]认为，在关节镜下滑囊切除术和肩胛骨成形术后，患者的症状有显著改善。平均随访2.9年，20名患者中的18名（90%）报告疼痛和功能比术前基线值有所改善，其中西安大略肩袖指数（WORC）的中位数从术前的35提高到术后的86.4。最近，Menge等人[47]的研究显示，74名SSS患者中有60名（81%）进行了滑囊切除术和肩胛骨成形术，取得了良好的结果。术前至术后各结果评分均显著改善：SF-12PCS由39.2分提高到45.4分，ASES从52.6分提高到75.8分，QuickDASH从40.2分下降到24.2分。术前精神状态评分越低、症状持续时间越长、年龄越大，术后结局评分越低[47]。

开放手术

1950年，Milch第一次记录了3名SSS患者的手术技术和部分肩胛骨切除术的结果[48]。从那时起，有大量研究显示肩胛骨内上角切除术的良好结局，特别是那些倾向解剖结构变异或骨骼病变的患者[7, 12, 43, 49-53]。事实上，Arntz和Matsen[7]报告了14名SSS患者中的12名（86%）因骨形态异常或肩胛胸壁不协调而接受了开放肩胛骨内上角切除术，结局良好。值得注意的是，研究人员还对切除的骨进行了组织学检查，没有发现异常，这与其他研究者的发现不一致[28, 41, 50]。

无影像学或手术证据的骨异常但有症状的患者可以单纯切除滑囊而不切除肩胛骨内上角。McCluskey和Bigliani[54]报道了9名SSS患者中有8名（89%）在单独的上锯滑囊切除术后获得了良好的结果。Nicholson和Duckworth[41]跟踪了17名患者，在滑囊切除术后平均2.5年，17名患者中有5名（29.4%）接受了额外的肩胛骨内上角切除术。研究者注意到，肩胛骨内上角切除允许更完整的滑囊切除，同时减轻了骨撞击。患者症状缓解，表现为ASES有显著改善。然而，较少的样本量限制了各组之间的比较分析。

虽然不太常见，但在肩胛骨下角的滑囊炎也可能发生，并且是对患者困扰最大的部位。Sisto和Jobe[55]报道了4名职业棒球投手在优势侧肩胛骨内下角进行开放切除术后取得的良好成绩，他们的投球恢复到职业水平，而且没有进一步的问题。

（陈翰）

参考文献

1. Burkhart SS, Morgan CD, Kibler WB. The disabled throwing shoulder: spectrum of pathology. Arthroscopy, 2003, 19(6): 641–661.
2. Warth RJ, Spiegl UJ, Millett PJ. Scapulothoracic bursitis and snapping scapula syndrome: a critical review of current evidence. Am J Sports Med, 2015, 43(1): 236–245.
3. Kuhn JE. Disorders of the shoulder: diagnosis and management. Philadelphia: Lippincott Williams & Wilkins, 1999.
4. Kuhn JE, Plancher KD, Hawkins RJ. Symptomatic scapulothoracic crepitus and bursitis. J Am Acad Orthop Surg, 1998, 6(5): 267–273.
5. Grunfeld G. Beitrag zur Genese des Skapularkrachens und der Ska-puloargeraushe. Arch Orthop J Unfall Chir, 1927, 24: 610–615.
6. Frank RM, Ramirez JM, Chalmers P, et al. Scapulothoracic anatomy and snapping scapula syndrome. Anat Res Int, 2013, 2013(3):635628.
7. Arntz C, Matsen F. Partial scapulectomy for dis-

abling scapulothoracic snapping. Orthop Trans, 1990, 14: 252–253.

8. Frank DK, Wenk E, Stern JC, et al. A cadaveric study of the motor nerves to the levator scapulae muscle. Otolaryngol Head Neck Surg, 1998, 117(6): 671–680.

9. Datir A, James SLJ, Ali K, et al. MRI of soft-tissue masses: the relationship between lesion size, depth, and diagnosis. Clin Radiol, 2008, 63(4): 373–380.

10. Haney TC. Subscapular elastofibroma in a young pitcher. A case report. Am J Sports Med, 1990, 18(6): 642–644.

11. Boyle MJ, Misur P, Youn SM, et al. The superomedial bare area of the costal scapula surface: a possible cause of snapping scapula syndrome. Surg Radiol Anat, 2013, 35(2): 95–98.

12. Carlson HL, Haig AJ, Stewart DC. Snapping scapula syndrome: three case reports and an analysis of the literature. Arch Phys Med Rehabil, 1997, 78(5): 506–511.

13. Spiegl UJ, Petri M, Smith SW, et al. Association between scapula bony morphology and snapping scapula syndrome. J Shoulder Elbow Surg, 2015, 24(8): 1289–1295.

14. Milch H. Snapping scapula. Clin Orthop, 1961, 20: 139–150.

15. Wood VE, Verska JM. The snapping scapula in association with the thoracic outlet syndrome. Arch Surg, 1989, 124(11): 1335–1337.

16. Higuchi T, Ogose A, Hotta T, et al. Clinical and imaging features of distended scapulothoracic bursitis: spontaneously regressed pseudotumoral lesion. J Comput Assist Tomogr, 2004, 28(2): 223–228.

17. Ciullo J. Subscapular bursitis: treatment of "snapping scapula" or "wash-board" syndrome. Arthroscopy, 1992, 8: 412–413.

18. Cobey MC. The rolling scapula. Clin Orthop Relat Res, 1968, 60: 193–194.

19. Codman E. The shoulder. Malabar: Krieger Publishing, 1984.

20. Kibler WB, Chandler TJ. Range of motion in junior tennis players participating in an injury risk modification program. J Sci Med Sport, 2003, 6(1): 51–62.

21. Galate JF, Blue JM, Gaines RW. Osteochondroma of the scapula. Mo Med, 1995, 92(2): 95–97.

22. Cinar BM, Akpinar S, Derincek A, et al. Elastofibroma dorsi: an unusual cause of shoulder pain. Acta Orthop Traumatol Turc, 2009, 43(5): 431–435.

23. Brown C. Compressive, invasive referred pain to the shoulder. Clin Orthop Relat Res, 1983, 173: 55–62.

24. Makin GJ, Brown WF, Ebers GC. C_7 radiculopathy: importance of scapular winging in clinical diagnosis. J Neurol Neurosurg Psychiatry, 1986, 49(6): 640–644.

25. Priest JD, Nagel DA. Tennis shoulder. Am J Sports Med, 1976, 4(1): 28–42.

26. Borstad JD, Ludewig PM. The effect of long versus short pectoralis minor resting length on scapular kinematics in healthy individuals. J Orthop Sports Phys Ther, 2005, 35(4): 227–238.

27. Muraki T, Aoki M, Izumi T, et al. Lengthening of the pectoralis minor muscle during passive shoulder motions and stretching techniques: a cadaveric biomechanical study. Phys Ther, 2009, 89(4): 333–341.

28. O'Holleran J, Millett PJ, Warner JJ. Textbook of arthroscopy. Philadelphia: WB Saunders, 2004.

29. Millett PJ, Pacheco IH, Gobezie R. Management of recalcitrant scapulothoracic bursitis: endoscopic scapulothoracic bursectomy and scapuloplasty. Tech Should Elbow Surg, 2006, 7: 200–205.

30. Gaskill T, Millett PJ. Snapping scapula syndrome: diagnosis and management. J Am Acad Orthop Surg, 2013, 21(4): 214–224.
31. Millett PJ, Gaskill TR, Horan MP, et al. Technique and outcomes of arthroscopic scapulothoracic bursectomy and partial scapulectomy. Arthroscopy, 2012, 28(12): 1776–1783.
32. Mozes G, Bickels J, Ovadia D, et al. The use of three-dimensional computed tomography in evaluating snapping scapula syndrome. Orthopedics, 1999, 22(11): 1029–1033.
33. Ken O, Hatori M, Kokubun S. The MRI features and treatment of scapulothoracic bursitis: report of four cases. Ups J Med Sci, 2004, 109(1): 57–64.
34. Srikumaran U, Wells JH, Freehill MT, et al. Scapular winging: a great masquerader of shoulder disorders: AAOS exhibit selection. J Bone Joint Surg Am, 2014, 96(14): e122.
35. Percy EC, Birbrager D, Pitt MJ. Snapping scapula: a review of the literature and presentation of 14 patients. Can J Surg, 1988, 31(4): 248–250.
36. Hodler J, Gilula LA, Ditsios KT, et al. Fluoroscopically guided scapulothoracic injections. Am J Roentgenol, 2003, 181(5): 1232–1234.
37. Lesprit E, Huec JC, Moinard M, et al. Snapping scapula syndrome: conservative and surgical treatment. Eur J Orthop Surg Traumatol, 2001, 11: 51–54.
38. Manske RC, Reiman MP, Stovak ML. Nonoperative and operative management of snapping scapula. Am J Sports Med, 2004, 32(6): 1554–1565.
39. Pearse EO, Bruguera J, Massoud SN, et al. Arthroscopic management of the painful snapping scapula. Arthroscopy, 2006, 22(7): 755–761.
40. Groh G, Simoni MDM, Allen T, et al. Treatment of snapping scapula with a periscapular muscle strengthening program. J Shoulder Elbow Surg, 1996, 5(2): S6.
41. Nicholson GP, Duckworth MA. Scapulothoracic bursectomy for snapping scapula syndrome. J Shoulder Elbow Surg, 2002, 11(1): 80–85.
42. Kuhne M, Boniquit N, Ghodadra N, et al. The snapping scapula: diagnosis and treatment. Arthroscopy, 2009, 25(11): 1298–1311.
43. Lehtinen JT, Macy JC, Cassinelli E, et al. The painful scapulothoracic articulation: surgical management. Clin Orthop Relat Res, 2004, 423: 99–105.
44. van Riet R, Bell S. Scapulothoracic arthroscopy. Tech Should Elbow Surg, 2006, 7: 143–146.
45. Harper GD, McIroy S, Bayley JI, et al. Arthroscopic partial resection of the scapula for snapping scapula: a new technique. J Shoulder Elbow Surg, 1999, 8(1): 53–57.
46. Blond L, Rechter S. Arthroscopic treatment for snapping scapula: a prospective case series. Eur J Orthop Surg Traumatol, 2014, 24(2): 159–164.
47. Menge TJ, Horan MP, Tahal DS, et al. Arthroscopic treatment of snapping scapula syndrome: outcomes at minimum of 2 years. Arthroscopy, 2017, 33(4):726–732.
48. Milch H. Partial scapulectomy for snapping of the scapula. J Bone Joint Surg Am, 1950, 32A(3): 561–566.
49. Cameron HU. Snapping scapulae: a report of three cases. Eur J Rheumatol Inflamm, 1984, 7(2): 66–67.
50. Morse BJ, Ebraheim NA, Jackson WT. Partial scapulectomy for snapping scapula syndrome. Orthop Rev, 1993, 22(10): 1141–1144.
51. Oizumi N, Suenaga N, Minami A. Snapping scapula caused by abnormal angulation of the superior angle of the scapula. J Shoulder Elbow Surg, 2004, 13(1): 115–118.
52. Parsons TA. The snapping scapula and subscapular exostoses. J Bone Joint Surg Br, 1973, 55(2):

345–349.
53. Ross AE, Owens BD, DeBerardino TM. Open scapula resection in beach-chair position for treatment of snapping scapula. Am J Orthop (Belle Mead NJ), 2009, 38(5): 249–251.
54. McCluskey G, Bigliani L. Surgical management of refractory scapulothoracic bursitis, Orthop Trans, 1990, 14: 252–253.
55. Sisto DJ, Jobe FW.The operative treatment of scapulothoracic bursitis in professional pitchers. Am J Sports Med, 1986, 14(3): 192–194.

第15章　肩胛骨骨折

Donald Lee, Schuyler Halverson

肩胛骨骨折在所有骨折中仅占1%，涉及肩胛骨的肩部骨折少于5%[1, 2]。肩胛骨像一个复杂的脚手架一样，为很多肌肉提供了附着点，每一个骨性区域都有自身的骨折发生率和临床显著性。肩胛骨骨折发生率由高到低依次是体部（45%）、盂颈（25%）、盂窝（10%）、肩峰（8%）、喙突（7%）和肩胛冈（5%）[3]。大部分肩胛骨骨折保守治疗已经足够[4]，需要手术治疗的肩胛骨骨折患病率和整体患病率明显不同，需要手术的骨折一般为肩胛骨周围区域的多发骨折。通过对90例手术的分析发现，71%的骨折涉及肩胛骨内上缘，68%涉及盂颈，23%涉及肩胛冈，22%涉及冈盂切迹，17%涉及关节内，没有单独的肩峰或喙突骨折手术，虽然文献记录了一系列的肩峰和喙突骨折手术[5-8]。值得注意的是，肩胛骨内上缘是最常见的需要手术的骨折部位，这是因为它是骨折常见点，而不是说这个部位本身是一个手术指征。这些解剖部位为下面进一步的分类、治疗和结局提供了一个基本框架。

分类

肩胛骨体骨折

1996年OTA分类的初始版本及2007年的修订版以肩胛骨骨折是否累及关节为标准，确定了A、B、C的分类形式[9, 10]。由于肩胛骨伴多个关节面和突起，解剖结构复杂，这种分类方法没能得到广泛的应用。为了解决这个问题，OTA和AO基金组织合作制订了一套综合的、更加深入的分类系统，它囊括了所有的肩胛骨骨折，将肩胛骨分为3部分：盂窝（fossa，F）、各个突起（processes，P）和体部（body，B）[10-12]（图15.1）。盂窝包括关节盂和盂缘，以及肩胛上切迹外侧的颈部。突起包括肩峰（位于盂外侧）和喙突（位于盂上方）。体部位于关节盂平面的内侧，头端起自肩胛上切迹外侧缘。分类系统描述了体部和盂窝的特征。

在基础分类系统中，B1指简单骨折，即体部有≤2个骨折出口点，B2指复杂体部骨折，即体部有≥3个骨折出口点。在深

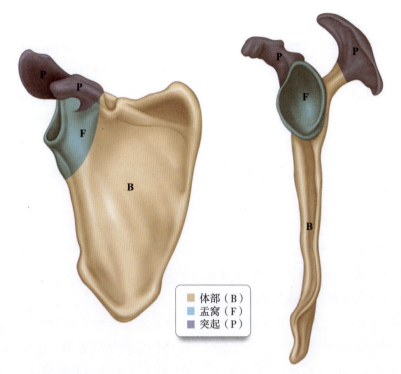

图15.1 肩胛骨体、盂窝和突起骨折的AO/OTA分类系统

入分类系统中，体部分为外侧缘（l，位于下关节缘和肩胛骨下角之间）、上缘（s，位于肩胛切迹和肩胛骨上角之间）、内侧缘（m，位于肩胛骨上下角之间）、中心部（c，没有涉及边缘），以及位于上盂缘和喙突基部外侧称为盂边（g）的小块区域。在深入分类系统编码中，肩胛骨体骨折，第一个字母为B，其后括号内标注涉及的所有分区，例如B（ml）指走行于肩胛骨内外侧缘之间的骨折。

在基础分类系统中，盂窝骨折分为：F0指关节外骨折，骨折断端与体部不再相连；F1指位于盂窝边缘、横向或斜向的简单骨折；F2指关节内多碎片骨折。深入分类系统以上下盂突的连线及其垂直平分线将关节盂分成四个象限。简单盂缘骨折

中，1指前端，2指后端，3指简单横向或短斜向。1或2的骨折若在垂直中线下，用a表示，若涉及上下象限用b表示，c表示同时涉及前后端且在垂直中线以下。1和2分类由包含了大部分骨折碎片的一侧确定。3的骨折中a表示垂直中线下，b代表垂直中线，c代表垂直中线上。复杂关节盂骨折若有≥2个骨折出口点，用4表示；如果骨折在中心，边缘无出口点，则用5表示。

涉及突起的骨折，P1指喙突骨折，P2指肩峰骨折，P3指两者均有。

若骨折平面是混合的，则将各代码结合起来。例如，之前描述的B（ml）骨折加上关节盂和体部分离，则编码应改为F0.B（ml）。若肩胛骨体上部骨折并涉及关节内粉碎性骨折及喙突骨折，则编码为

F2.B（mls）.P1。

在使用AO/OTA基础分类系统讨论肩胛骨体骨折时，外科医生的同意率为82%，整体Kappa系数为0.75。对于体部骨折，基础分类系统的测试者间信度kappa系数和整体同意率分别为0.57~0.59与49%~82%，盂窝骨折为0.79与90%，突起骨折为0.49~0.53与72%~81%[11, 13, 14]。当用深入分类系统描述涉及体部下缘、内侧缘、上缘的骨折时，Kappa系数分别为0.73、0.71、0.62，整体同意率分别为72%、61%、5%[12]。在深入分类系统讨论盂窝骨折关节内骨折的同意率为86%~100%，这些结果是用三维CT分析临床骨折类型得到的[11, 12, 15]。新AO/OTA分类系统相较于原OTA分类系统有更好的整体同意率和Kappa系数，新系统分别为81%与0.53，旧系统分别为57%与0.47[14]。

盂窝骨折

Ideberg分类系统[16]经Heggland[17]改良，用来对肩胛骨关节内骨折（图15.2）进行分类。1型骨折涉及前侧盂缘，1A指骨折碎片≤5 mm，1B指骨折碎片>5 mm。2~6型均涉及完全的关节盂骨折，而不仅仅是盂缘骨折。各型的骨折平面不同，2型骨折出口在盂颈下方，3型骨折出口在喙突基部上方。4型骨折涉及肩胛颈和体部，骨折平面由肩胛冈下方穿行至内侧缘。5型骨折结合了4型的水平骨折面和2型骨折（a）或3型骨折（b），或者2型和3型骨折（c）。6型骨折指严重盂窝粉碎性骨折，或者指1A混合1B骨折。1型骨折占了关节盂骨折的绝大部分（85%：1A 50%，1B 35%），并且与脱位（66%）、半脱位（22%）、其他骨骼损伤（44%）、其他神经损伤（6%）密切相关。2~5型骨折的发生率依次为3%、1%、6%和5%，并发其他骨骼损伤的发生率分别为66%、100%、0%和60%。2型骨折伴半脱位的发生率为33%，尚无其他的伴脱位或神经损伤的报告[18]。

盂颈骨折

盂颈骨折分类不是基于骨折线位置，而是根据骨折碎片的移位情况（图15.3）[19]。1型骨折指无移位或轻微移位，2型骨折是指移位≥1 cm和/或成角≥40°[20, 21]。盂颈骨折的描述中可能会用到以下术语：解剖颈（指骨折出口在喙突上外侧）、外科颈（指骨折出口在喙突内侧）和下颈部（指骨折线在肩胛冈以下，出口沿着肩胛骨内侧缘）。

喙突骨折

Ogawa等人最初将喙突骨折分成5类，后来基于骨折与喙锁韧带关系将骨折简化成2类[7, 22]。1型骨折位于韧带后方，2型骨折位于韧带前方（图15.4）。1型骨折与关节盂上部骨折的相关性为32%，并且与肩关节脱臼和肩袖损伤密切相关，而2型骨折与锁骨远端骨折密切相关。90%的喙突骨折与肩锁关节脱位相关，不管是何种类型。

第 15 章　肩胛骨骨折 · 161

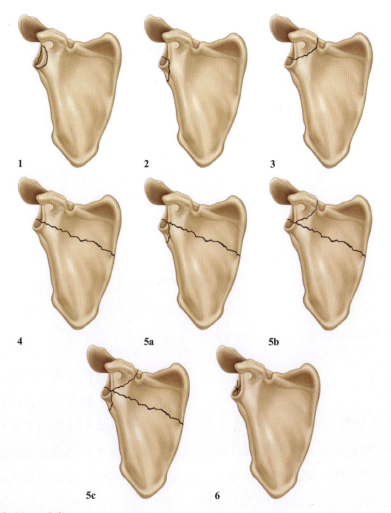

图 15.2　盂窝骨折 Ideberg 分类

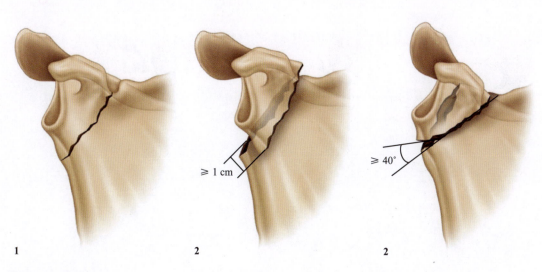

图 15.3　盂颈骨折分类

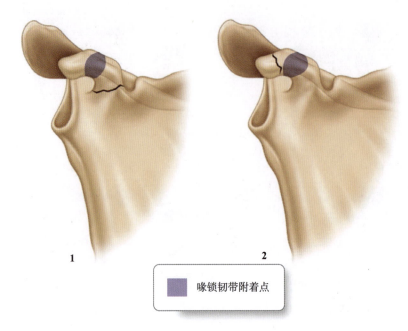

图 15.4 喙突骨折 Ogawa 分类

肩峰骨折

Kuhn 等人[23]将肩峰骨折分为 3 类（图 15.5）。1 型骨折是指有轻微错位的骨折，1A 骨折指由肌肉拉伤导致的撕脱性骨折，1B 指由直接创伤导致的骨折。2 型和 3 型骨折是指在任何方向上存在错位的骨折，以及它俩的区别在于是否伴有肩峰下空间狭窄。该分类系统指出了应力骨折的可能性，但是由于应力骨折的损伤机制与其他骨折完全不同，与类风湿性关节炎密切相关，不适用于大部分人群，因此并没有将

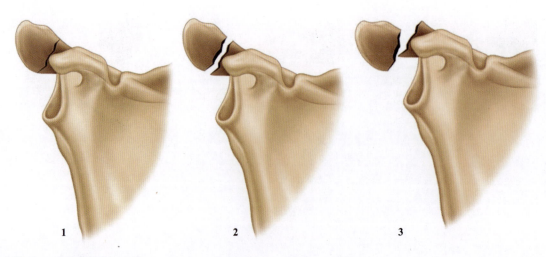

图 15.5 肩峰骨折 Kuhn 分类

其专门设置成一类。

Kuhn分类系统的1A骨折通常不必经手术治疗，很快就会恢复，但有骨不连的报告。1B骨折恢复后一般不遗留肩功能问题，但同侧肩损伤会延缓愈合过程。2型和3型骨折与肩部和臂丛损伤密切相关。2型骨折不需手术治疗，尽管有相关损伤，但所有患者的临床结局都为优良。3型骨折是唯一的结局为次优的类型，所有患者都因机械性阻挡导致活动范围受限。应力骨折尽管没有被专门分成一类，但Kuhn指出其通常保守治疗效果差，易造成痛性骨不连。

肩上方悬吊复合体损伤与肩胛骨外侧悬吊系统骨折

肩胛骨骨折有50%伴有锁骨骨折[24]。浮肩指同侧锁骨和关节盂骨折造成肩部不稳定。在逐步了解了喙肩韧带、喙锁韧带和肩锁韧带的重要性后，浮肩的定义调整为肩上方悬吊复合体（SSSC）的双处断裂[25, 26]（图15.6）。SSSC是指协同维持肩部稳定性的多个部位，它是由远端锁骨、肩锁韧带、肩峰、关节盂、喙突、喙锁韧带构成的一个环。目前没有广泛应用的SSSC分类方法，关于SSSC损伤的诊断在临床上比较困难。

要认识到，前面章节提到的骨折分类很少单独出现，描述一个患者的肩损伤要同时使用多个分类系统，非常冗长。SSSC在描述远端锁骨或肩锁韧带时有不足，Lambert等人[27]制订了一套针对肩胛骨外侧悬吊系统（LSSS）的深入分类系统。LSSS包括远端锁骨、肩峰、喙突、肩胛冈和关节盂，分为3类。S0型的LSSS完整，整体的支持结构没有断裂。S1型的LSSS不完全断裂，为单部位断裂，它可以进一步分为S1a（喙锁韧带外侧锁骨骨折）、S1b（肩锁关节不完全分离）和S1c（肩峰骨折、肩胛冈骨折或喙突基部骨折，涉及或不涉及关节盂）（图15.7）。

S2型的LSSS完全断裂，即存在多处断裂，它进一步分为S2a（喙锁韧带内侧锁骨骨折）、S2b（肩锁关节完全分离伴喙锁韧带断裂）和S2c（肩峰骨折、肩胛冈骨折或喙突基部骨折，涉及或不涉及关节盂）。

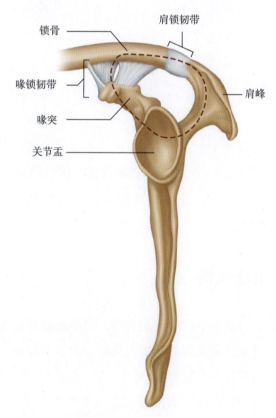

图15.6　SSSC示意图

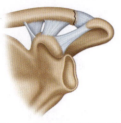 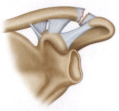

S1a = 喙锁韧带外侧锁骨骨折   S1b = 肩锁关节不完全分离

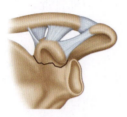 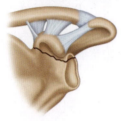

S1c = 喙突基部骨折（涉及或不涉及关节盂）

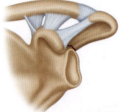 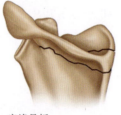

或肩胛冈骨折、肩峰骨折

图 15.7 LSSS 分类示意图

LSSS 分类系统在外科医生中的整体同意率为 47%，Kappa 指数为 0.54[27]。使用该分类系统可以更准确地区分肩伤中 LSSS 是否完整，准确率为 93%，Kappa 指数为 0.63。

相关损伤

除了罕见的撕脱骨折，肩胛骨骨折需要高能量机制，常发生在 35～42 岁男性患者的机动车事故中[3, 28-32]。基于损伤机制，肩胛骨骨折患者的并发损伤率高达 95%，平均有 3.9 处其他重大损伤[29, 30]。多项针对并发损伤的研究结果相互矛盾。肩胛骨骨折与上肢、胸、骨盆、神经血管损伤，以及胸腹简明外伤量表（AIS）、创伤严重度评分（ISS）相关[29-37]。尽管有相矛盾的病例，但仍有几项值得注意的发现。肩胛骨骨折与 ISS 高得分相关，但与其他没有肩胛骨骨折却 ISS 得分相同的患者相比，除了同侧上肢伤和胸外伤增加，其他损伤、住院时间、重症监护收治没有不同[29-31]。另外，肩胛骨骨折相对于其他多发伤，可能与更低的死亡率相关，一个可能的原因是，相比不涉及肩胛骨的直接外伤，肩胛骨丰富的肌肉组织保护了其下的生命器官[38]。肩胛骨骨折患者最常见的死亡原因是肺并发症，通常是因肋骨骨折引起肺组织挫伤、患者呼吸变浅变小（不敢正常呼吸以免引发锐痛），导致致命肺炎发生[30]。

影像学评估

对疑似肩胛骨骨折的评估涉及 3 个主要的影像学体位。正位片可以显示关节盂、肩胛颈、肩胛骨体外侧部和外侧缘、肩胛冈。Y 位片可以显示肩胛骨体。腋位片可以显示肩峰、肩锁关节、喙突和关节盂前后缘。Velpeau 位虽然可以代替腋位来评估肩脱位，但是不能像腋位一样很好地显示肩胛骨的解剖结构。标准胸部 X 线片可以显示内侧肩胛骨体和缘，但是不能很好地独立筛查儿童肩胛骨骨折[39]。尽管有很多其他的体位发表，但很少证实其有临床相关性。Bhatia 位是个例外，它通过喙突上下柱的正交视图，可显示喙突的复杂骨折[40]。

CT 在诊断肩胛骨骨折中的作用目前还有争议。一项针对外科医生使用 X 线片或 CT 图像诊断肩胛骨骨折的能力的比较研究发现，肩胛骨骨折分类的测试者间信度没有提高，有些主要依赖 CT 诊断的骨折准确率更差[41]。但对于复杂骨折或可能需要手术的骨折，CT 不管是对诊断还是后续手术都有指导意义[5, 42-46]（图 15.8）。现在 CT 被广泛应用于高能创伤患者的初期评估中，这个争议也变得没那么重要。

手术指征

最早的一例肩胛骨骨折手术固定记录是在 1910 年，但直到 20 世纪 90 年代才确立了其手术指征，这很大程度上归因于研究者对骨折类型的深入了解和对 CT 的使用[42, 47]。目前，对于大多数患者，肩胛骨骨折的非手术处理仍是适用的，通常为悬吊制动 2 周，之后进行活动度训练。不管骨折部位如何，90% 以上的患者结局是非常好的[48-55]。

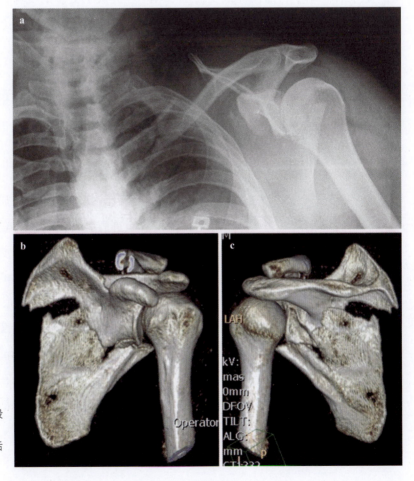

图 15.8 （a）X 线片，正位，复杂肩胛骨骨折伴锁骨中段骨折 （b）三维 CT，正位，同一骨折 （c）三维 CT，后位，同一骨折

保守治疗偶尔会造成有症状的骨折畸形愈合、不愈合或骨折错位[24, 56-59]。

很多研究者都制订了手术干预的标准，但很少超越专家意见建立有大量证据支持的、全面的适应证指南[1, 24, 60-62]。因此，临床实践和已出版的适应证指南相关性低[63]。绝对适应证只有开放伤和肩胛骨体在肋骨间穿入胸腔，两者都十分罕见，所以不包含在下述讨论中[64-68]。

Bauer 等人[69]总结出对有较大错位的肩峰、喙突、关节盂、解剖颈骨折或外科颈不稳定骨折应当使用切开复位内固定术（ORIF），但是没有具体定义什么是较大错位。表 15.1 总结了目前循证最支持的 ORIF 指征，下面将对每种类型做具体讨论。

表 15.1　肩胛骨骨折 ORIF 指征

关节内关节盂骨折	涉及 >25% 关节盂，伴肱骨脱位[70]或关节塌陷 >5 mm[71]
关节外盂颈骨折	成角 >40° 或错位 >1 cm[24]
关节外肩胛骨体骨折	明显错位，无统一的测量标准
肩峰骨折	下方错位 >1 cm，痛性不愈合[23]
喙突骨折	错位 >1 cm，痛性不愈合[72]
肩上方悬吊复合体损伤	SSSC 双点断裂
罕见原因	胸腔内异物 开放骨折

关节盂骨折

作为关节内骨折，关节盂骨折如果影响了关节吻合度（盂窝骨折）和关节稳定性（盂缘骨折），则需要手术治疗。

盂窝骨折的手术治疗可以预防创伤后僵硬及肩部活动时疼痛[1]。Mayo[71]报道了 ORIF 治疗关节错位 >5 mm 或造成肱骨头脱位的盂窝骨折的结果。患者包括 Ideberg 1~4 型骨折，82% 的患者长期结局非常好，18% 的患者对结局不满意，大多因为其他相关损伤。该标准已经过临床及生物力学研究证实，但也有其他文献认为标准应为 >2 mm 或 >3 mm[51, 61, 63, 73-77]。

盂缘骨折通常是肱骨头创伤性脱位造成的，因此手术指征为关节稳定性受影响[1]。标准包括缘错位 >10 mm，前缘 >1/4 被累及或后缘 >1/3 被累及[70]。尽管这些指征最初是基于专家的意见，但是相关研究提供了更多的支持，研究发现使用了这些标准的结局是可接受的[78-80]。

盂颈骨折

盂颈骨折是不稳定的，因为盂肱关节失去悬吊附着，不再与中轴骨有稳固的联系。关于到底是关节盂向内侧移位还是肩胛骨向外侧移位的争辩越来越少，因为最近有几项非常好的研究通过轴位影像证实是肩胛骨向外侧移位[81, 82]。肩胛骨向外侧移位造成了肩峰和肱骨头在肩外展时发生撞击，改变了肩袖的生物力学机制，导致几乎所有的结局都很差[1, 83, 84]。多个文献分别独立提出，为避免撞击出现，盂颈可允许的最大错位为 1 cm[20, 24]。另外，关节盂不管是在水平面还是在冠状面，旋转 >40° 会导致明显的疼痛和活动度降低，因此是另外一个手术指征[24]。用 X 线检查来评估关节盂旋转非常不可靠，必须使用 CT，有时需要采用三维重建。

肩胛骨体骨折

99%单纯肩胛骨体骨折采取了保守治疗，其中86%功能结局好或非常好[48]。多项研究发现经保守治疗的单纯肩胛骨体骨折不管与对侧还是与普通人群相比，都没有明显差异，但可能有罕见的症状性骨折畸形愈合存在[4, 51, 55, 85-88]。目前对肩胛骨体骨折的手术指征尚没有一致意见，但是应当对患者个体进行分析。一些文献提出将错位1 cm作为指征，但是其他文献发现保守处理<2 cm的错位并没有造成功能问题，并提议将错位>2.5 cm或成角畸形>45°作为手术指征[20, 51, 89]。幸运的是，需要手术的肩胛骨体骨折结局非常好，1%的患者需要ORIF，功能结局100%都非常好[48]。另有一些罕见的肩胛骨体骨折指征，包括骨折穿透胸腔、从关节内穿至盂肱关节、骨折畸形愈合再手术及不愈合再手术[64-67, 85-87]。

肩峰和喙突骨折

介绍肩胛骨突出部位骨折手术的文献比较少，目前没有绝对适应证。提议指征包括骨折线扩张至冈盂切迹、痛性不愈合、任何方向错位>1 cm、肩峰向下错位或存在同侧其他需要手术的肩胛骨骨折[6, 7, 23, 62, 72]。少数几个文献报告了肩胛骨突出部位骨折的临床结局，所有患者（除了一项案例研究）的结局都非常好，骨折愈合且恢复了全范围的无痛活动[6-8, 72, 90, 91]。

复合骨折

对于复合骨折，如果其中任何一个部位的骨折需要手术，或者复合骨折切断了SSSC、LSSS，则都需要进行手术。例如，盂颈和锁骨复合骨折，若喙锁韧带断裂，或者喙锁韧带完整，但是盂颈骨折达到了前面描述的手术指征：>1 cm错位或>40°成角，则需要进行手术。如果喙锁韧带完整，但是满足了在第9章中描述的指征标准，则仅需对锁骨进行手术。另外一个例子，肩峰和喙突骨折，若喙突骨折在喙锁韧带内侧，即对SSSC造成了双点切断，则为Ogawa 2型骨折，需要进行手术治疗。

手术干预

所有肩胛骨骨折的一个相同点是很难找到足够厚的皮质骨来做手术固定，因为成人的部分肩胛骨厚度小于2 mm，不能接受螺钉固定。Burke等人[92]描绘了肩胛骨不同部位的平均骨厚度，如盂窝25 mm，外侧缘9.7 mm，肩胛冈8.3 mm，肩胛骨体中心部位3 mm。基于这些测量，肩胛骨适宜做内固定的部位包括盂颈、肩胛冈、外侧缘和喙突。

骨折部位不同，内固定方法各异。盂颈骨折可以用3.5 mm厚的骨盆轮廓重建钢板，或者用轮廓与关节盂后侧及肩胛骨外侧缘吻合的预制肩胛骨钢板。盂颈骨折也可以使用2块钢板，一块沿着肩胛骨外侧缘，一块沿着肩胛冈。盂缘骨折使用碎片间加压螺钉，可以经皮植入或开放切口植入，关节镜下软组织缝合。若为高度粉碎性骨折则不能做内固定，可以移除骨块然后做骨移植。盂窝骨折通常使用碎片间加压螺钉或预制重建钢板。SSSC双点断裂需要预制锁骨钢板，用上述方法修复第二断裂部位。肩峰骨折需要使用空心螺钉张力带技术或预制肩峰钢板进行固定。喙突骨折可以使用碎片间加压螺钉固定，若碎片太小，可将其切除。

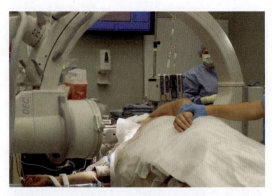

图15.9 患者侧卧位，使用绷带固定体位。造影仪C形臂可以放置在患者上方，以便在术中观察骨折和植入物位置

手术入路

尽管有很多改良式，但肩胛骨的主要固定手术入路包括前路、后路、上路和关节镜。表15.2列出了基于骨折部位的推荐入路。总体上，患者处于侧卧位，允许前后入路结合。造影仪可直接放置在患者上方，以便在术中显示骨折和植入物位置（图15.9）。若只需要前路，患者可为仰卧位或沙滩椅体位。

表15.2 不同骨折部位的推荐手术入路

关节内关节盂骨折	
盂窝前方	三角肌胸肌前路
盂窝上方	上方三角肌分离
盂窝后方	后路
关节外肩胛骨体骨折	
盂窝下方	改良Judet
肩胛骨体外侧	改良Judet
肩胛骨体中心	标准Judet
肩胛冈	后路
肩胛骨多个缘	标准Judet
肩峰骨折	后路延伸到肩峰
喙突骨折	三角肌胸肌前路
锁骨骨折	上方与骨折平行处

三角肌胸肌前路及横锁入路

三角肌胸肌前路入路（图15.10a）可针对前盂缘骨折（Ideberg 1a）、关节内盂窝骨折、上盂窝骨折、喙突骨折和伴锁骨骨折的Ideberg 3骨折。皮肤切口起自喙突上方，靠近锁骨中段，然后向远端、外侧、斜向延伸越过三角肌胸肌间隙至三角肌止点。三角肌胸肌间隙确定以后，头静脉可牵拉至内侧或外侧，后者更好，因为手术方向是向内侧的。沿联合肌腱外侧切开锁骨胸筋膜，近端靠近但没有越过喙肩韧带。如有必要可在此时暴露喙突。确认并结扎肱骨前下回旋动脉。将肩胛下肌从肱骨小结节上松解开，暴露前关节囊，抬高前关节囊和骨膜，暴露其下的关节盂。松解肩袖间隙后手术视野会更好[93]。对于锁骨骨折，可在锁骨长轴下方、骨折部位正上方做水平切口（图15.10b）。需要注意保护锁骨上神经，切开颈阔肌，骨膜下剥离锁骨（图15.10c）。

和覆盖其上的筋膜抬离肩胛冈，以用于修补。切开菱形肌和冈下肌、小圆肌之间的筋膜，暴露肩胛骨内侧缘。如需暴露肩峰骨折，需要向前外侧延长切口。三角肌和冈下肌的间隙位于肩胛冈下[93]。

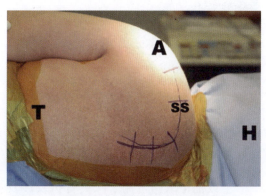

图15.11　肩胛骨后路入路切口画线。H代表肱骨头，A代表后侧肩峰，SS代表肩胛冈，T代表胸廓

标准Judet入路是从内侧向外侧将冈下肌和小圆肌抬离冈下窝，显露肩胛骨体和肩胛颈[94]（图15.12）。改良Judet入路可通过冈下肌和小圆肌的间隙来暴露盂颈[95]。另外，可通过切开冈下肌和小圆肌的肌腱来暴露关节内关节盂骨折，如有必要，可切开后关节囊。直接比较标准Judet和改良Judet，可以看到两者都可以很好地暴露全部的肩胛骨内侧缘和外侧缘，改良Judet的暴露表面仅为标准Judet的20%[96]。这主要是因为标准Judet几乎从冈下窝完全切断了冈下肌，但是这并没有实际益处，因为其下的骨组织太薄弱，无法允许钢钉固定。一例肩胛骨体骨折（图15.8）合并锁骨骨折使用的是标准Judet结合前上路入路（图15.13）。

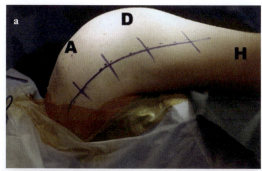
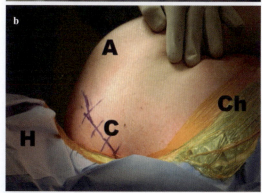
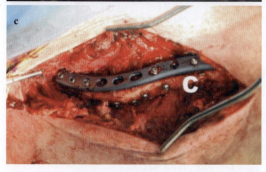

图15.10　（a）三角肌胸肌前路入路切口画线。A代表肩峰，D代表三角肌，H代表肱骨　（b）锁骨骨折手术切口画线。H代表肱骨头，C代表锁骨，A代表肩峰，Ch代表胸壁　（c）锁骨骨折固定术中照片。C代表锁骨

后路入路

后路入路（图15.11）可以处理后盂缘骨折（Ideberg 1b）、关节内盂窝骨折（Ideberg 2~4）、盂颈骨折、肩峰骨折、肩胛骨体骨折和肩胛冈骨折。切口从肩峰后外侧角水平切开，与肩胛冈平行，然后沿肩胛骨内侧缘垂直向上。仔细将三角肌、斜方肌

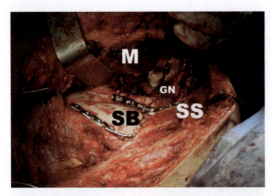

图15.12 后关节囊标准Judet手术照片。将冈下肌和冈上肌（M）抬离肩胛冈（SS）、肩胛骨体（SB）、盂颈（GN）。用骨盆轮廓重建钢板来固定肩胛骨体骨折

上或前上入路

上或前上入路可用于喙突骨折及涉及喙突的上盂窝骨折和锁骨骨折。锁骨骨折的皮肤切口可以水平，在锁骨下方与锁骨平行（图15.8b、c），或者在损伤处沿Langer线使用军刀状切口。分离前、中三角肌，如有必要，可以翻开部分三角肌，以暴露肩峰前部和锁骨。打开肩袖间隙，暴露关节盂[93]。

关节镜

关节镜对盂缘骨折（Ideberg 1a、1b、6）是有益的，可使用标准后位和前上位入口进镜[97]。因为关节囊韧带结构通常附着在骨折碎片上，贯穿盂唇的不可吸收缝线可以允许复位操作及骨折固定。如果附着部位的软组织完整性不好时，可以使用缝线锚。另外，当大片关节内骨折碎片无法用缝线固定时，如微小错位的Idberg 2、3型骨折[98-102]，关节镜可用于协助经皮螺钉复位。

（陈倩倩）

参考文献

1. Hardegger FH, Simpson LA, Weber BG. The operative treatment of scapular fractures. J Bone Joint Surg Br, 1984, 66(5): 725–731.
2. Goss TP. Scapular fractures and dislocations: diagnosis and treatment. J Am Acad Orthop Surg, 1995, 3(1): 22–33.
3. McGahan JP, Rab GT, Dublin A. Fractures of the scapula. J Trauma, 1980, 20(10): 880–883.
4. Dimitroulias A, Molinero KG, Krenk DE, et al. Outcomes of nonoperatively treated displaced scapular body fractures. Clin Orthop Relat Res, 2011, 469(5): 1459–1465.
5. Armitage BM. Mapping of scapular fractures with three-dimensional computed tomography. J Bone Jt Surg, 2009, 91(9): 2222.
6. Ogawa K, Naniwa T. Fractures of the acromion and the lateral scapular spine. J Shoulder Elbow Surg, 1997, 6(6): 544–548.
7. Ogawa K, Yoshida A, Takahashi M, et al. Fractures of the coracoid process. J Bone Joint Surg Br, 1997, 79(1): 17–19.
8. Nissen CW. The acromion: fractures and os acromiale. Oper Tech Sports Med, 2004, 12(1): 32–34.
9. OTA. Fracture and dislocation compendium. J Orthop Trauma, 1996, 10: 1–154.
10. Marsh JL, Slongo TF, Agel J, et al. Fracture and dislocation classification compendium—2007: Orthopaedic Trauma Association classification, database and outcomes committee. J Orthop Trauma,

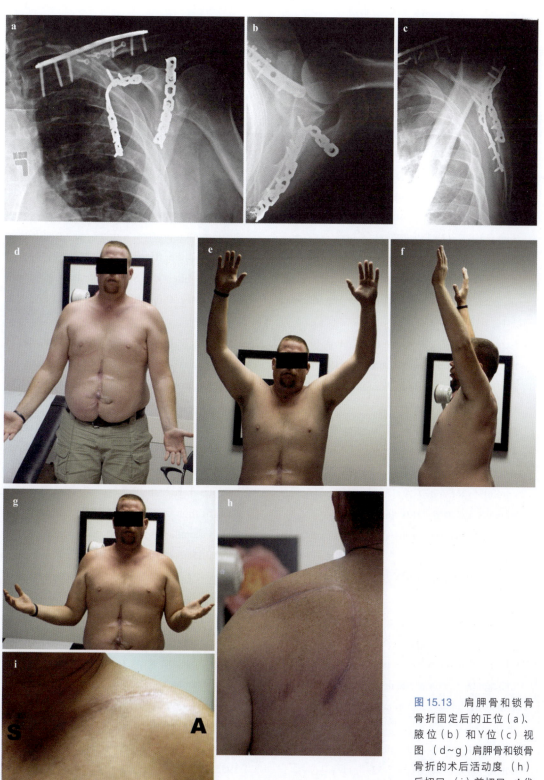

图 15.13 肩胛骨和锁骨骨折固定后的正位（a）、腋位（b）和Y位（c）视图（d~g）肩胛骨和锁骨骨折的术后活动度（h）后切口（i）前切口，A代表肩峰，S代表胸骨切迹

2007, 21(10 Suppl): S1–S133.

11. Jaeger M, Lambert S, Südkamp NP, et al. The AO Foundation and Orthopaedic Trauma Association (AO/OTA) scapula fracture classification system: focus on glenoid fossa involvement. J Shoulder Elbow Surg, 2013, 22(4): 512–520.

12. Audigé L, Kellam JF, Lambert S, et al. The AO foundation and Orthopaedic Trauma Association (AO/OTA) scapula fracture classification system: focus on body involvement. J Shoulder Elbow Surg, 2014, 23(2): 189–196

13. Harvey E, Audigé L, Herscovici D, et al. Development and validation of the new international classification for scapula fractures. J Orthop Trauma, 2012, 26(6): 364–369.

14. Neuhaus V, Bot AGJ, Guitton TG, et al. Scapula fractures: Interobserver reliability of classification and treatment. J Orthop Trauma, 2014, 28(3): 124–129.

15. ter Meulen DP, Janssen SJ, Hageman MGJS, et al. Quantitative three-dimensional computed tomography analysis of glenoid fracture patterns according to the AO/OTA classification. J Shoulder Elbow Surg, 2016, 25(2): 269–275.

16. Ideberg R. Surgery of the shoulder. Philadelphia: Decker, 1984.

17. Heggland EJ, Parker RD. Simultaneous bilateral glenoid fractures associated with glenohumeral subluxation/dislocation in a weightlifter. Orthopedics, 1997, 20(12): 1180–1184.

18. Ideberg R, Grevsten S, Larsson S. Epidemiology of scapular fractures: incidence and classification of 338 fractures. Acta Orthop Scand, 1995, 66(5): 395–397.

19. Goss TP. Fractures of the glenoid neck. J Shoulder Elbow Surg, 1994, 3(1): 42–52.

20. Nordqvist A, Petersson C. Fracture of the body, neck, or spine of the scapula: a long-term follow-up study. Clin Orthop Relat Res, 1992, 283: 139–144.

21. Zdravkovic D, Damholt VV. Comminuted and severely displaced fractures of the scapula. Acta Orthop Scand, 1974, 45(1): 60–65.

22. Ogawa K, Toyama Y, Ishige S, et al. Fracture of the coracoid process: its classification and pathomechanism. Nihon Seikeigeka Gakkai Zasshi, 1990, 64(10): 909–919.

23. Kuhn JE, Blasier RB, Carpenter JE. Fractures of the acromion process: a proposed classification system. J Orthop Trauma, 1994, 8(1): 6–13.

24. Ada JR, Miller ME. Scapular fractures: analysis of 113 cases. Clin Orthop Relat Res, 1991, 269: 174–180.

25. Herscovici D, Fiennes AG, Allgöwer M, et al. The floating shoulder: ipsilateral clavicle and scapular neck fractures. J Bone Joint Surg Br, 1992, 74(3): 362–364.

26. Goss TP. Double disruptions of the superior shoulder suspensory complex. J Orthop Trauma, 1993, 7(2): 99–106.

27. Lambert S, Kellam JF, Jaeger M, et al. Focussed classification of scapula fractures: failure of the lateral scapula suspension system. Injury, 2013, 44(11): 1507–1513.

28. Imatani RJ. Fractures of the scapula: a review of 53 fractures. J Trauma, 1975, 15(6): 473–478.

29. Baldwin KD, Ohman-Strickland P, Mehta S, et al. Scapula fractures: a marker for concomitant injury? A retrospective review of data in the National Trauma Database. J Trauma, 2008, 65(2): 430–435.

30. Thompson DA, Flynn TC, Miller PW, Fischer RP. The significance of scapula fractures. J Trauma, 1985, 25(10): 974–977.

31. Veysi VT, Mittal R, Agarwal S, et al. Multiple trauma and scapula fractures: so what? J Trauma,

2003, 55(6): 1145–1147.
32. Stephens NG, Morgan AS, Corvo P, et al. Significance of scapular fracture in the blunttrauma patient? Ann Emerg Med, 1995, 26(4): 439–442.
33. Akaraborworn O, Sangthong B, Thongkhao K, et al. Scapular fractures and concomitant injuries. Chin J Traumatol, 2012, 15(5): 297–299.
34. Lunsjo K, Tadros A, Czechowski J. Scapular fractures and associated injuries in blunt trauma: a prospective study. J Bone J Surg Br, 2006.
35. Dinopoulos H, Giannoudis PV. Scapula fracture in Polytrauma patients. J Bone Joint Surg Br, 2003, 85: 559.
36. Boerger TO, Limb D. Suprascapular nerve injury at the spinoglenoid notch after glenoid neck fracture. J Shoulder Elbow Surg, 2000, 9(3): 236–237.
37. Heim KA, Lantry JM, Burke CS, et al. Early results of scapular fractures treated operatively at a level one trauma center. Eur J Trauma Emerg Surg, 2008, 34(1): 55–59.
38. Weening B, Walton C, Cole PA, et al. Lower mortality in patients with scapular fractures. J Trauma, 2005, 59(6): 1477–1481.
39. Yanchar NL, Woo K, Brennan M, et al. Chest x-ray as a screening tool for blunt thoracic trauma in children. J Trauma Acute Care Surg, 2013, 75(4): 613–619.
40. Bhatia DN, Dasgupta B, Rao N. Orthogonal radiographic technique for radiographic visualization of coracoid process fractures and pericoracoid fracture extensions. J Orthop Trauma, 2013, 27(5): e118–e121.
41. McAdams TR, Blevins FT, Martin TP, et al. The role of plain films and computed tomography in the evaluation of scapular neck fractures. J Orthop Trauma, 2002, 16(1): 7–11.
42. Bartoníček J, Cronier P. History of the treatment of scapula fractures. Arch Orthop Trauma Surg, 2010, 130(1): 83–92.
43. Bartoníček J, Frič V. Scapular body fractures: results of operative treatment. Int Orthop, 2011, 35(5): 747–753.
44. Anavian J, Conflitti JM, Khanna G, et al. A reliable radiographic measurement technique for extra-articular scapular fractures. Clin Orthop Relat Res, 2011, 469(12): 3371–3378.
45. Chan CM, Chung CT, Lan HHC. Scapular fracture complicating suprascapular neuropathy: the role of computed tomography with 3D reconstruction. J Chin Med Assoc, 2009, 72(6): 340–342.
46. Bartoníček J, Tuček M, Klika D, et al. Pathoanatomy and computed tomography classification of glenoid fossa fractures based on ninety patients. Int Orthop, 2016, 40(11): 2383–2392.
47. Bartoníček J, Kozánek M, Jupiter JB. Early history of scapular fractures. Int Orthop, 2016, 40(1): 213–222.
48. Zlowodzki M, Bhandari M, Zelle BA, et al. Treatment of scapula fractures: systematic review of 520 fractures in 22 case series. J Orthop Trauma, 2006, 20(3): 230–233.
49. Edwards SG, Whittle AP, Wood GW. Nonoperative treatment of ipsilateral fractures of the scapula and clavicle. J Bone Joint Surg Am, 2000, 82(6): 774–780.
50. Ramos L, Mencía R, Alonso A, et al. Conservative treatment of ipsilateral fractures of the scapula and clavicle. J Trauma, 1997, 42(2): 239–242.
51. Jones CB, Sietsema DL. Analysis of operative versus nonoperative treatment of displaced scapular fractures. Clin Orthop Relat Res, 2011, 469(12): 3379–3389.
52. Schofer MD, Sehrt AC, Timmesfeld N, et al. Fractures of the scapula: long-term results after conservative treatment. Arch Orthop Trauma Surg, 2009, 129(11): 1511–1519.

53. van Noort A, van Kampen A. Fractures of the scapula surgical neck: outcome after conservative treatment in 13 cases. Arch Orthop Trauma Surg, 2005, 125(10): 696–700.

54. McKoy BE, Bensen CV, Hartsock LA. Fractures about the shoulder: conservative management. Orthop Clin North Am, 2000, 31(2): 205–216.

55. Gosens T, Speigner B, Minekus J. Fracture of the scapular body: functional outcome after conservative treatment. J Shoulder Elbow Surg, 2009, 18(3): 443–448.

56. Harris RD, Harris JH. The prevalence and significance of missed scapular fractures in blunt chest trauma. Am J Roentgenol, 1998, 151(4): 747–750.

57. Armstrong CP, van der Spuy J. The fractured scapula: importance and management based on a series of 62 patients. Injury, 1984, 15(5): 324–329.

58. Charlton WP, Kharazzi D, Alpert S, et al. Unstable nonunion of the scapula: a case report. J Shoulder Elbow Surg, 2003, 12(5): 517–519.

59. Anavian J, Khanna G, Plocher EK, et al. Progressive displacement of scapula fractures. J Trauma, 2010, 69(1): 156–161.

60. Cole PA, Gauger EM, Herrera DA, et al. Radiographic follow-up of 84 operatively treated scapula neck and body fractures. Injury, 2012, 43(3): 327–333.

61. Anavian J, Gauger EM, Schroder LK, et al. Surgical and functional outcomes after operative management of complex and displaced intra-articular glenoid fractures. J Bone Joint Surg Am, 2012, 94(7): 645–653.

62. Lantry JM, Roberts CS, Giannoudis PV. Operative treatment of scapular fractures: a systematic review. Injury, 2008, 39(3): 271–283.

63. Mulder FJ, van Suchtelen M, Menendez ME, et al. A comparison of actual and theoretical treatments of glenoid fractures. Injury, 2015, 46(4): 699–702.

64. Blue JM, Anglen JO, Helikson MA. Fracture of the scapula with intrathoracic penetration. J Bone Joint Surg Am, 1997, 79: 1076–1078.

65. Porte AN, Wirtzfeld DA, Mann C. Intrathoracic scapular impaction: an unusual complication of scapular fractures. Can J Surg, 2009, 52(3): E62–E63.

66. Schwartzbach CC, Seoudi H, Ross AE, et al. Fracture of the scapula with intrathoracic penetration in a skeletally mature patient: a case report. J Bone Joint Surg Am, 2006, 88(12): 2735–2738.

67. Report C. Intrathoracic displacement of a scapular fracture. J Bone Joint Surg Am, 2012, 16: 16–18.

68. Stepanovic ZL, Milisavljevic SS, Prodanovic NS, et al. Open scapulothoracic dissociation. J Trauma Acute Care Surg, 2015, 79(4): 698–700.

69. Bauer G, Fleischmann W, Dussler E. Displaced scapular fractures: indication and long-term results of open reduction and internal fixation. Arch Orthop Trauma Surg, 1995, 114(4): 215–219.

70. de Palma A. Surgery of the shoulder. 3rd ed. Philadelphia: Lippincott, 1983.

71. Mayo KA, Benirschke SK, Mast JW. Displaced fractures of the glenoid fossa. Results of open reduction and internal fixation. Clin Orthop Relat Res, 1998, 347: 122–130.

72. Anavian J, Wijdicks CA, Schroder LK, et al. Surgery for scapula process fractures: good outcome in 26 patients. Acta Orthop, 2009, 80(3): 344–350.

73. Soslowsky LJ, Flatow EL, Bigliani LU, et al. Articular geometry of the glenohumeral joint. Clin Orthop Relat Res, 1992, 285: 181–190.

74. Sen RK, Sud S, Saini G, et al. Glenoid fossa fractures: outcome of operative and nonoperative treatment. Indian J Orthop, 2014, 48(1): 14–19.

75. Goss TP. Fractures of the glenoid cavity. J Bone Joint Surg Am, 1992, 74: 299–305.

76. Kavanagh B, Bradway J, Cofield R. Open reduc-

tion and internal fixation of displaced intra-articular fractures of the glenoid fossa. J Bone Joint Surg Am, 1993, 75(4): 479–484.
77. Schandelmaier P, Blauth M, Schneider C, et al. Fractures of the glenoid treated by operation: a 5- to 23-year follow-up of 22 cases. J Bone Joint Surg Br, 2002, 84(2): 173–177.
78. Niggebrugge AHP, van Heusden HA, Bode PJ, et al. Dislocated intra-articular fracture of anterior rim of glenoid treated by open reduction and internal fixation. Injury, 1993, 24(2): 130–131.
79. van Oostveen DPH, Temmerman OPP, Burger BJ, et al. Glenoid fractures: a review of pathology, classification, treatment and results. Acta Orthop Belg, 2014, 80(1): 88–98.
80. Scheibel M, Magosch P, Lichtenberg S, et al. Open reconstruction of anterior glenoid rim fractures. Knee Surg Sports Traumatol Arthrosc, 2004, 12(6): 568–573.
81. Zuckerman SL, Song Y, Obremskey WT. Understanding the concept of Medialization in scapula fractures. J Orthop Trauma, 2012, 26(6): 350–357.
82. Patterson JMM, Galatz L, Streubel PN, et al. CT evaluation of extraarticular glenoid neck fractures: does the glenoid medialize or does the scapula lateralize? J Orthop Trauma, 2012, 26: 360–363.
83. Pace AM, Stuart R, Brownlow H. Outcome of glenoid neck fractures. J Shoulder Elbow Surg, 2005, 14(6): 585–590.
84. Romero J, Schai P, Imhoff AB. Scapular neck fracture—the influence of permanent malalignment of the glenoid neck clinical outcome. Arch Orthop Trauma Surg, 2001, 121(6): 313–316.
85. Cole PA, Talbot M, Schroder LK, et al. Extraarticular malunions of the scapula: a comparison of functional outcome before and after reconstruction. J Orthop Trauma, 2011, 25(11): 649–656.
86. Gauger EM, Ludewig PM, Wijdicks CA, et al. Pre- and postoperative function after scapula malunion reconstruction: a novel kinematic technique. J Orthop Trauma, 2013, 27(8): e186–e191.
87. Martin SD, Weiland AJ. Missed scapular fracture after trauma. A case report and a 23-year follow-up report. Clin Orthop Relat Res, 1994, 299: 259–262.
88. Sorenson SM, Armstrong AD. Scapular Malunion in a Vietnam War Veteran: Superior Medial Angle of the Scapula Impinging on the Clavicle. JBJS, 2015, 5(4): 1–4.
89. Jones CB, Cornelius JP, Sietsema DL, et al. Modified judet approach and minifragment fixation of scapular body and glenoid neck fractures. J Orthop Trauma, 2009, 23(8): 558–564.
90. Guiral J, Real JL, Curto JM. Isolated fracture of the coracoid process of the scapula. Acta Orthop Belg, 1996, 62(1): 10–12.
91. Vaienti E, Pogliacomi F. Delayed diagnosis of isolated coracoid process fractures: results of 9 cases treated conservatively. Acta Biomed, 2012, 83(2): 138–146.
92. Burke CS, Roberts CS, Nyland JA, et al. Scapular thickness-implications for fracture fixation. J Shoulder Elbow Surg, 2006, 15(5): 645–648.
93. Lee DH. Operative techniques: shoulder and elbow surgery. 1st ed. Philadelphia: Elsevier, 2011.
94. Judet R. Traitement chirsurgical dos fractures de l'onoplate, indication operatuires. Acta Orthop Belg, 1964, 30: 673–678.
95. Obremskey WT, Lyman JR. A modified judet approach to the scapula. J Orthop Trauma, 2004, 18(10): 696–699.
96. Harmer LS, Phelps KD, Crickard CV, et al. A comparison of exposure between the classic and modified judet approach to the scapula. J Orthop Trauma, 2015, 30(5): 1.
97. Bauer T, Abadie O, Hardy P. Arthroscopic treat-

ment of glenoid fractures. Arthroscopy, 2006, 22(5): 569.

98. Marsland D, Ahmed HA. Arthroscopically assisted fixation of glenoid fractures: a cadaver study to show potential applications of percutaneous screw insertion and anatomic risks. J Shoulder Elbow Surg, 2011, 20(3): 481–490.

99. Qu F, Yuan B, Qi W, et al. Arthroscopic fixation of comminuted glenoid frac-tures using cannulated screws and suture anchors. Medicine (Baltimore), 2015, 94(49): e1923.

100. Tauber M, Moursy M, Eppel M, et al. Arthroscopic screw fixation of large anterior glenoid fractures. Knee Surg Sports Traumatol Arthrosc, 2008, 16(3): 326–332.

101. Yang HB, Wang D, He XJ. Arthroscopic-assisted reduction and percutaneous cannulated screw fixation for Ideberg type III glenoid fractures: a minimum 2-year follow-up of 18 cases. Am J Sports Med, 2011, 39(9): 1923–1928.

102. Gras F, Marintschev I, Aurich M, et al. Percutaneous navigated screw fixation of glenoid fractures. Arch Orthop Trauma Surg, 2013, 133(5): 627–633.

第16章 肩胛骨运动障碍的康复

Ann M. Cools, Todd S. Ellenbecker, Lori A. Michener

引言

肩胛骨运动障碍有多种原因，包括骨性结构障碍（如锁骨骨折）、神经障碍（如胸长神经或副神经麻痹）或肌肉功能障碍（如软组织延展性受限，肌肉力量弱、抑制或不平衡）[1]。肩胛骨康复的临床思路应基于患者的临床评估、上肢和肩胛骨的运动学和肌肉功能改变、肩胛骨运动障碍生物力学机制及医生对肩颈疼痛慢性功能障碍的最新理解。肩胛骨康复计划的制订应基于肩胛骨位置和运动模式的关键损伤、症状改变测试，以及客观临床检查和额外临床测量确定的动态稳定性。肩胛骨临床评估应包括所有可能导致运动障碍的局部和远端因素。动力链的近端，如脊柱的活动度和稳定性及下肢的功能在肩部康复中是很关键的，特别是对于那些依赖下肢和脊柱将力量传递到上肢的患者。过头类项目运动员还应查看远端因素，如肘部力量和活动度、前臂旋前或旋后。由于观察到的肩胛骨运动障碍也许是正常的个体差异[2,3]，因此肩胛骨运动障碍必须与实际的临床症状和患者主诉相关联。不同的矫正手法，即症状改变测试，如肩胛骨辅助试验（SAT）和肩胛骨复位测试（SRT）可以通过矫正肩胛骨位置和运动来改变患者症状[1,4,5]。肩部症状调整手段（SSMP）也包括一些矫正手法，可以确认肩胛胸壁复合体的功能障碍，以此作为治疗策略的依据。临床人员还应意识到慢性肩部疼痛和功能障碍患者可能存在中枢敏感化[7]。

肩胛骨治疗的目标是恢复与患者症状相关的肩胛骨位置和运动模式，覆盖了肩部大部分的动力链[8]。柔韧性不足和肌肉功能障碍都需要进行处理（图16.1，摘自Cools等人[9]的文章）。本章旨在描述肩胛骨周围柔韧性和肌肉功能障碍的治疗策略和方法。其次，着重介绍过头类项目运动员肩胛骨运动障碍的高阶康复。最后，讨论肩胛骨康复后的效果和结局。

柔韧性不足的治疗

肩胛骨位置和盂肱关节活动度相关性的研究对治疗肩关节活动度下降及肩胛

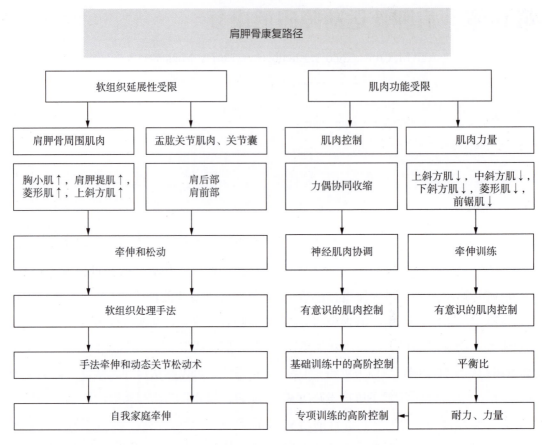

图16.1 肩胛骨康复路径图

功能障碍的临床人员有重要意义。Laudner等人[10]报告了40名职业棒球投手的肩关节后部紧张（水平内收活动度受限）与以肩胛骨前置为特征的肩胛骨功能障碍存在相关性。另外，Ludewig和Reynolds[11]的文献回顾描述了粘连性关节囊炎和肩关节僵硬患者存在肩胛骨上旋和后倾的变化。Vermeulen等人[12]的研究显示增加盂肱关节活动度的物理治疗可以改善肩胛骨生物力学。因此，本章前面提到的肩胛骨功能障碍患者评估应包括盂肱关节活动度客观定量测试，以确定它在肩胛骨功能障碍中的潜在作用。这包括在肩外展90°固定肩胛骨的情况下，使用量角器和倾角计进行外旋和内旋测量[13]（图16.2）。另外，由于过头类项目运动员的水平内收和肩胛骨功能异常存在潜在关系，因此水平手臂内收测量也很重要[10]（图16.3）。关于优秀过头类项目运动员的正常活动度模式，骨科和运动医学的文献阐述非常多[14-18]。这些研究提供了重要的框架，指导临床人员认识正常的肩活动度模式，辨认可能影响肩胛骨机制的活动度受限患者。

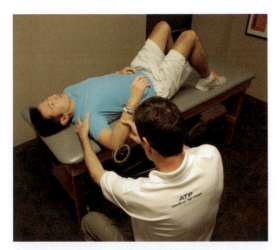

图16.2　固定肩胛骨，测量盂肱关节的内旋

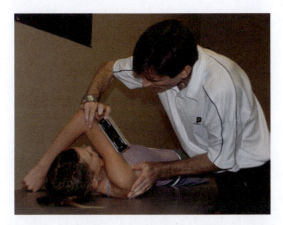

图16.3　固定肩胛骨，利用数字倾角计测量水平内收活动度

其他评估包括针对胸部肌肉柔韧性的测量[19]。Kluemper等人[20]和Lynch等人[21]使用双正方形法测量游泳运动员在站立位的肩前移和肩胛骨位置的双侧差异。这种方法可以快速识别肩前移姿势，也可以在仰卧位进行测量。Ellenbecker等人[22]使用此方法发现优秀网球运动员的利手肩前移增加。肩前移增加的个体可以通过干预来改善胸部柔韧性，如仰卧位泡沫轴上肩胛骨后缩牵伸（有或无治疗师辅助）（图16.4）及墙角牵伸[21, 23]。研究表明，侧卧牵伸可以对肩内旋活动度产生短期和长期的改善效果[24, 25]，缓解肩后部紧张，推荐在临床上使用（图16.5）。McClure等人[26]、Moore等人[27]和Ellenbecker等人[28]支持使用手臂内收（水平内收）牵伸，后来的研究显示使用弹力带做3组30s收缩、放松后，内旋角度增加了8°（图16.6）。最近的临床研究[29]中，治疗师在牵伸时对肩和肩胛骨外侧缘施加内向固定的效果更好，显示了在手臂内收牵伸时固定肩胛骨的重要性（图16.7）。

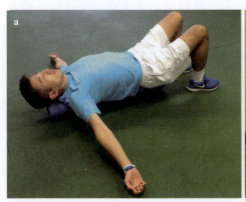 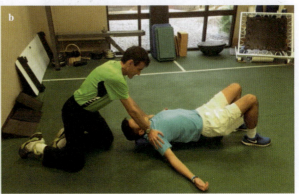

图16.4　泡沫轴上胸肌牵伸伴（a）或不伴（b）治疗师加压

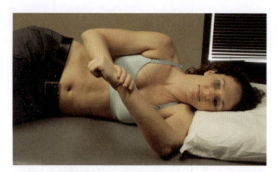

图16.5　侧卧牵伸

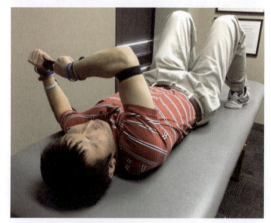

图16.6　患者使用弹力带做自主水平内收

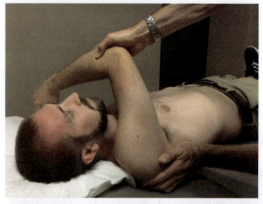

图16.7　固定肩胛骨行手臂水平内收牵伸

肌肉功能障碍的治疗

在肩胛骨训练的早期阶段，为了改善本体感觉，使肩胛骨静态位置正常化，有意识的肌肉控制也许是必要的。优先考虑患者对肩胛骨运动方向的主动控制，首先是治疗师辅助患者，其后患者自己练习。根据主要的肩胛骨运动障碍类型，应当将其向后倾、上旋、外旋的方向矫正。一项肩胛骨三维运动分析显示，正常的受试者可以习得稳定的后倾和上旋动作[30]。另外de Mey等人[31]的研究显示，运动前让患者有意识地矫正肩胛骨位置可以使动态肩关节训练中的目标肌群特别是中斜方肌和下斜方肌有更高的肌电活动。有头前倾、含胸、肩胛带前伸的患者，将肩胛骨位置矫正和脊柱姿势结合起来尤为重要。鼓励患者每天重复练习，强调改变姿势习惯。记忆唤起方法对于形成习惯可能是有用的[9]。

基于对患者的观察和客观检查，治疗师要决定训练是集中于功能性运动中肩胛背神经损伤的神经肌肉控制（力偶激活和共同收缩）还是肩胛骨肌群中的单个肌肉力量及平衡训练。两个方法最基本的不同是训练的选择。若着重于运动控制，应选择低负荷的功能性动作，主要是不同平面的抬臂训练，因为训练的主要目标是优化日常活动中的神经肌肉控制。研究提示单个肌肉的高强度训练不能使神经系统适应运动优化策略[2]。运动控制训练应当主要强调动作的质量和耐力，在康复高阶时期，还应加入能量传递和吸收[1, 2]。可以在基础姿势、动作和训练中练习肩胛骨肌群共同收缩（如刺激性向下滑动、双侧外旋、胸椎伸展）。由于肩胛带功能包括开链和闭链活动，训练时要兼顾两者，训练肩胛骨能在保持承重位置的前提下完成上肢承重和非承重任务。这些必须与患者的功能性诉求一致。Kibler等人[32]描述了早期康复的开链肩胛骨控制训练。他们的文章描述了低位划船、下滑动、割草机及抢劫姿势训练，可激活关键肩胛骨稳定肌肉，但不对肩关节造成过多应力，适用于非手术治疗早期及术后康复。一般认为闭链活动可以改善动态盂肱和肩胛胸壁稳定性，激活关节内和关节周围本体感受器，促进肩袖和肩胛骨稳定肌群的共同收缩。但应当注意，俯卧撑、滑墙闭链训练主要用来激活肩胛骨前侧肌群，如前锯肌和胸小肌，应谨慎选择这些练习，以免激活本来就短缩或过度活跃的肌肉[33]。在早期，额外的贴扎和佩戴支具可以助力进阶，但目前文献对于这些干预效果的结论还不统一[34]。也可以考虑使用神经肌肉电刺激疗法（NMES）。对前锯肌和下斜方肌进行NMES可以增加健康肩关节的肩峰肱骨距离，提示对于有肩峰下疼痛综合征的患者作用较好[35]。

如果发现肌肉力量下降或失衡严重，需要进行高负荷、针对特定肌群的训练，以恢复肌肉力量及肌肉内和肌肉间的平衡。这些训练是针对特定肌群的分离训练，较少在功能位（如俯卧位和侧卧位）[36, 37]。功能性训练如抬臂总会或多或少地激活所有的肩胛骨肌肉，无法分离特定肌群。若一块肌肉力量弱而另一块过度活跃，需要最小化激活过度活跃的肌肉，恢复肌肉间平衡。当肌肉平衡恢复后，可以进行肩胛骨肌群整体的力量训练。

练习选择可能基于很多标准，如文献中的一般指南、特定训练方案的结局研究证据、治疗师的个人喜好、患者诉求和期待功能的相关性。对健康人和上肢疼痛或功能障碍患者的肌电活动研究为颈肩疼痛伴肩胛骨功能障碍患者选择治疗方案提供了基础。研究显示特定的肩胛骨肌肉功能障碍与肩痛或颈痛相关，对健康人的研究证实了基于治疗目标选择训练的合理性。重点训练特定肌肉激活模式可能改善肩胛骨的动作质量，并恢复理想的运动模式。假设肩胛骨功能障碍和异常肩胛骨肌群激活模式的变异性很大，训练应当首先着重恢复肌肉平衡。根据现有文献和临床经验，过度活跃的肌肉经常是上斜方肌、菱形肌、胸小肌和肩胛提肌，而活动不足的肌肉可能是上斜方肌、菱形肌、中斜方肌、下斜方肌及前锯肌[38-40]。目前上斜方肌和菱形肌在肩胛骨功能障碍中的作用还不明确，但是上肢疼痛和功能障碍的患者可能同时存在过度收缩和力量下降[11, 41]。了解了失衡状况后，可根据肌肉平衡比（更多或更少的肌肉活动）来选择训练。表16.1是根据现有证据[41, 42]和临床经验得到的临床相关平衡比和最适宜的训练。

从临床角度看，运动控制障碍、肌肉失衡及过度活跃并不容易通过客观检查或测量发现，通常是治疗师依靠视诊来确认正常和异常的肩胛骨位置和运动。使用肩胛骨内侧缘作为标志，可确认3种肩胛骨位置异常。主要表现为肩胛骨内侧缘下方突出（Ⅰ型），可能是肩胛骨过度前倾导致的。其机制可能是胸小肌柔韧性不足和/或

表 16.1　根据临床相关平衡比选择训练

过度活跃的肌肉	活动不足的肌肉	临床相关平衡比	建议训练	参考文献
胸小肌	前锯肌	胸小肌/前锯肌	站位前锯肌出拳	[33]
	中斜方肌	胸小肌/中斜方肌	抬臂加外旋	[43]
	下斜方肌	胸小肌/下斜方肌	抬臂加外旋	[43]
	菱形肌	胸小肌/菱形肌	抬臂加外旋	[43]
上斜方肌	前锯肌	上斜方肌/前锯肌	肘俯卧撑	[37]
			仰卧位前锯肌出拳	[44]
			抬臂加外旋	[43]
			滑墙	[43]
	中斜方肌或下斜方肌	上斜方肌/中斜方肌或上斜方肌/下斜方肌	抬臂加外旋	[43]
			侧卧位前屈	[36]
			侧卧位外旋	[36]
			俯卧位水平外展加外旋	[36]
			俯卧位伸展	[36]
			俯卧90°外展位外旋	[45]
	菱形肌	上斜方肌/菱形肌	抬臂加外旋	[43]
肩胛提肌	前锯肌	肩胛提肌/前锯肌	滑墙	[43]
	上斜方肌	肩胛提肌/上斜方肌	杠铃上举耸肩	[46]
	中斜方肌、下斜方肌或菱形肌	肩胛提肌/中斜方肌、肩胛提肌/下斜方肌或肩胛提肌/菱形肌	过头后缩	[46]
菱形肌	前锯肌	菱形肌/前锯肌	滑墙	[43]

负责后倾的力偶，即下斜方肌和/或前锯肌功能障碍。Ⅰ型的训练重点是激活前锯肌和下斜方肌。包含外旋成分的训练可以增加下斜方肌的活动[36, 43]。若整个内侧缘突起（Ⅱ型），表明肩胛骨过度内旋。训练应集中在肩胛骨外旋，激活斜方肌和前锯肌力偶。肩外展90°位，在水平面做肩胛骨后缩训练可增加肩胛骨外旋，并激活斜方肌及前锯肌，可在开链（如水平外展加外旋）和闭链（如俯卧至侧卧臀桥）进行练习。若主要表现为肩胛骨内侧缘上部突出（Ⅲ型），则是因为肩胛骨过度下旋。机制可能是肩胛提肌或菱形肌紧张，或者上旋力偶（包括上斜方肌和前锯肌）功能障碍，稳定性主要来自中、下斜方肌。应着重促进上旋，手臂尽量举高使肩胛骨处于最大上旋，如过头耸肩和肩胛骨后缩[46]。

康复训练应始终包含动力链的近端和远端。通过对侧腿站立或四点跪位伸腿制造对角模式，对前锯肌和中、下斜方肌活动有积极的影响[47, 48]。加入躯干旋转也能促进良好的肩胛骨位置，如后倾、外旋；增加下斜方肌活动，降低上/下斜方肌比[49]。将上肢功能性模式融入肩胛骨训练，如肘、前臂、腕和手的活动。

尽管肩胛骨在正常肩部功能中的作用是公认的，任何上肢的康复方案都应包含与肩胛骨相关的干预，但是仍有很多的不确定问题，因此临床人员和研究者在解读现有研究和临床指南时应该保持评判态度。首先，肩痛和肩胛骨运动障碍的因果关系仍不清楚。仍不知道肩胛骨运动学改变是颈肩病理的代偿还是贡献因素。调查肩胛骨运动障碍是否是危险因素的前瞻性研究，其结果是相互冲突的[50-52]。根据最近的一个疼痛适应理论，在疼痛时肌肉内和肌肉间的活动会重新分布，短期可能有益（避免进一步疼痛或伤害），但对痛觉敏感的组织可能有长期不利的力学效应[53]。由这个理论看，肩胛骨肌肉功能障碍可能是颈肩疼痛的结果。第二，许多健康人也存在肩胛骨运动障碍[54]，过头类项目运动员的两侧肩胛骨不对称是正常的[1]，视诊发现的肩胛骨位置和运动"异常"可能只是正常的运动学差异，反映了个体在完成任务时采取的不同协调模式[2]。因此，应正确地看待可能的肩胛骨运动障碍，将活动异常与症状联系起来[6]。第三，在制订针对肩胛骨的运动处方时，应考虑到包含盂肱关节的成分。在大部分肩胛骨训练中，由于有外旋和内旋，因此肩袖高度激活。不可能也没必要把肩胛骨训练和盂肱关节训练分开，更重要的是把上肢动力链的两个部分以协调的方式整合起来。

过头类项目运动员的肩胛骨康复

文献中有过头类项目运动员存在肩胛骨功能障碍的证据。Oyama等人[55]的研究发现过头类项目运动员优势侧上肢有更多的肩胛骨上旋、前倾与内旋。另外，优势侧的肩胛带普遍更前伸。Cools等人[56]在优秀的少年网球运动员中也发现了类似的肩胛骨位置与肩胛骨肌肉力量差异，或优势侧和非优势侧不对称。肌电研究显示网球发球、触地球[57-58]及其他过头投掷类动作[59]对肌肉的要求很高。这些研究表明肩胛骨肌群需要良好的位置和稳定性，特别是在引臂后期、减速期。推荐着重在肩外展、外旋90°位置时（引臂后期）及加速晚期进行随球动作的训练。Ellenbecker等人[60]的描述性研究展现了两项在过头类项目运动员中常用的、可以中度至高度募集前锯肌、后侧肩袖及下斜方肌，并且使用生物力学运动模式刺激这些肌肉的增进式训练（见图16.8和16.9）。训练重点是低强度、高重复。Carter等人[61]的研究显示经过8周的弹力带和增进式肩袖和肩胛骨稳定训练，肩部力量和投掷速度提升。图16.10是随球动作专项训练，对投掷运动员的优势侧进行弹力带阻力和节律稳定训练。还需要进一步的研究来探明肩胛骨稳定训练对提升运动表现和预防损伤的影响。

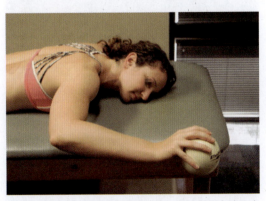

图16.8　90/90增强式放抓球训练，增强后侧肩袖及肩胛骨肌群激活

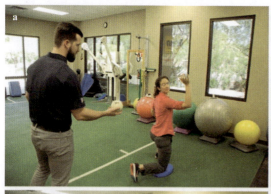
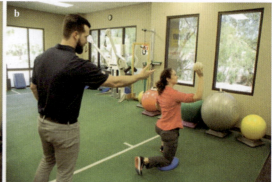
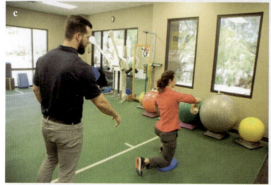
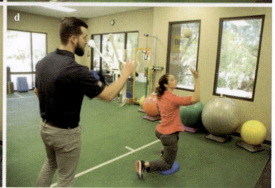

图16.9　90/90反手接球增强式训练

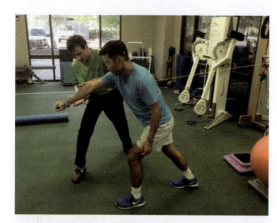

图16.10　使用弹力带并保持节律性稳定来进行肩胛骨前伸训练，模仿投掷动作的随球阶段

进行肩胛骨针对性训练后的结局

肩胛骨针对性训练的有效性研究是有限的[34]。缺乏证据表明肩胛骨针对性训练比普通照护和非肩胛骨针对性训练优越。

5项随机临床试验[62-66]研究了针对肩痛患者的多种肩胛骨针对性训练。干预包括力量训练、运动控制、相关肩胛骨软组织牵伸及肩胛骨松动。总体来说，证据指示肩胛骨针对性训练可以改善肩胛骨肌肉的功能和力量，但是患者自评对疼痛和肩部功能的改善有限、甚至没有效果。

一般会推荐使用肩胛骨针对性训练来改善相关的功能障碍，但各训练方案间没有优次之分。5项研究[62-66]均评价了肩胛骨针对性训练的有效性，但只有2项结果显示效优。值得关注的是，Celik等人[63]报告对冻结肩患者进行肩胛骨重点康复，第6周时短期疼痛改善了，但是治疗效果的优越性在第12周时没有维持住。Struyf等人[66]报告经过治疗，肩峰下疼痛综合征患者的自评结局是有改善的。Struyf的肩胛骨针对性训练整合了肌肉功能训练、牵伸及肩胛骨松动，效果优于着重盂肱关节的训练项目。Mulligan等人[65]最近的研究报告了肩胛骨稳定训练的排列顺序是重要的。肩胛骨稳定训练的第1周，患者的自评结局倾向于有较大的改善。总体来说，针对肩痛患者的肩胛骨针对性训练效果优于普通照护和非肩胛骨针对性训练效果的证据是有限的。

还需要进一步的研究来确定肩胛骨损伤与肩胛骨和盂肱关节的肌肉运动缺陷及功能丧失是否有关。肩胛骨针对性训练可以改善肩胛骨力量，但这些改变没有影响患者的自评结局。应进一步探究需要治疗的功能障碍关键临界值及与患者自评结局提升相关的功能障碍改善临界值。

（陈倩倩）

参考文献

1. Kibler WB, Sciascia AD. The shoulder at risk: scapular dyskinesis and altered glenohumeral rotation. Oper Tech Sports Med, 2016, 24(3): 162–169.
2. Mcquade KJ, Borstad J, de Oliveira AS. Critical and theoretical perspective on scapular stabilization: what does it really mean, and are we on the right track? Phys Ther, 2016, 96(8): 1162–1169.
3. Wright AA, Wassinger CA, Frank M, et al. Diagnostic accuracy of scapular physical examination tests for shoulder disorders: a systematic review. Br J Sports Med, 2013, 47: 886–892.
4. Rabin A, Irrgang JJ, Fitzgerald GK, et al. The intertester reliability of the scapular assistance test. J Orthop Sports Phys Ther, 2006, 36: 653–660.
5. Tate AR, McClure PW, Kareha S, et al. Effect of the scapula reposition test on shoulder impingement symptoms and elevation strength in overhead athletes. J Orthop Sports Phys Ther, 2008, 38: 4–11.
6. Lewis J. Rotator cuff related shoulder pain: assessment, management and uncertainties. Man Ther, 2016, 23: 57–68.
7. Struyf F, Geraets J, Noten S, et al. A multivariable prediction model for the Chronification of non-traumatic shoulder pain: a systematic review. Pain Physician, 2016, 19: 1–10.
8. Kibler WB, Ludewig PM, McClure PW, et al. Clinical implications of scapular dyskinesis in shoulder injury: the 2013 consensus statement from the "scapular summit". Br J Sports Med, 2013, 47: 877–885.
9. Cools AM, Struyf F, de Mey K, et al. Rehabilitation of scapular dyskinesis: from the office worker to the elite overhead athlete. Br J Sports Med, 2014, 48: 692–697.
10. Laudner KG, Moline MT, Meister K. The relationship between forward scapular posture and posterior shoulder tightness among baseball players. Am J Sports Med, 2010, 38: 2106–2112.
11. Ludewig PM, Reynolds JF. The association of scapular kinematics and glenohumeral joint pathologies. J Orthop Sports Phys Ther, 2009, 39: 90–104.
12. Vermeulen HM, Stokdijk M, Eilers PH, et al. Measurement of three dimensional shoulder movement patterns with an electromagnetic tracking device in patients with a frozen shoulder. Ann Rheum Dis, 2002, 61: 115–120.
13. Wilk KE, Reinold MM, Macrina LC, et al. Glenohumeral internal rotation measurements differ depending on stabilization techniques. Sports Health, 2009, 1: 131–136.
14. Ellenbecker TS, Roetert EP. Age specific isoki-

netic glenohumeral internal and external rotation strength in elite junior tennis players. J Sci Med Sport, 2003, 6: 63–70.

15. Ellenbecker TS, Roetert EP, Bailie DS, et al. Glenohumeral joint total rotation range of motion in elite tennis players and baseball pitchers. Med Sci Sports Exerc, 2002, 34: 2052–2056.

16. Manske R, Wilk KE, Davies G, et al. Glenohumeral motion deficits: friend or foe? Int J Sports Phys Ther, 2013, 8(5): 537–553.

17. Shanley E, Rauh MJ, Michener LA, et al. Shoulder range of motion measures as risk factors for shoulder and elbow injuries in high school softball and baseball players. Am J Sports Med, 2011, 39: 1997–2006.

18. Wilk KE, Macrina LC, Fleisig GS, et al. Correlation of glenohumeral internal rotation deficit and total rotational motion to shoulder injuries in professional baseball pitchers. Am J Sports Med, 2011, 39: 329–335.

19. Reiman M, Manske R. Functional testing in human performance. Champaign: Human Kinetics Publishers, 2009.

20. Kluemper M, Uhl TL, Hazelrigg A. Effect of stretching and strengthening shoulder muscles on forward shoulder posture in competitive swimmers. J Sport Rehabil, 2006, 15: 58–70.

21. Lynch SS, Thigpen CA, Mihalik JP, et al. The effects of an exercise intervention on forward head and rounded shoulder postures in elite swimmers. Br J Sports Med, 2010, 44: 376–381.

22. Ellenbecker TS, Kovacs M. A bilateral comparison of anterior shoulder position in elite junior tennis players. J Orthop Sports Phys Ther, 2010, 40: A47.

23. Wang CH, McClure P, Pratt NE, et al. Stretching and strengthening exercises: their effect on three-dimensional scapular kinematics. Arch Phys Med Rehabil, 1999, 80: 923–929.

24. Laudner KG, Sipes RC, Wilson JT. The acute effects of sleeper stretches on shoulder range of motion. J Athl Train, 2008, 43: 359–363.

25. Manske RC, Meschke M, Porter A, et al. A randomized controlled single-blinded comparison of stretching versus stretching and joint mobilization for posterior shoulder tightness measured by internal rotation motion loss. Sports Health, 2010, 2: 94–100.

26. McClure P, Balaicuis J, Heiland D, et al. A randomized controlled comparison of stretching procedures for posterior shoulder tightness. J Orthop Sports Phys Ther, 2007, 37: 108–114.

27. Moore SD, Laudner KG, Mcloda TA, et al. The immediate effects of muscle energy technique on posterior shoulder tightness: a randomized controlled trial. J Ortop Sports Phys Ther, 2011, 41: 400–407.

28. Ellenbecker TS, Manske R, Sueyoshi T, et al. The acute effects of a contract-relax horizontal cross body adduction stretch on shoulder internal rotation range of motion using a stretch strap. J Orthop Sports Phys Ther, 2016, 46: A37.

29. Salamh PA, Kolber MJ, Hanney WJ. Effect of scapular stabilization during horizontal adduction stretching on passive internal rotation and posterior shoulder tightness in young women volleyball athletes: a randomized controlled trial. Arch Phys Med Rehabil, 2015, 96: 349–356.

30. Mottram SL, Woledge RC, Morrissey D. Motion analysis study of a scapular orientation exercise and subjects' ability to learn the exercise. Man Ther, 2007, 14: 13–18.

31. de Mey K, Danneels LA, Cagnie B, et al. Conscious correction of scapular orientation in overhead athletes performing selected shoulder rehabilitation exercises: the effect on trapezius muscle activation measured by surface electromyography.

J Orthop Sports Phys Ther, 2013, 43: 3–10.

32. Kibler WB, Sciascia AD, Uhl TL, et al. Electromyographic analysis of specific exercises for scapular control in early phases of shoulder rehabilitation. Am J Sports Med, 2008, 36: 1789–1798.

33. Castelein B, Cagnie B, Parlevliet T, et al. Serratus anterior or pectoralis minor: which muscle has the upper hand during protraction exercises? Man Ther, 2016, 22: 158–164.

34. Reijneveld EA, Noten S, Michener LA, et al. Clinical outcomes of a scapular-focused treatment in patients with subacromial pain syndrome: a systematic review. Br J Sports Med, 2017, 51(5): 436–441.

35. Bdaiwi AH, Mackenzie TA, Herrington L, et al. Acromiohumeral distance during neuromuscular electrical stimulation of the lower trapezius and serratus anterior muscles in healthy participants. J Athl Train, 2015, 50: 713–718.

36. Cools AM, Dewitte V, Lanszweert F, et al. Rehabilitation of scapular muscle balance—which exercises to prescribe? Am J Sports Med, 2007, 35: 1744–1751.

37. Ludewig PM, Hoff MS, Osowski EE, et al. Relative balance of serratus anterior and upper trapezius muscle activity during push-up exercises. Am J Sports Med, 2004, 32: 484–493.

38. Castelein B, Cagnie B, Parlevliet T, et al. Scapulothoracic muscle activity during elevation exercises measured with surface and fine wire EMG: a comparative study between patients with subacromial impingement syndrome and healthy controls. Man Ther, 2016, 23: 33–39.

39. Michener LA, Sharma S, Cools AM, et al. Relative scapular muscle activity ratios are altered in subacromial pain syndrome. J Shoulder Elbow Surg, 2016, 25(11): 1861–1867.

40. Struyf F, Cagnie B, Cools AM, et al. Scapulothoracic muscle activity and recruitment timing in patients with shoulder impingement symptoms and glenohumeral instability. J Electromyogr Kinesiol, 2014, 24: 277–284.

41. Castelein B, Cagnie B, Cools AM. Analysis of the recruitment of superficial and deep scapular muscles in patients with chronic shoulder and neck pain, and implications for rehabilitation exercises. Belgium: Ghent University, 2016.

42. Schory A, Bidinger E, Wolf J, et al. A systematic review of the exercises that produce optimal muscle ratios of the scapular stabilizers in normal shoulders. Int J SPorts Phys Ther, 2016, 11: 321–336.

43. Castelein B, Cagnie B, Parlevliet T, et al. Superficial and deep scapulothoracic muscle electromyographic activity during elevation exercises in the scapular plane. J Orthop Sports Phys Ther, 2016, 46: 184–193.

44. Uhl TL, Muir TA, Lawson L. Electromyographical assessment of passive, active assistive, and active shoulder rehabilitation exercises. PM R, 2010, 2(2): 132–141.

45. Ekstrom RA, Donatelli RA, Soderberg GL. Surface electromyographic analysis of exercises for the trapezius and serratus anterior muscles. J Orthop Sports Phys Ther, 2003, 33: 247–258.

46. Castelein B, Cools AM, Parlevliet T, et al. Modifying the shoulder joint position during shrugging and retraction exercises alters the activation of the medial scapular muscles. Man Ther, 2016, 21: 250–255.

47. de Mey K, Danneels L, Cagnie B, et al. Kinetic chain influences on upper and lower trapezius muscle activation during eight variations of a scapular retraction exercise in overhead athletes. J Sci Med Sport, 2013, 16: 65–70.

48. Maenhout A, van Praet K, Pizzi L, et al. Electro-

myographic analysis of knee push up plus variations: what is the influence of the kinetic chain on scapular muscle activity? Br J Sports Med, 2010, 44: 1010–1015.

49. Yamauchi T, Hasegawa S, Matsumura A, et al. The effect of trunk rotation during shoulder exercises on the activity of the scapular muscle and scapular kinematics. J Shoulder Elbow Surg, 2015, 24: 955–964.

50. Clarsen B, Bahr R, Andersson SH, et al. Reduced glenohumeral rotation, external rotation weakness and scapular dyskinesis are risk factors for shoulder injuries among elite male handball players: a prospective cohort study. Br J Sports Med, 2014, 48: 1327–1333.

51. Kawasaki T, Yamakawa J, Kaketa T, et al. Does scapular dyskinesis affect top rugby players during a game season? J Shoulder Elbow Surg, 2012, 21: 709–714.

52. Struyf F, Nijs J, Meeus M, et al. Does scapular positioning predict shoulder pain in recreational overhead athletes? Int J Sports Med, 2014, 35: 75–82.

53. Hodges PW, Tucker K. Moving differently in pain: a new theory to explain the adaptation to pain. Pain, 2011, 152: S90–S98.

54. Uhl TL, Kibler WB, Gecewich B, et al. Evaluation of clinical assessment methods for scapular dyskinesis. Arthroscopy, 2009, 25: 1240–1248.

55. Oyama S, Myers JB, Wassinger CA, et al. Asymmetric resting scapular posture in healthy overhead athletes. J Athl Train, 2008, 43: 565–570.

56. Cools AM, Palmans T, Johansson FR. Age-related, sport-specific adaptions of the shoulder girdle in elite adolescent tennis players. J Athl Train, 2014, 49: 647–653.

57. Kovacs M, Ellenbecker TS. An 8-stage model for evaluating the tennis serve: implications for performance enhancement and injury prevention. Sports Health, 2011, 3: 504–513.

58. Ryu RK, Mccormick J, Jobe FW, et al. An electromyographic analysis of shoulder function in tennis players. Am J Sports Med, 1988, 16: 481–485.

59. Digiovine NM, Jobe FW, Pink M, et al. An electromyographic analysis of the upper extremity in pitching. J Shoulder Elbow Surg, 1992, 1: 15–25.

60. Ellenbecker TS, Sueyoshi T, Bailie DS. Muscular activation during plyometric exercises in 90 degrees of glenohumeral joint abduction. Sports Health, 2015, 7: 75–79.

61. Carter AB, Kaminski TW, Douex AT Jr, et al. Effects of high volume upper extremity plyometric training on throwing velocity and functional strength ratios of the shoulder rotators in collegiate baseball players. J Strength Cond Res, 2007, 21(1): 208–215.

62. Baskurt Z, Baskurt F, Gelecek N, et al. The effectiveness of scapular stabilization exercise in the patients with subacromial impingement syndrome. J Back Musculoskelet Rehabil, 2011, 24: 173–179.

63. Celik D. Comparison of the outcomes of two different exercise programs on frozen shoulder. Acta Orthop Traumatol Turc, 2010, 44: 285–292.

64. Moezy A, Sepehrifar S, Solaymani-Dodaran M. The effects of scapular stabilization based exercise therapy on pain, posture, flexibility and shoulder mobility in patients with shoulder impingement syndrome: a controlled randomized clinical trial. Med J Islam Repub Iran, 2014, 28: 87.

65. Mulligan EP, Huang M, Dickson T, et al. The effect of Axioscapular and rotator cuff exercise training sequence in patients with subacromial impingement syndrome: a randomized crossover trial. Int J Sports Phys Ther, 2016, 11: 94–107.

66. Struyf F, Nijs J, Mollekens S, et al. Scapular-focused treatment in patients with shoulder impingement syndrome: a randomized clinical trial. Clin Rheumatol, 2013, 32: 73–85.

第17章 复杂型肩胛骨功能障碍的康复：考虑疼痛和运动模式改变

Aaron D. Sciascia, Robin Cromwell, Tim L. Uhl

引言

肩胛骨功能障碍在前几章已经详细描述过。大多数关于肩胛骨运动改变的讨论都集中在翼状肩胛[1]和肩胛骨弹响[2]上。翼状肩胛是指患者无论是在休息时还是在手臂运动时，肩胛骨内侧缘均呈不对称突出[1]。肩胛肌功能障碍和/或肩胛骨位置不平衡往往导致肩关节功能异常。既往文献表明肩胛骨功能障碍主要是周围神经病变影响到胸长神经、肩胛背神经、副神经及其支配的肌肉组织，或潜在的神经肌肉问题（如肌营养不良）引起的[3-6]。最近的文献已经证明由于肩胛骨骨结构、脊柱关节和肩关节复合体、运动表现和组织弹性的改变，引发肩胛骨错位或肩胛骨运动模式改变，导致肩关节疼痛[7-10]。

复杂型肩胛骨功能障碍的特征是多种因素导致的明显的肩胛骨运动障碍和手臂功能受限，引起中度至重度疼痛。最典型的因素包括神经损伤（胸长神经或副神经麻痹）、创伤性损伤（一个或多个肩胛肌撕脱）、未治疗的损伤慢性化或慢性软组织功能障碍。神经源性的肩胛骨功能障碍可通过康复治疗恢复一定程度的手臂功能。但若保守治疗失败，应该考虑手术治疗，如肌肉转移手术[11]。由于解剖结构被破坏，肩胛肌撕脱患者通常需要手术复位，达到减轻疼痛和改善功能的目的[9]。有长期肩胛骨功能障碍而无明确神经或创伤原因的患者是医生面对的最大挑战。目前针对复杂型肩胛骨功能障碍尚无标准化的治疗方法，且治疗方法也并非适合每位患者。与典型的肌骨损伤康复治疗相比，慢性功能障碍引起的疼痛和失代偿给医生带来了更大的挑战。患者有可能不仅有生物力学和解剖学上的改变，还有疼痛信号处理上的改变。这类患者往往需要个性化治疗，医生在制订和实施康复治疗方案时必须兼顾康复治疗的科学性和艺术性。

应用个体化照护首先要对引起疼痛和功能障碍的原因进行彻底评估，从患者的角度找到具体的受限因素并确定优先级。如果疼痛的原因或患者的需求没有完全确定，那么不良结果可能会持续出现。本章将介绍疼痛信号处理改变的概念及其对肩胛骨功能的影响，详细介绍动力链康复治疗方法和针对复杂型肩胛骨功能障碍的改良动力链康复治疗方法。

运动训练之外的考虑

最近的研究已证实痛知觉和心理因素都可导致身体功能障碍。慢性损伤可导致神经肽的长期释放，神经肽的释放可导致脊髓上的疼痛处理改变，从而导致超敏反应产生[12, 13]。这种超敏反应被称为中枢敏感化，其特征是将疼痛反应放大，即使是程度较低的伤害性刺激，患者也更容易感受到高强度疼痛，甚至是比真正受影响区域更大的躯体疼痛[13]。就算在疼痛刺激被移除或组织损伤愈合后，疼痛也会持续很长时间。这种现象及疼痛处理的其他改变（外周敏化或没有疼痛敏化）已在实验和临床症状中得到证实[14, 15]。此外，损伤可能会导致混合性疼痛，痛反应并非是患者疼痛的唯一原因。

最近，研究发现心理因素可能会影响肩部受伤患者的疼痛感觉[14-18]。一个可能的因素是患者倾向于将疼痛夸张化、灾难化。疼痛灾难化的特征是对实际或预期的疼痛刺激产生更夸张的负面心理状态。患者通常持续意识到疼痛，有疼痛不会消失的无助感，以及对运动感到恐惧，害怕运动会加剧疼痛。为了区分这两种因素，可以将中枢敏感化和疼痛灾难化简单描述为：中枢敏感化是由于大脑对痛觉的神经可塑性[13]，使身体做出反应，疼痛灾难化是指

一个人如何根据以前的经验来处理疼痛。

慢性复杂型肩胛骨功能障碍患者在疼痛处理过程中可能会经历这些变化。然而，医生若仅仅采用传统的康复治疗方法（如理疗或运动疗法），可能效果欠佳。疼痛处理发生改变的患者可以采用以下两种治疗方法的任一种[20, 21]：治疗由运动引起的疼痛和功能障碍，或者治疗静态疼痛。由运动引起的疼痛，即患者只在主动运动或被动运动时感到疼痛。有可能是解剖学和生理学缺陷导致了这种感觉。在这种情况下，可以尝试传统康复治疗方法，如使用抗炎药和理疗控制疼痛，并给予治疗性运动，以减轻疼痛、缓解功能障碍。如果传统康复方法不能减轻疼痛，则需要考虑其他措施，如非麻醉性处方药物，通过阻断离子通道将神经冲动传递到大脑来减轻神经源性疼痛。将疼痛的阈值调大，让系统安静下来，以便运动疗法发挥作用[22]。

静态疼痛患者可能具有中枢敏感化或疼痛灾难化的特征。这些患者可能会受益于神经疼痛宣教[23]。疼痛宣教教育患者关于疼痛的感知和可能发生的身体反应。当教育是基于疼痛的神经生理学（每个人的大脑如何感知疼痛），而不是集中于传统的解剖学和生物力学（如原因是组织撕裂）时，这种方法似乎会更有效[24, 25]。这些方案可能对慢性复杂型肩胛骨功能障碍患者有帮助，因为这些患者可能表现出与慢性肩痛患者相似的特征[14, 16, 17]。然而，值得注意的是，一些研究者发现，神经疼痛宣教结合其他干预手段（如手法治疗或有氧

运动），治疗效果更佳[26, 27]。

为了对患者产生积极的影响，治疗复杂型肩胛骨功能障碍可能需要评估疼痛感觉水平，可以用问卷调查和定量的感觉测试做最初的评估。问卷类如疼痛检测问卷（painDETECT questionnaire）[28]、简明疼痛量表（brief pain inventory）[29]和疼痛灾难化程度量表（PCS）[19]可以用来获得患者的疼痛感觉。定量的感觉测试可以通过机械性装置和触觉装置来进行。使用机械性装置设置不同温度和力量引发疼痛反应[14, 16, 17]，触觉装置包括单纤维、刷子、振动和尖或钝的针设备等[30]。

如果在休息时出现疼痛，应首先尝试神经疼痛宣教和药物干预。相反，如果患者因活动引起疼痛，则应采取传统的运动疗法。然而，对于复杂型肩胛骨功能障碍，典型的康复手段（以长杠杆的手臂运动为特征）常常无效。建议医生遵循动力链疗法，因为患者可能会更加适合整体训练。然而，疼痛和复杂功能障碍的存在可能会限制动力链疗法的效果。在这些情况下，可以尝试使用神经疼痛宣教弥补。通常可以对动力链练习进行调整，允许较少的自由度方向；或者利用更多的闭链练习，以减少对高激惹组织的刺激。

理解动力链疗法

不同于以保护愈合组织、减少疼痛为主要治疗目标的传统急性期治疗方法，动力链疗法的特点是将身体作为一个整体来治疗，不专门针对受伤关节的局部症状[31, 32]。该方法通常作为一个框架，将身体的各个部分按顺序配合来完成一个动态任务。根据定义，动力链是身体各个部分协调有序地激活、调动和稳定，以产生一个动态活动[33]。

针对肩部损伤的动力链康复框架主要侧重于三个关键部分[32]。第一，患者在运动过程中是直立的，而非仰卧或俯卧，尽可能地模拟功能需求。第二，缩短肩膀和躯干上的杠杆臂，以减轻受伤手臂的负荷。第三，使用腿部和躯干来激活肩胛骨和肩部肌肉，以启动手臂运动，这是运动的典型神经模式[34, 35]。这个框架后来扩大到包括一系列的渐进目标[31]：① 正确的姿势排列，② 在所有相关节段建立适当的运动，③ 通过加强下肢、躯干运动来促进肩胛骨运动，④ 运用夸张的肩胛骨后缩来控制过度的前伸，⑤ 早期运用闭链运动，⑥ 多平面运动。

首先，鼓励医生为患者建立正确的姿势对线。通过肌肉再教育、软组织活动和脊柱或肋骨松动等合理的、渐进的治疗计划，可以帮助患者建立正确的姿势，恢复骨骼节段的稳定性和灵活性。由于核心力量是动力链的驱动力，因此在康复治疗中应尽早开始局部和整体的肌肉再教育和核心肌群强化，以达到最佳的稳定性和发力[36]。在动力链疗法的第一阶段，软组织问题，即上肢和下肢的灵活性也应该得到解决。若不改善这些问题，可能会阻碍治疗，导致治疗过程延迟。良好的胸椎节段性活动和胸廓活动是手臂运动时肩胛骨可随之运动的必要条件。缺乏良好的骨骼排列、足够的软组织灵活性和核心稳定性会阻碍肩胛肌的正常活动。

下一个步骤是直接治疗肩胛骨。上、下斜方肌纤维与前锯肌和菱形肌保证了肩胛胸壁的基本稳定和运动。下斜方肌对抗前锯肌，起稳定肩胛骨的作用。局部解剖显示，下斜方肌纤维在手臂抬高过程中长度变化最小，因此其功能是在手臂上抬时，在前锯肌带动肩胛骨上旋的同时防止前锯肌将肩胛骨向胸壁外侧和前侧拉动[37, 38]。前锯肌在手臂抬高时参与肩胛骨的所有三维运动，在稳定肩胛骨内侧缘和下角防止肩胛骨翘起[39]的同时，促进肩胛骨上旋、后倾和外旋。

手臂过顶功能的实现需要肩胛骨后倾和外旋，以此优化肩部肌肉激活，同时躯干和髋部肌肉协同工作。这种动力链激活模式有助于肩胛骨上的肌肉得到最大的激活[32]。这种完整的顺序允许回缩的肩胛骨作为肩袖起点的稳定基础，允许最佳的关节面压迫[40, 41]。因此，实施结合下肢稳定性和肌肉激活的肩胛骨稳定训练是合适的。

康复治疗的后期为功能阶段，主要目标是加强盂肱关节的力量。开链运动试图通过长杠杆臂分离肩袖，在单平面运动范围内进行，这可能会造成关节的剪切力，从而激惹肌肉。这些练习在非功能位的卧位或侧卧位进行，适当减弱动力链的激活[42-44]。只有当动力链环节得到优化后，才能采用传统的强化措施。但是，这些措施也应加以调整，使动力链环节成为一个整体，而不是孤立地模拟正常的功能。下文提供了一个动力链练习的范例（图17.1~17.7）。

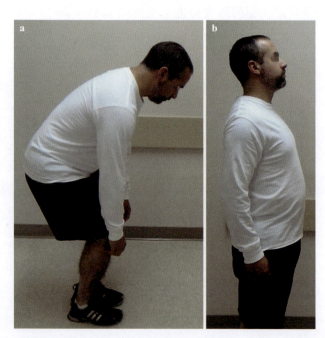

图17.1 胸骨提升：从躯干和膝盖轻微弯曲开始（a），在保持手臂放在身体一侧的同时，患者被要求站直，收缩肩胛骨（b）

第 17 章 复杂型肩胛骨功能障碍的康复：考虑疼痛和运动模式改变 · 193

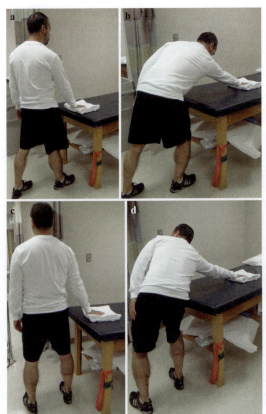

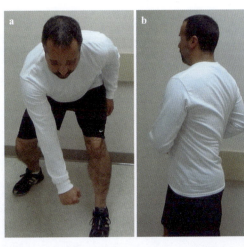

图17.4 非制动时进行割草机练习。起始位置不变，但是手臂轻微弯曲，指向对侧的膝盖（a），接着患者将身体重心向后移动，躯干轻微旋转，促进肩胛骨后缩（b）

图17.2 站立位桌上滑行，可帮助屈曲（a、b）和外展（c、d）。做任一方向运动时，患者将手放在毛巾上，躯干带动手臂

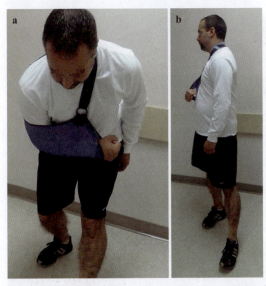

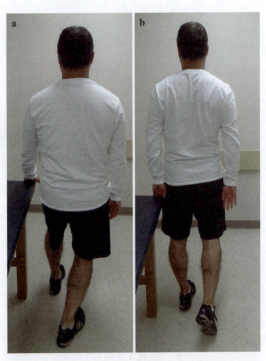

图17.3 在早期制动时即可以开始割草机练习。指导患者跨步站立，一条腿向前伸，躯干弯曲（a）。然后患者将身体重心向后移动，躯干轻微旋转，促进肩胛骨后缩（b）

图17.5 站立式低位划船：患侧手臂抵住坚实的表面（如桌子或其他物体的一侧），髋部、膝盖微微弯曲（a）。指示患者伸展髋部和手臂，促进肩胛骨后缩（b）

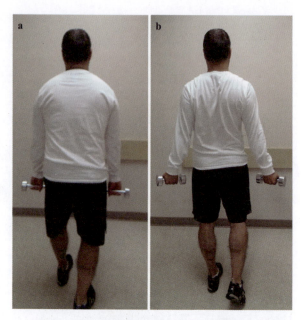

图 17.6 用 0.9～1.4 千克的哑铃替换桌子，可以进阶站立式低位划船（a）。患者伸展髋部和手臂，同时外旋手臂以获得肩胛骨后缩（b）

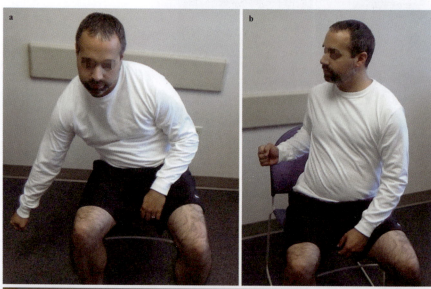

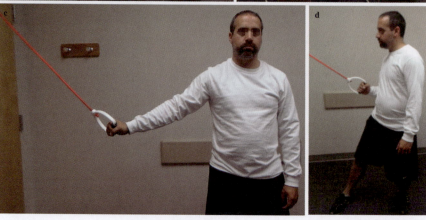

图 17.7 击剑式练习最初是在手臂稍微外展的情况下进行的（a）。指导患者转动躯干、内收手臂来获得肩胛骨后缩和下降（b）。这项练习可进展为使用弹力带站立进行（c）。指导患者在旋转躯干和手臂内收的同时向外侧迈步，以获得肩胛骨后缩和下降（d）

改良动力链疗法

虽然上述治疗肩胛骨功能障碍的康复治疗框架和康复目标有助于医生将患者身体作为一个整体进行治疗，但在某些情况下，需要调整动力链康复治疗框架，以帮助患者克服其功能缺陷。特别是没有特定原因的复杂型肩胛骨功能障碍患者，其可能无法通过动力链康复计划立即改善症状。慢性复杂型肩胛骨功能障碍患者常出现以下症状和临床表现：

- 肥大或过度活跃的上斜方肌，通常被认为是过早激活并在某些情况下持续激活的少数几种肌肉之一，如手臂抬高时伴随耸肩，从而限制流畅和全范围的活动。
- 手臂抬高时，单一下斜方肌或前锯肌或两者同时激活受限，造成内侧缘和下角翘起（肩胛骨过度前倾和内旋）。
- 胸小肌和背阔肌紧张。
- 肩袖萎缩。
- 手臂活动引起疼痛，可能伴有非骨赘引起的肩胛骨下可闻及的弹响声或摩擦声（重新定位以减轻疼痛）。
- 对疼痛过敏，如复杂的区域疼痛综合征或其他疼痛集中特征。
- 肩胛骨在手臂运动过程中可表现为可观察到的、无法控制的痉挛性运动。

针对肩胛骨功能障碍的这些临床表现，我们分析得出以下解释。

当患有慢性复杂型肩胛骨功能障碍的患者试图活动手臂时，肱骨头不能集中在盂窝内。肱骨头无法在关节盂内居中，提示可能存在盂窝挤压对位欠佳。如果盂窝挤压不能正常发挥作用，就可能发生肩袖萎缩。盂窝正常挤压时也是盂肱关节功能最好的时候，身体试图通过替代模式带动肩胛骨以完成预期的任务。文献表明，在抬高手臂的动作中，上斜方肌的激活增加，以补偿肩袖功能障碍或减少的盂窝挤压对位。此外，胸大肌、胸小肌和背阔肌在长期存在功能障碍的情况下可能会不恰当地作为稳定肌使用。这些肌肉的重复使用可能会增加肌筋膜触发点引起的肌肉疼痛[45]。胸大肌和胸小肌收缩可以改变肩胛骨的位置，使其更加前倾和内旋[7]。背阔肌过于紧张限制肱骨抬高和外旋[46]。久而久之，由于这些组织一直灵活性较差，不正常的肩胛骨运动模式最终成为固定模式，因此导致运动控制的改变。肩胛骨和手臂的这类运动模式并不常见，可能会产生肩胛下滑囊炎（肩胛骨弹响）、慢性疼痛、痉挛和异常运动时机等负面结果。对于复杂型肩胛骨功能障碍患者来说，整体设计动力链疗法可能比较困难，需要进行调整，以限制运动过程中使用的身体部位数量。医生必须考虑所有可能导致这些改变的因素，现将常见的肩胛骨功能缺陷和改良动力链疗法详述如下[31,32]。

近端不足

以动力链为基础的上肢康复治疗需要

增强核心功能，为综合康复提供基础[31, 32]。综合康复治疗主要利用核心功能，在整个运动过程中使用腿、髋部和躯干带动手臂。理想情况下，康复计划首先应注重发展核心力量和稳定，以优化解剖结构。下一步是将核心功能与肩部正确的协调任务结合起来。最后，患者应该从单个任务进展到复杂的任务，充分引导运动系统，以实现最佳功能，从而减少冗余的动作[33]。

慢性复杂型肩胛骨功能障碍患者即使核心稳定性已经形成，也往往不能立即开始执行常规的动态任务。例如，要求患者进行一项需要单独抬高手臂的运动，可能会加重他们目前的症状，因为该动作需要较长的杠杆臂，这在动力链的下肢部分未激活时更为严重。在这个过程中，这些患者似乎缺乏适当移动肩胛骨的本体感觉-运动觉。克服这一问题的第一个调整是将有意识的肩胛骨矫正作为基础练习（图17.8）。如果这项技术不成功，结合镜子为肩胛骨定位提供视觉反馈，可使用运动控制和运动再教育的原则[47, 48]。视觉结果将有助于患者获得关于肩胛骨位置的实时反馈。

大多数姿势问题可以通过改善肌肉系统的灵活性和/或身体结构的活动度来解决。通过标准的静态、动态和/或弹力拉伸，可以提高上肢和下肢的灵活性。根据之前研究以上肢运动为主的运动员的肌肉灵活性缺陷的结果，下肢肌肉群应以腘绳肌、髋屈肌、髋内收肌、髋旋转肌和腓肠肌、比目鱼肌为目标。改善下肢肌肉灵活性与改善下肢运动模式和提高整体运动成绩有关[49-52]。胸小肌、背阔肌和肩部后面的肌肉应该是上肢的重点[53-56]。医生在治疗慢性复杂型肩胛骨功能障碍患者的肩关节或周围软组织僵硬时，应考虑拉伸时的施加时间和负荷[57]。这些患者的肩胛骨和肩部肌肉在伸展到自然极限时通常是高度敏感的，尤其是当被拉伸的肢体承受的压力大小及维持拉伸的时间没有被考虑在内的时候。在这些情况下，使用长时间持续拉伸的原则，并计算到达末端范围的总时间可能是有用的[57, 58]。

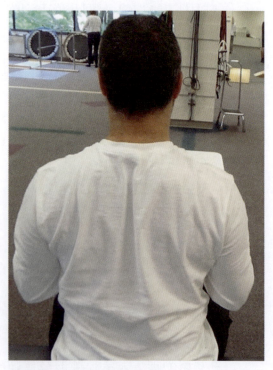

图17.8 在进行任何手臂运动之前，指示患者有意识地后缩肩胛骨

促进肩胛骨运动

肩胛骨周围肌肉，如前锯肌和下斜方肌是早期康复治疗的重点。前面描述的动力链疗法提倡早期训练，包括躯干和髋部肌群，有利于肌肉由近端到远端逐渐激活。针对复杂型肩胛骨功能障碍患者，这种方法可能需要调整、改良。首先，肩胛骨旋转发生在手臂抬高期间；然而，在肩胛骨肌肉功能的再教育中，我们发现单独的平移更为有益。许多患者有着较差的肩胛骨位置和本体感觉。因此，专注于简单的平移动作首先可以增强意识，同时激活肩胛骨肌肉组织。以闭链方式进行这些练习，可促进本体感觉，降低自由度，减少对受刺激肩胛骨肌肉组织的需求[59]。

上肢闭链练习可促进关节协调和协同激活周围肌肉组织，具有稳定结构的能力[60, 61]。这包括将远端部分（手或肘）放在固定的表面上，如桌子或可移动球上，促进肱骨向肩胛骨压缩。闭链练习是一种较好的恢复和提高本体感觉的康复方法。上肢闭链练习的一个例子是，患者被要求在坐位时将手臂支撑在桌子上，而不是在站立时进行肩胛骨后缩和肱骨外旋（在身侧）（图17.9）。坐位去除了原本来自下肢的运动，但仍然可以在练习中使用躯干和核心。这一基本原理遵循Bernstein确立的理论：自由度越小，运动系统在过渡到需要更大自由度的更具功能性的运动之前，会优化基本运动[62, 63]。

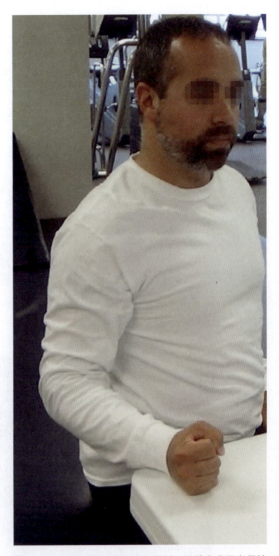

图17.9 手臂支撑的外旋动作举例。手臂在桌子上保持不动，躯干向外侧旋转

一旦患者通过简单的练习得到功能改善，便进阶到复杂的动力链运动，如坐位支撑手臂上抬（图17.10），最终鼓励站立位手臂活动。利用躯干和/或下肢来促进肩胛骨的协调运动是一种理想的方法，它模拟了动力链的激活次序。躯干伸展时，盂肱关节受到的应力最小，可促进肩胛骨后缩（图17.11）。

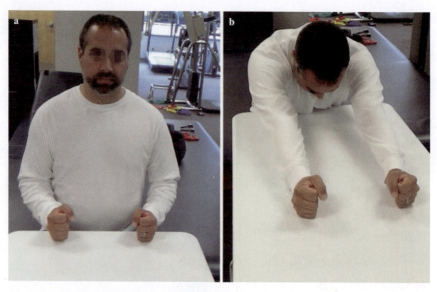

图17.10 坐位（a），指示患者躯干带动手臂上抬（b）

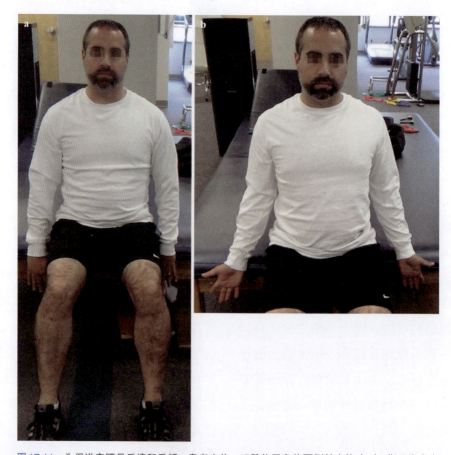

图17.11 为促进肩胛骨后缩和后倾，患者坐位，双臂位于身体两侧并内旋（a），指示患者坐直，双臂向外侧旋转（b）

当患者由于肩胛骨功能障碍而手臂运动困难时，必须使用其他躯体部分进行功能代偿。这需要扩大运动自由度。具体来说，利用躯干运动来实现手臂上抬，克服肩胛骨和肩部的功能障碍。

随着肩关节治疗进程的推进，当已准备好进行肩关节运动和负重时，可以引入同侧和对侧腿部动作激活的运动模式。

作为改良动力链康复治疗框架的最后一个部分，医生应尝试使用水平面治疗方式，它有助于加强肩胛骨后缩和前伸（图17.12）。研究已证明，通过保持近端固定，髋关节和躯干肌肉可在某具体活动中得到更有效的激活，而这种激活先于手臂运动的发生[64]。这种康复方式除了可以产生和传递力量到远端躯体，还可以为手臂运动提供稳定基础[65]。康复计划也应该鼓励刺激适当的本体感觉反馈，这样患者才能恢复到他们想要的功能水平[31, 32, 60]。

案例分析

分享两个案例研究，来说明复杂型肩胛骨功能障碍患者的康复方案设计。

案例1：一名15岁的女性运动员（篮球和足球）来到医生办公室，抱怨右侧的肩部和肩胛骨疼痛已经持续了约12个月。她报告说没有任何已知的损伤。她的肩部症状开始于无疼痛的弹响，几个月后发展为更明显的卡顿，并且手臂在运动时出现疼痛。她不能在活动中使用手臂来保持平衡，因为当手臂屈曲和外展时伴有疼痛。

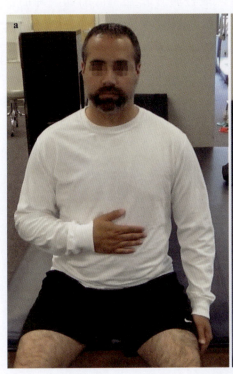
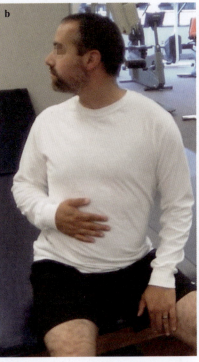

图17.12 为促进肩胛骨后缩和下降，患者取坐位，手臂横过躯干，类似于悬吊的姿势（a），指示患者旋转躯干并向后看（b）

医生给她做了MRI，发现她的肩胛骨上可能存在盂唇损伤和肿物。肌电图检查不明显，提示无神经累及。患者和她的父母选择手术切除肩胛下滑囊，因为它被认为是导致这种现象的原因，但他们没有考虑可能存在的盂唇病变。手术后，患者的弹响和卡顿减少了；然而，肩胛骨运动出现障碍。她回归足球运动，但在篮球运动时疼痛加剧，情况变得更加严重。她不得不停止运动，选择向另一位医生寻求帮助。

在第二名医生对她的首次检查中，记录了以下检查结果：

- 严重的肩胛骨运动障碍，伴随多种不同的运动模式。
- 姿势异常，包括右侧肩胛带前旋及肩向下倾斜，右侧肩胛骨前倾、上抬，头前伸，骨盆后旋伴腰椎前凸、颈椎和胸椎变平。
- 在没有严重肩胛骨肌张力障碍的情况下，右臂无法前屈、外展超过75°。
- 下斜方肌无力，徒手肌力测试等级3（共5级）。
- 背阔肌、胸小肌和上斜方肌有明显的疼痛和紧张感。
- 单腿下蹲动作测试髋部肌力不足。
- 盂唇和肩袖检查阴性。

第二名医生将其诊断为肩胛骨肌张力障碍伴下斜方肌肌力不足。

最初的治疗包括常用的动力链练习，如附录中的动作。随访6周后，患者的核心力量和稳定性得到改善，主动活动范围扩大，肩胛骨肌张力障碍减轻。然而，肩胛骨的控制能力仍然很差，疼痛仍在持续。医生担心该患者的运动控制没有改善、运动模式可能根深蒂固，因此利用表面肌电图检验了肌肉的激活模式和强度。

表面肌电图结果显示，手臂下降时背阔肌过度激活，同时下斜方肌激活。除了这些明显的肌肉激活变化，患者的肩胛骨在手臂上抬和降低的过程中打战，肩胛骨功能障碍问题突出。此外，患者出现冈下肌萎缩。这些发现导致治疗团队改进了基于动力链的训练计划。为了使神经肌肉活动的神经通路恢复到更典型的模式，医生要求患者在运动过程中坐下，通过闭链手臂支撑来使手臂解除负荷，从而改变训练方式。例如，要求患者坐正，同时收缩核心肌肉以稳定身体的中心部分。指示患者有意识地将肩胛骨置于后缩和下降的位置，手臂支撑在前面的一个平台上，同时指示患者用手臂做小的顺时针圆周运动（图17.13）。该练习用于改善前锯肌、菱形肌、下斜方肌和肩袖的激活次序，同时试图抑制上斜方肌和背阔肌的激活。接下来，患者坐位，支撑平台放置在她的身侧。使用与上个练习相同的躯干的姿势，然后将手臂横过躯干（类似于戴着吊带），并保持手臂姿势。患者被指示在保持手臂位置的同时向外侧转动躯干（图17.9）。这个练习的目的是通过重力帮助肩胛骨后缩、下降和躯干旋转，促进下斜方肌激活。进阶动作如图17.14、17.15和17.16所示。

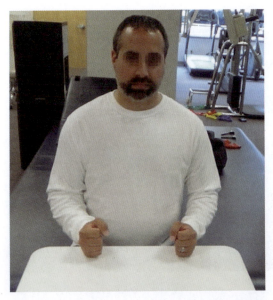

图17.13 患者坐位，双臂放在桌子上。指示患者将肩部的运动最小化，同时一只手做圆周运动3~5次，每次10~20秒

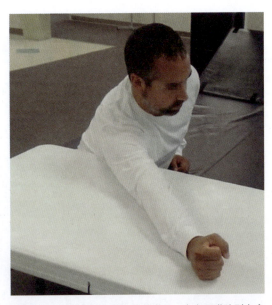

图17.14 随着闭链手臂上抬的进展，患者可进阶到在肩胛骨平面进行有支撑的手臂上抬

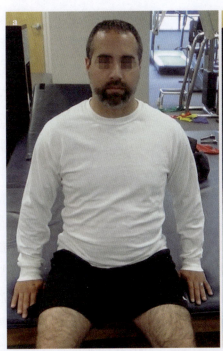

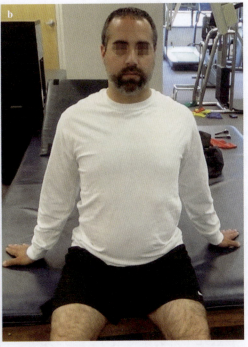

图17.15 患者坐位，胸骨提升始于躯干微微弯曲，手臂放在床上内旋（a）。手臂保持在身体两侧，指示患者挺胸坐直并外旋手臂，以此辅助肩胛骨后缩（b）

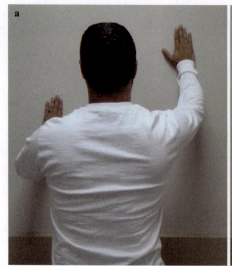
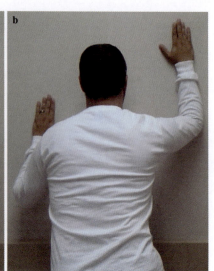

图17.16 不对称手部俯卧撑，手在墙上，位置一上一下（a），指示患者将身体向前移动，直到前臂接触到墙面（b）

在本例中，复杂型肩胛骨功能障碍患者通常不能使用基于动力链的大动作。对练习的修改旨在继续将身体视为一个整体，这一点通过躯干的补充运动表现出来。患者对手臂的卸载反应良好，并通过重力和躯干灵活性，连同限制手臂的活动范围，共同促进肩胛骨运动。当发生较小范围的肩部和肩胛骨运动时，她不仅感觉疼痛减轻，也发现肩胛骨肌张力障碍减少。

案例2：一名46岁男性患者，右侧肩胛骨剧烈疼痛，无法使用右臂进行前屈或过头运动。他最初是在日常工作中尝试切割钢螺栓时受伤的。在切割过程中，工具滑脱导致患者的手臂被强行从身体上分离。他立刻感到右肩胛骨内侧有爆裂声和灼痛感。他接受了许多医生的评估，被诊断为撞击综合征、肩袖肌腱炎和颈椎神经根病。经过几个月的康复治疗，疼痛几乎没有减轻，他被转到我这里，被诊断为肩胛骨肌肉撕脱[9]。他选择了手术治疗，结果显示，他的下斜方肌和菱形肌均脱离肩胛骨。实施肌肉再附着术后，患者进行了约8个月的物理治疗[9]。

在手术干预及术后康复后，患者的疼痛减轻；然而，患者害怕再次出现疼痛，出现运动恐惧，不敢前屈手臂。在手术18个月后的一次随访中，患者说："我只有想象要移动手臂时才能移动手臂。当我不假思索地移动手臂时，肩和腋下痛到让我无法呼吸。"他还报告了低水平伤害性超敏反应。

根据他的陈述，我决定下一个治疗方法基于运动控制原则，主要是神经成像。患者的身体感知和疼痛处理之间可能存在脱节，类似于截肢者感觉到幻肢痛[66]。在同一次随访中，患者站立位，在他面前有两面全身镜，一面镜子垂直于他的身体。垂直的镜子挡住了患者的视线，使他无法看到患侧手臂，而只能看到健侧手臂。患者被要求把注意力集中在镜子中健侧肢体的反射上，从镜子中看起来他好像在看自己的整个身体。当患者表示图像看起来完整时，指示他将双臂向前抬起到90°的位置。在重复12次之后，要求他在舒适的情况下尽可能地抬高双臂，超出肩膀水平。

通过使用镜子，患者可以将双臂同时抬高到约110°的位置，过程中几乎没有疼痛。当镜子被取走后，患者又开始受到限制，在疼痛出现前只能做5次手臂抬高。指导患者进行类似的治疗，每天20分钟，每周5天，直到3个月后的下一次随访。在后续随访中，患者的手臂可以完全抬高（160°），几乎没有疼痛，也没有使用镜子。

痛觉和疼痛反应受大脑地图的调控。大脑地图是大脑处理信息的区域，处理后将信息发送到适当的结构上，执行经外部和内部刺激后的激活反应[66, 67]。在上述案例中，镜像技术通过改变患者对身体图像的感知来消除或减少疼痛。基于大脑地图负责处理感官输入及产生图像[66]这个观点，疼痛和身体图像被认为是紧密相关的。由于大脑地图的设计是为了完成这两项任务，因此我们有理由认为两项任务间是互相影响的。曾经，疼痛被认为是单向地从受伤区域传播到大脑；然而，在上面的例子中，似乎发生了相反的情况，大脑将疼痛投射到身体上，这颠覆了单向通路的概念。身体感知通常不被认为是一种控制疼痛和功能的干预方法，因为大多数治疗肌肉、骨骼疾病的医生只指导患者进行受累肢体的单侧、同侧活动，同时关注肌肉收缩感觉和全身运动，几乎不涉及非受累

侧。身体图像概念表明，作为神经肌肉再教育的一部分，双侧运动可能是有益的[67, 68]。从理论上讲，在动态任务中看到自己双侧肢体的能力将帮助患者重新训练大脑，使其感知到一个合适的、平衡的身体图像，从而改善身体功能。

总结

复杂型肩胛骨功能障碍的康复治疗采用以动力链为基础的治疗方案，该方案可通过一系列合理的治疗措施解决患者特定的内部连接缺陷，有助于恢复从近端到远端肌肉激活的自然顺序。该方案的重点是训练肌肉的易化、灵活性、力量和本体感觉，并结合动力链的耐力训练。具体来讲，在整个康复计划中，设计模拟肩胛肱骨复合体负荷应力的功能锻炼应以一种合乎逻辑的方式逐步进行。在康复治疗结束时，预防性或前瞻性的练习也应作为治疗方法的一部分，提升患者应对未来的负荷应力的能力。

附录

康复进阶：功能性肩部康复要求逐渐提高肩关节的功能水平，最终使肩部恢复最大活动。在熟悉神经肌肉系统和具有机械性能良好的动力链的情况下，可进行进阶康复治疗。还需重视脊柱姿势和髋部肌肉的活动，以促进肩胛骨和盂肱关节的运动。力量提升是建立在功能运动模式之上的。

基本动力链示例方案诀窍：通过灵活使用多个节段来增加自由度。例如，扩大躯干屈曲以达到最终伸展，使肩胛骨可以很容易地利用重力下降，旋转躯干以促进肩胛骨后缩，侧屈躯干以帮助更好的旋转，使用快速牵张反射来改善肌肉收缩能力。

注意：即使是相同的练习和问题，也可能需要根据患者的情况给予提示。

- 胸骨提升（图17.1）。
- 站立位桌上滑行（图17.2）。
- 交叉站立使用吊带进行割草机练习，后移重心使躯干旋转（图17.3）。
- 站立位割草机练习（图17.4）。
- 低位划船（图17.5）。
- 保持手臂靠近身体，从低位划船到外旋，通过躯干伸展帮助脊柱活动（图17.6）。
- 进阶到击剑式练习（图17.7）。

改良动力链示例方案诀窍：通过限制活动节段的数量来减小自由度，即相比于站立位，用坐位减少活动范围，允许激活主要肌肉，通过闭链运动卸载手臂的重量。

- 有意识地纠正肩胛骨位置自我纠正（图17.8）。
- 使用桌子支撑实现躯干带动外旋（图17.9）。
- 闭链手臂上抬（图17.10）。
- 躯干伸展促进肩胛骨后缩（图17.11）。
- 躯干旋转促进肩胛骨后缩（图17.12）。
- 搅拌锅的动作（图17.13）。
- 在肩胛骨平面闭链手臂上抬（图17.14）。
- 坐位胸骨提升（图17.15）。
- 不对称手部俯卧撑（图17.16）。

（张鑫）

参考文献

1. Kuhn JE, Plancher K, Hawkins R. Scapular winging. J Am Acad Orthop Surg, 1995, 3: 319–325.
2. Kuhne M, Boniquit N, Ghodadra N, et al. The snapping scapula: diagnosis and treatment. Arthroscopy, 2009, 25(11): 1298–1311.
3. Bigliani LU, Perez-Sanz IR, Wolfe IN. Treatment of trapezius paralysis. J Bone Joint Surg Am, 1985, 67: 871–877.
4. Herzmark MH. Traumatic paralysis of the serratus anterior relieved by transplantation of the rhomboidei. J Bone Joint Surg Am, 1951, 33: 235–238.
5. Steinman S, Wood M. Pectoralis major transfer for serratus anterior paralysis. J Shoulder Elbow Surg, 2003, 12: 555–560.
6. Wright TA. Accessory spinal nerve injury. Clin Orthop Relat Res, 1975, 108: 15–18.
7. Borstad JD, Ludewig PM. The effect of long versus short pectoralis minor resting length on scapular kinematics in healthy individuals. J Orthop Sports Phys Ther, 2005, 35(4): 227–238.
8. Gumina S, Carbone S, Postacchini F. Scapular dyskinesis and SICK scapula syndrome in patients with chronic type III acromioclavicular dislocation. Arthroscopy, 2009, 25(1): 40–45.
9. Kibler WB, Sciascia AD, Uhl TL. Medial scapular muscle detachment: clinical presentation and surgical treatment. J Shoulder Elbow Surg, 2014, 23(1): 58–67.
10. Ludewig PM, Cook TM. Alterations in shoulder kinematics and associated muscle activity in people with symptoms of shoulder impingement. Phys

Ther, 2000, 80(3): 276–291.

11. Kibler WB. Sports medicine surgery. Philadelphia: Elsevier Saunders, 2010.

12. Gottrup H, Kristensen AD, Bach FW, et al. After sensations in experimental and clinical hypersensitivity. Pain, 2003, 103: 57–64.

13. Latremoliere A, Woolf CJ. Central sensitization: a generator of pain hypersensitivity by central neural plasticity. J Pain, 2009, 10(9): 895–926.

14. Coronado RA, Simon CB, Valencia C, et al. Experimental pain responses support peripheral and central sensitization in patients with unilateral shoulder pain. Clin J Pain, 2014, 30(2): 143–151.

15. Gwilym SE, Oag HCL, Tracey I, et al. Evidence that central sensitisation is present in patients with shoulder impingement syndrome and influences the outcome after surgery. J Bone Joint Surg Br, 2011, 93(4): 498–502.

16. Valencia C, Fillingim RB, Bishop M, et al. Investigation of central pain processing in postoperative shoulder pain and disability. Clin J Pain, 2014, 30(9): 775–786.

17. Valencia C, Kindler LL, Fillingim RB, et al. Investigation of central pain processing in shoulder pain: converging results from 2 musculoskeletal pain models. J Pain, 2012, 13(1): 81–89.

18. Wylie JD, Suter T, Potter MQ, et al. Mental health has a stronger association with patient-reported shoulder pain and function than tear size in patients with full-thickness rotator cuff tears. J Bone Joint Surg Am, 2016, 98: 251–256.

19. Sullivan MJL, Bishop S, Pivik J. The pain catastrophizing scale: development and validation. Psychol Assess, 1995, 7: 524–532.

20. Dean BJ, Gwilym SE, Carr AJ. Why does my shoulder hurt? A review of the neuroanatomical and biochemical basis of shoulder pain. Br J Sports Med, 2013, 47(17): 1095–1104.

21. Malfait AM, Schnitzer TJ. Towards a mechanism-based approach to pain management in osteoarthritis. Nat Rev Rheumatol, 2013, 9: 654–664.

22. Louw A, Puentedura EJ. Therapeutic neuroscience education. Story City: Pain Institute and International Spine, 2013.

23. Louw A, Puentedura EJ, Zimney K, et al. Know pain, know gain? A perspective on pain neuroscience education in physical therapy. J Orthop Sport Phys Ther, 2016, 46(3): 131–134.

24. Louw A, Diener I, Butler DS, et al. The effect of neuroscience education on pain, disability, anxiety, and stress in chronic musculoskeletal pain. Arch Phys Med Rehabil, 2011, 92: 2041–2056.

25. Louw A, Diener I, Landers MR, et al. Preoperative pain neuroscience education for lumbar radiculopathy. Spine, 2014, 39(18): 1449–1457.

26. Brage K, Ris I, Falla D, et al. Pain education combined with neck-and aerobic training is more effective at relieving chronic neck pain than pain education alone: a preliminary randomized controlled trial. Man Ther, 2015, 20(5): 686–693.

27. Girbes EL, Meeus M, Baert I, et al. Balancing"hands-on" with "hands-off" physical therapy interventions for the treatment of central sensitization pain in osteoarthritis. Man Ther, 2015, 20(2): 349–352.

28. Freynhagen R, Baron R, Gockel U, et al. PainDETECT: a new screening questionnaire to identify neuropathic components in patients with back pain. Curr Med Res Opin, 2006, 22(10): 1911–1920.

29. Cleeland CS, Ryan KM. Pain assessment: global use of the brief pain inventory. Ann Acad Med Singap, 1994, 23(2): 129–138.

30. Backonja M, Attal N, Baron R, et al. Value of quantitative sensory testing in neurological and

pain disorders: NeuPSIG consensus. Pain, 2013, 154: 1807–1819.
31. Sciascia AD, Cromwell R. Kinetic chain rehabilitation: a theoretical framework. Rehabil Res Pract, 2012, 2012: 853037.
32. McMullen J, Uhl TL. A kinetic chain approach for shoulder rehabilitation. J Athl Train, 2000, 35(3): 329–337.
33. Sciascia AD, Thigpen CA, Namdari S, et al. Kinetic chain abnormalities in the athletic shoulder. Sports Med Arthrosc Rev, 2012, 20(1): 16–21.
34. Bouisset S, Zattara M. A sequence of postural movements precedes voluntary movement. Neurosci Lett, 1981, 22: 263–270.
35. Hodges PW, Richardson CA. Feedforward contraction of transversus abdominus is not influenced by the direction of arm movement. Exp Brain Res, 1997, 114: 362–370.
36. Kibler WB, Press J, Sciascia AD. The role of core stability in athletic function. Sports Med, 2006, 36(3): 189–198.
37. Bagg SD, Forrest WJ. A biomechanical analysis of scapular rotation during arm abduction in the scapular plane. Am J Phys Med Rehabil, 1988, 67: 238–245.
38. Johnson G, Bogduk N, Nowitzke A, et al. Anatomy and actions of the trapezius muscle. Clin Biomech, 1994, 9: 44–50.
39. Ludewig PM, Cook TM, Nawoczenski DA. Three-dimensional scapular orientation and muscle activity at selected positions of humeral elevation. J Orthop Sports Phys Ther, 1996, 24(2): 57–65.
40. Lippitt S, Matsen FA 3rd. Mechanisms of glenohumeral joint stability. Clin Orthop Relat Res, 1993, 291: 20–28.
41. Lippitt S, Vanderhooft JE, Harris SL, et al. Glenohumeral stability from concavity-compression: a quantitative analysis. J Shoulder Elbow Surg, 1993, 2(1): 27–35.
42. Ballantyne BT, O'Hare SJ, Paschall JL, et al. Electromyographic activity of selected shoulder muscles in commonly used therapeutic exercises. Phys Ther, 1993, 73(10): 668–677.
43. Blackburn TA, WD ML, White B, et al. EMG analysis of posterior rotator cuff exercises. Athletic Training, 1990, 25(1): 40–45.
44. Townsend H, Jobe FW, Pink M, et al. Electromyographic analysis of the glenohumeral muscles during a baseball rehabilitation program. Am J Sports Med, 1991, 19: 264–272.
45. Han SC, Harrison P. Myofascial pain syndrome and trigger-point management. Reg Anesth, 1997, 22: 89–101.
46. Borstad JD, Briggs MS. Reproducibility of a measurement for latissimus dorsi muscle length. Physiother Theory Pract, 2010, 26(3): 195–203.
47. Sanchez FJN, Gonzalez JG. Influence of three accuracy levels of knowledge of results on motor skill acquisition. J Hum Sport Exerc, 2010, 5(3): 476–484.
48. Sidaway B, Bates J, Occhiogrosso B, et al. Interaction of feedback frequency and task difficulty in children's motor skill learning. Phys Ther, 2012, 92: 948–957.
49. Bandy WD, Irion JM, Briggler M. The effect of static stretch and dynamic range of motion training on the flexibility of the hamstring muscles. J Orthop Sports Phys Ther, 1998, 27: 295–300.
50. Higgs F, Winter SL. The effect of a four-week proprioceptive neuromuscular facilitation stretching program on isokinetic torque production. J Strength Cond Res, 2009, 23: 1442–1447.
51. Ross MD. Effect of a 15-day pragmatic hamstring stretching program on hamstring flexibility and single hop for distance test performance. Res

Sports Med, 2007, 15: 271–281.

52. Worrell TW, Smith TL, Winegardner J. Effect of hamstring stretching on hamstring muscle performance. J Orthop Sports Phys Ther, 1994, 20(3): 154–159.

53. Lephart SM, Smoliga JM, Myers JB, et al. An eight-week golf-specific exercise program improves physcial characteristics, swing mechanics, and golf performance in recreational golfers. J Strength Cond Res, 2007, 21(3): 860–869.

54. Robb AJ, Fleisig GS, Wilk KE, et al. Passive ranges of motion of the hips and their relationship with pitching biomechanics and ball velocity in professional baseball pitchers. Am J Sports Med, 2010, 38(12): 2487–2493.

55. Tsai YS, Sell TC, Smoliga JM, et al. A comparison of physical characteristics and swing mechanincs between golfers with and without a history of low back pain. J Orthop Sports Phys Ther, 2010, 40(7): 430–438.

56. Vad VB, Bhat AL, Basrai D, et al. Low back pain in professional golfers: the role of associated hip and low back range-of-motion deficits. Am J Sports Med, 2004, 32(2): 494–497.

57. Jacobs CA, Sciascia AD. Factors that influence the efficacy of stretching programs for patients with Hypomobility. Sports Health, 2011, 3(6): 520–523.

58. Kelley MJ, McClure PW, Leggin BG. Frozen shoulder: evidence and a proposed model guiding rehabilitation. J Orthop Sports Phys Ther, 2009, 39(2): 135–148.

59. Wise MB, Uhl TL, Mattacola CG, et al. The effect of limb support on muscle activation during shoulder exercises. J Shoulder Elbow Surg, 2004, 13: 614–620.

60. Lephart SM, Henry TJ. The physiological basis for open and closed kinetic chain rehabilitation for the upper extremity. J Sport Rehabil, 1996, 5: 71–87.

61. Uhl TL, Carver TJ, Mattacola CG, et al. Shoulder musculature activation during upper extremity weight-bearing exercise. J Orthop Sports Phys Ther, 2003, 33(3): 109–117.

62. Bernstein N. The coordination and regulation of movement. London: Pergamon, 1967.

63. Sporns O, Edelman GM. Solving Bernstein's problem: a proposal for the development of coordinated movement by selection. Child Dev, 1993, 64: 960–981.

64. Zattara M, Bouisset S. Posturo-kinetic organization during the early phase of voluntary upper limb movement. J Neurol Neurosurg Psychiatry, 1988, 51: 956–965.

65. Cordo PJ, Nashner LM. Properties of postural adjustments associated with rapid arm movements. J Neurophysiol, 1982, 47(2): 287–308.

66. Ramachandran VS, Rogers-Ramachandran D. Synaesthesia in phantom limbs induced with mirrors. Proc Biol Sci, 1996, 263(1369): 377–386.

67. Ramachandran VS, Altschuler EL. The use of visual feedback, in particular mirror visual feedback, in restoring brain function. Brain, 2009, 132: 1693–1710.

68. Zult T, Goodall S, Thomas K, et al. Mirror training augments the cross-education of strength and affects inhibitory paths. Med Sci Sports Exerc, 2016, 48(6): 1001–1013.